ADVANCE PRAISE FOR *DOOM*

"Humans have so many ways to suffer awful collective disasters—from earthquakes to warfare to plagues—that one would think we would have developed better ways of responding socially, economically, and politically. But it seems our primary means of coping is psychological: to appreciate watching the suffering from a safe distance. In his sweeping, synthetic, engaging book *Doom*, master historian Niall Ferguson explains why and offers a path forward for better, safer, and saner responses the next time we face catastrophe."
—Nicholas Christakis, Sterling Professor of Social and
Natural Science, Yale University

"*Doom* is an important contribution at a vital time for us all. This engaging book is a lot more than a highly readable history of catastrophes. Its insightful multidisciplinary approach provides us with critical insights into the attributes of disasters and—with a sharp analysis of bureaucratic and political structures, lack of policy imagination, social networks, and online influences—offers actionable response measures. It is a must-read if we are to develop political and social structures that can navigate a lot better through inevitably hard-to-predict catastrophes that threaten wide-scale pain and suffering."   —Mohamed A. El-Erian, president, Queens' College,
University of Cambridge, and author of *When Markets Collide*
and *The Only Game in Town*

"Post-COVID, lots of 'experts' are arguing about what went wrong and why. Niall Ferguson is grappling with a more important truth—that we can't prevent catastrophe, but we can build a world far more resilient to it. Doing so requires both history and humility. This book will give readers a healthy dose of both."   —Rana Foroohar, associate business editor, *Financial Times*

DOOM

DOOM

THE POLITICS
OF CATASTROPHE

Niall Ferguson

PENGUIN PRESS

NEW YORK

2021

PENGUIN PRESS
An imprint of Penguin Random House LLC
penguinrandomhouse.com

LIBRARY OF CONGRESS CATALOGING-IN-PUBLICATION DATA
Names: Ferguson, Niall, author.
Title: Doom : the politics of catastrophe / Niall Ferguson.
Description: 1st [edition]. | New York : Penguin Press, 2021. |
Includes bibliographical references and index.
Identifiers: LCCN 2020043578 (print) | LCCN 2020043579 (ebook) |
ISBN 9780593297377 (hardcover) | ISBN 9780593297384 (ebook)
Subjects: LCSH: COVID-19 (Disease)—History. |
COVID-19 (Disease)—Political aspects. |
Epidemics—Political aspects. | Political leadership.
Classification: LCC RA644.C67 F47 2021 (print) |
LCC RA644.C67 (ebook) | DDC 362.1962/414—dc23
LC record available at https://lccn.loc.gov/2020043578
LC ebook record available at https://lccn.loc.gov/2020043579

Printed in the United States of America
1st Printing

Book design by Daniel Lagin

For Molly, Ayaan,
Felix, Freya, Lachlan, Thomas, and Campbell

Contents

———

Introduction

This is not a history of our perplexing postmodern plague, nor a general history of pandemics. This is a general history of catastrophe—of all kinds of disasters, from the geological to the geopolitical, from the biological to the technological. For how else are we to see our disaster—or any disaster—in a proper perspective?

Chapter 1
THE MEANING OF DEATH

Though life expectancy has hugely improved in the modern era, death remains inevitable and is, in absolute terms, more common than ever. Yet we have become estranged from death. Ultimately, not only are we as individuals doomed, but so is the human race itself. All the world religions and a number of secular ideologies have sought to make this eschaton seem more imminent (as well as immanent) than it really is. What we have to fear is a big disaster, not doomsday. Of the big disasters in human history, the biggest have been pandemics and wars.

Chapter 2
CYCLES AND TRAGEDIES

Catastrophe is innately unpredictable because most disasters (from earthquakes to wars) are not normally distributed, but randomly or according to power laws. Cyclical theories of history cannot get around that. Disasters are more like tragedies: those who try to predict them are unlikely to be heeded. In addition to predicting more disasters than actually happen, Cassandras are up against a bewildering array of cognitive biases. In the end, faced with uncertainty, most people just decide to ignore the possibility that they as individuals will be victims of catastrophe. "The bells of hell go ting-a-ling-a-ling for you but not for me," a ditty sung by British soldiers in World War I, is humanity's signature tune.

Chapter 3
GRAY RHINOS, BLACK SWANS, AND DRAGON KINGS   69

Disasters are often foreseen (gray rhinos), yet even some predicted disasters can appear completely unexpected when they strike (black swans). A few have consequences beyond excess mortality that set them apart (dragon kings). Disasters are not either "natural" or "man-made." Decisions to locate settlements near potential disaster zones—by a volcano, on a fault line, next to a river subject to severe flooding—are what make most natural disasters in some respects man-made. In terms of loss of life, more big disasters happen in Asia than elsewhere. The great American disaster has been, by Asian standards, not all that disastrous.

Chapter 4
NETWORLD   105

The decisive determinant of the scale of a disaster is whether or not there is contagion. Social network structure is therefore as important as the innate properties of a pathogen or anything else (such as an idea) that can be virally spread. People worked out the efficacy of quarantines, social distancing, and other measures now referred to as "non-pharmaceutical interventions" long before they properly understood the true nature of the diseases they sought to counter, from smallpox to bubonic plague. The essence of such measures is to modify network structures to make it less of a small world. Such modifications can be spontaneous behavioral adaptations, but they usually need to be hierarchically mandated.

Chapter 5
THE SCIENCE DELUSION   141

The nineteenth century was a time of major advances, especially in bacteriology. But we should not succumb to a Whig interpretation of medical history. Empire forced the pace of research into infectious diseases, but it also forced the pace of the globalization of the world economy, creating new opportunities for diseases, not all of which submitted to vaccination or therapy. The 1918 influenza was a grim revelation of the limits of science. Breakthroughs in our understanding of risks can be offset by increased network integration and fragility.

Chapter 6
THE PSYCHOLOGY OF POLITICAL INCOMPETENCE

We tend to attribute too much of the responsibility for political disasters, as well as military ones, to incompetent leaders. It was a pleasing argument of the Indian economist Amartya Sen that famines were caused by unaccountable governments and avoidable market failures, not food shortages per se, and that democracy was the best cure for famines. That theory may well explain some of the worst famines in the century and a half from the 1840s to the 1990s. But why should Sen's law apply only to famines? Why not to the most man-made of disasters, wars? It is a paradox that the transition from empires to more or less democratic nation-states was attended by so much death and destruction.

Chapter 7
FROM THE BOOGIE WOOGIE
FLU TO EBOLA IN TOWN

In 1957, the rational response to a new and deadly strain of flu seemed to be a combination of pursuing natural herd immunity and selective vaccination. There were no lockdowns and no school closures, despite the fact that the Asian flu in 1957 was about as dangerous as COVID-19 in 2020. The success of Eisenhower's response reflected not only the nimbleness of the federal government of those days but also the Cold War context of much-improved international cooperation on issues of public health. Yet the successes of the 1950s, '60s, and '70s were deceptive. HIV/AIDS revealed the weaknesses of both national and international agencies. So, in their different ways, did SARS, MERS, and Ebola.

Chapter 8
THE FRACTAL GEOMETRY OF DISASTER

Accidents will happen, from the *Titanic* to *Challenger* to Chernobyl. Small disasters are like microcosms of big ones, but because they are less complex, we can understand them more easily. The common feature of all disasters, whether sinking ships or exploding nuclear reactors, is the combination of operator error and managerial error. Often the point of failure in a disaster is not at the top (the "blunt end") or at the point of contact (the "sharp end") but within middle management—a favorite theme of the physicist Richard Feynman and an insight with general applicability.

Chapter 9
THE PLAGUES

Like so many past pandemics, COVID-19 originated in China. But the varied impact of the disease on the rest of the world's countries confounded expectations. Far from being well prepared for a pandemic, the United States and the United Kingdom fared badly. It was countries such as Taiwan and South Korea that had learned the right lessons from SARS and MERS. It was tempting to blame Anglo-American travails on the incompetence of populist leaders. However, something more profound had gone wrong. The public health bureaucracy in each case had failed. And the role of the internet platforms in disseminating fake news about COVID-19 led to poor and sometimes downright harmful adaptations in public behavior.

Chapter 10
THE ECONOMIC CONSEQUENCES OF THE PLAGUE

The shift from complacency to panic in mid-March 2020 led to economically crushing lockdowns in many countries. Were they the right solutions to the problem posed by COVID-19? The answer is probably not, but that did not make it smart for the United States to attempt a return to normality that summer (the dumb reopening) without adequate testing and tracing. The predictable result was a second, smaller wave and a "tortoise-shaped" recovery. Less predictable was the near-revolutionary political eruption over the issue of racism, which bore striking resemblances to mass movements precipitated by previous pandemics.

Chapter 11
THE THREE-BODY PROBLEM

The COVID-19 crisis is widely regarded as dooming the United States to decline relative to China. This is probably wrong. The empires of our time—the United States, China, and the European Union—all made a mess of the pandemic in their different ways. But it is hard to see why the countries that handled it well would be eager to join Xi Jinping's imperial panopticon. In a number of respects, the crisis has shown the persistence of American power: in financial terms, in the race for a vaccine, and in the technological competition. Rumors of American doom are once again exaggerated. Perhaps because of this exaggeration, the risk of not just cold but hot war is rising.

Conclusion
FUTURE SHOCKS

We have no way of knowing what the next disaster will be. Our modest goal should be to make our societies and political systems more resilient—and ideally antifragile—than they currently are. That requires a better understanding of network structure and of bureaucratic dysfunction than we currently possess. Those who would acquiesce in a new totalitarianism of ubiquitous surveillance in the name of public safety have failed to appreciate that some of the worst disasters described in this book were caused by totalitarian regimes.

List of Illustrations

222 Maurice Hilleman talks with his research team as they study the Asian flu virus in a lab at Walter Reed Army Medical Center, Silver Spring, Maryland, 1957: Ed Clark/ The LIFE Picture Collection via Getty Images.

257 The *Hindenburg* on fire at the mooring mast in Lakehurst, New Jersey, May 6, 1937: National Archives, Records of the U.S. Information Agency (USIA).

264 The correlation between space shuttle O-ring incidents and temperatures at launch: Richard Feynman, *"What Do You Care What Other People Think?": Further Adventures of a Curious Character.* Copyright © 1988 by Gweneth Feynman and Ralph Leighton. Used by permission of W. W. Norton & Company, Inc.

278 Cesium-137 deposition levels across Europe following the Chernobyl nuclear disaster, May 10, 1986: Yu A. Izrael et al., "The Atlas of Caesium-137 Contamination of Europe After the Chernobyl Accident," Joint Study Project of the CEC/CIS Collaborative Programme on the Consequences of the Chernobyl Accident (n.d.), https://inis.iaea .org/collection/NCLCollectionStore/_Public/31/056/31056824.pdf.

291 Passenger flows from Wuhan before the January 23 lockdown of the city. From *The New York Times.* © 2020 The New York Times Company. All rights reserved. Used under license.

293 Observed and expected weekly excess mortality in the United States (all causes), 2017–20: Centers for Disease Control and Prevention.

297 COVID-19 in comparative perspective: Eskild Petersen et al., "Comparing SARS-CoV-2 with SARS-CoV and Influenza Pandemics," *Lancet Infectious Diseases* 20, no. 9 (September 2020), pp. E238–E244, https://doi.org/10.1016/S1473-3099(20)30484-9.

304 Patient 31 was a South Korean superspreader who passed COVID-19 to more than a thousand other people: Marco Hernandez, Simon Scarr, and Manas Sharma, "The Korean Clusters: How Coronavirus Cases Exploded in South Korean Churches and Hospitals," Reuters, March 20, 2020, https://graphics.reuters.com/CHINA-HEALTH -SOUTHKOREA-CLUSTERS/0100B5G33SB/index.html.

334 The U.S. unemployment rate since 1948: Federal Reserve Bank of St. Louis.

348 The one bipartisan issue. Percentages of Republicans and Democrats who say they have an "unfavorable" opinion of China: Pew Research Center, July 30, 2020.

350 U.S. dollar, nominal and real trade-weighted effective exchange rate since 1964: Bank for International Settlements.

DOOM

Introduction

Still, thou art blest, compar'd wi' me!
The present only toucheth thee:
But Och! I backward cast my e'e,
On prospects drear!
An' forward tho' I canna see,
I guess an' fear!

—Robert Burns, "To a Mouse"

CONFESSIONS OF A SUPERSPREADER

Never in our lifetimes, it seems, has there been greater uncertainty about the future—and greater ignorance of the past. At the beginning of 2020, very few people grasped the significance of the news coming out of Wuhan about a new coronavirus. When I first spoke and wrote publicly about the rising probability of a global pandemic, in the week ending January 26, 2020,[1] I was regarded as eccentric (certainly by the majority of the delegates at the World Economic Forum in Davos, who seemed oblivious to the danger). The conventional wisdom at that time, from Fox News to *The Washington Post,* was that the coronavirus posed a lesser threat to Americans than the usual winter wave of influenza. On February 2, I wrote, "We are now dealing with an epidemic in the world's most populous country, which has a significant chance of becoming a global pandemic. . . . The challenge is . . . to resist that strange fatalism that leads most of us not to cancel our travel plans and not to wear uncomfortable masks, even when a dangerous virus is spreading exponentially."[2] Looking back, I read those sentences as a veiled confession. I was traveling manically in January and February, as I had done for most of the previous twenty years. In January, I flew from London to Dallas, from Dallas to San Francisco, and from there to Hong Kong (January 8), Taipei (January 10), Singapore (January 13), Zurich (January 19), back to San Francisco (January 24), and then to Fort Lauderdale (January 27). I wore a mask once or twice but found it intolerable after an hour and took it off. In the course of February, I flew almost as frequently, though not so far: to New York, Sun Valley, Bozeman, Washington, D.C., and Lyford Cay. You may wonder what kind of life that was. I used to joke that the lecture circuit had turned me into an "international man of history." I realized only later that I might have been one of the "superspreaders" whose hyperactive travel schedules were spreading the virus from Asia to the rest of the world.

My weekly newspaper column in the first half of 2020 became a kind of plague diary, though I never mentioned the fact that I was ill for most of February, with a painful cough I could not shake off. (To get through lectures, I relied heavily on Scotch.) "Worry about grandparents," I wrote on February 29; "the mortality rate for people in their eighties is above 14 per cent, whereas it's close to zero for those under 40." I omitted the less comforting data on asthmatic men in their mid-fifties. I also left out the fact that I went to see a doctor twice, only to be told that—as more or less everywhere in the United States at that time—there were no tests available for COVID-19. All I knew was that it was serious, and not only for me and my family:

> Those who blithely say, "This is no worse than the flu" . . . are missing the point. . . .
>
> Uncertainty surrounds it because it is so difficult to detect in its early stages, when many carriers are both infectious and asymptomatic. We don't know for sure how many people have it, so we don't exactly know its reproduction number and its mortality rate. There's no vaccine and there's no cure.[3]

In another article, published in *The Wall Street Journal* on March 8, I wrote, "If the U.S. turns out to have proportionately as many cases as South Korea, it will soon have some 46,000 cases and more than 300 deaths—or 1,200 deaths if the U.S. mortality rate is as high as Italy's."[4] At that point, total confirmed cases in the United States stood at just 541; deaths at 22. We passed 46,000 cases on March 24 and 1,200 deaths on March 25, just over two weeks later.[5] On March 15 I noted, "John F. Kennedy airport was thronged yesterday with people doing what, since time immemorial, they have done in times of plague: fleeing the big city (and spreading the virus). . . . We are entering the panic phase of the pandemic."[6] That was the same day I myself flew, with my wife and my two youngest children, from California to Montana. I have been here ever since.

I wrote and thought about little else in the first half of 2020. Why this intense preoccupation? The answer is that, although my core competency is financial history, I have been keenly interested in the role of disease in history ever since studying the Hamburg cholera epidemic of 1892 as a graduate student more than thirty years ago. Richard Evans's meticulously detailed study of that episode introduced me to the idea that the mortality caused by a deadly pathogen is partly a reflection of the social and political order it attacks. It was the class structure as much as the bacterium *Vibrio cholerae* that killed people in Hamburg, Evans argued, because the entrenched power of the city's property owners had been an insuperable obstacle to improving the city's antiquated water and sewage systems. The mortality rate for the poor was thirteen times higher than for the rich.[7] Researching *The Pity of War* a few years later, I was struck by statistics that suggested the German army had collapsed in 1918 partly because of a surge of illness, possibly resulting from the Spanish influenza pandemic.[8] *The War of the World* delved more deeply into the history of the 1918–19 pandemic, showing how the First World War ended with twin pandemics—not only influenza but also the ideological contagion of Bolshevism.[9]

The work I did on empires in the 2000s also involved excursions into the history of contagious disease. No account of European settlement in the New World could have omitted the role that disease played in "thinning the *Indians,* to make room for the *English*," as John Archdale, the governor of Carolina in the 1690s, callously remarked. (The title of the second chapter of my book *Empire* was "White Plague.") I was also very struck by the terrible toll of tropical disease on British soldiers stationed far from home: a man's chances of surviving a tour of duty in Sierra Leone were pitifully low—1 in 2.[10] *Civilization* devoted an entire chapter to the role of modern medicine in the expansion of Western settlement and rule, showing how colonial regimes meaningfully improved our knowledge of and ability to control contagious diseases, without glossing over the brutal methods often employed.[11] *The Great Degeneration* explicitly warned of our growing vulnerability to "the . . . random mutation of viruses like influenza,"[12] while *The Square and the Tower* was essentially a history of the world based on the insight that "network structures are as important as viruses in determining the speed and extent of a contagion."[13]

As I write (in late October 2020), the COVID-19 pandemic is far from over. There have been nearly twenty-six million confirmed cases, a fraction of the total number infected with the SARS-CoV-2 virus, to judge by seroprevalence figures from around the world.[14] The death toll approaches 1.2 million, which is certainly an underestimate, as the statistics from a number of large countries (notably Iran and Russia) cannot be trusted. And the cumulative body count continues to rise globally at a rate of more than 3.5 percent a week—to say nothing of the number of people whose health has been permanently damaged, which no one has yet estimated. It seems increasingly likely that Lord Rees, Britain's astronomer royal, has won his bet with the Harvard psychologist Steven Pinker that "bioterror or bioerror will lead to one million casualties in a single event within a six month period starting no later than Dec 31 2020."[15] Some epidemiologists have argued that, without drastic social distancing and economic lockdowns, the ultimate death toll could have been between thirty and forty million.[16] Because of government restrictions and changes in public behavior, it will surely not be as high. Yet precisely these "non-pharmaceutical interventions" have inflicted a shock on the world economy far greater than that caused by the 2008–9 financial crisis—potentially as great as the shock of the Great Depression, but compressed into months, not years.

Why write history now, when the story is not yet over? The answer is that this is not a history of our perplexing postmodern plague, though two of the later chapters (9 and 10) offer a preliminary sketch of such a history. This is a general history of catastrophe—not just pandemics but all kinds of disasters, from the geological (earthquakes) to the geopolitical (wars), from the biological (pandemics) to the technological (nuclear accidents). Asteroid strikes, volcanic eruptions, extreme weather events, famines, catastrophic accidents, depressions, revolutions, wars, and genocides: all life—and much death—is here. For how else are we to see our disaster—any disaster—in a proper perspective?

THE ALLURE OF DOOM

The book's starting point is that we cannot study the history of catastrophes, natural or man-made—though the dichotomy, as we shall see, is somewhat false—apart from the history of economics, society, culture, and politics. Disasters are rarely entirely exogenous events, with the exception of a massive meteor strike, which hasn't happened in sixty-six million years, or an alien invasion, which hasn't happened at all. Even a catastrophic earthquake is only as catastrophic as the extent of urbanization along the fault line—or the shoreline, if it triggers a tsunami. A pandemic is made up of a new pathogen and the social networks that it attacks. We cannot understand the scale of the contagion by studying only the virus itself, because the virus will infect only as many people as social networks allow it to.[17] At the same time, a catastrophe lays bare the societies and states that it strikes. It is a moment of truth, of revelation, exposing some as fragile, others as resilient, and others as "antifragile"—able not just to withstand disaster but to be strengthened by it.[18] Disasters have profound economic, cultural, and political consequences, many of them counterintuitive.

All societies live under uncertainty. Even the earliest civilizations of which records remain were acutely aware of the vulnerability of *Homo sapiens*. Since human beings began recording their thoughts in art and literature, the possibility of an extinction event or "end time" has loomed large. As chapter 1 explains, the prospect of the Apocalypse—of a final, spectacular Day of Judgment—has been central to Christian theology since Jesus himself prophesied it. Muhammad incorporated into Islam the spectacular denouement described in the Book of Revelation. We find similar visions of destruction even in the more cyclical faiths of Hinduism and Buddhism—and indeed in ancient Norse mythology. Often, sometimes subconsciously, we modern humans interpret the disasters we encounter or experience in eschatological terms. Indeed, in some secular ideologies, notably Marxism, a secular apocalypse, in which capitalism collapses under the weight of its contradictions, is something as devoutly to be wished for as the "Rapture" of the evangelicals. There is something familiar about the vehemence with which the most radical prophets of disastrous climatic change demand drastic economic penance to avert the end of the world.

I first encountered the word "doom" as a boy in East Africa, where it was the brand name of a popular insecticide spray, nowadays occasionally used for religious purposes.[19] To my sons, *Doom* is a computer game. The word originates in the Old English *dóm,* Old Saxon *dóm,* and Old Norse *dómr,* meaning a formal judgment or sentence, usually of the adverse variety. "All unavoided is the doom of destiny," says Richard III. "What, will the line stretch out to th' crack of doom?" asks Macbeth. We dread doom, of course. Yet we are also fascinated by it—hence the abundant literature on the subject of "the last days of mankind" (the ironical title of Karl Kraus's great satirical play about World War I). Science fiction and cinema have portrayed our doom as a species countless times: a lethal pandemic is only one of the many ways mankind has been wiped out in the course of popular entertainment. It was revealing that, during the first phase of the COVID-19 lockdowns in the United States, one of the most frequently watched movies on Netflix was *Contagion,* the 2011 film by Steven Soderbergh about a (much worse) pandemic.[20] I found myself rewatching the BBC's 1975 drama *Survivors* and reading Margaret Atwood's MaddAddam trilogy with appalled fascination. Doom is alluring.

Yet what we have to fear is not the end of the world—which invariably disappoints the millennialists by failing to occur on schedule—but big disasters that most of us survive. These can take multiple forms. They vary enormously in scale. And even if they have been predicted, they cause a very distinctive kind of pandemonium. The petrifying yet squalid reality of catastrophe is rarely captured in literature. A rare exception is Louis-Ferdinand Céline's deeply cynical account of the German invasion of France in 1914 in *Voyage au bout de la nuit* (1932). "When you have no imagination, dying is small beer," observes Céline. "When you do have an imagination, dying is too much."[21] Few authors have better captured the chaos of a large disaster and the sheer terror and disorientation of the individual's experience. France survived the horrendous casualties of the opening phase of the First World War. Yet Céline's cynical, traumatized portrayal of French low life, from the outposts of French Equatorial Africa to the outskirts of Paris, seems to foretell the even greater calamity that lay ahead.

Strange Defeat was the title the historian Marc Bloch gave his account of France's collapse in the summer of 1940.[22] There have been many such strange defeats in history—disasters that were not difficult to foresee and yet precipitated collapse. In many respects, the American and British experiences of COVID-19 have both, in their different ways, been strange defeats, intelligible only as colossal failures by governments to make adequate preparations for a disaster they always knew to be a likely contingency. To blame this failure almost entirely on populist braggadocio would be facile. In terms of excess mortality, Belgium fared as badly, if not worse. Its prime minister for most of 2020 was a liberal woman, Sophie Wilmès.

Why do some societies and states respond to catastrophe so much better than others? Why do some fall apart, most hold together, and a few emerge stronger? Why does politics sometimes cause catastrophe? These are the central questions posed by *Doom*. The answers are far from obvious.

THE UNCERTAINTY OF CATASTROPHE

If only disasters were predictable, how much less perplexing life would be! For centuries, writers have sought to tease out predictability from the historical process by means of various cyclical theories—religious, demographic, generational, and monetary. In chapter 2, I consider these and ask how much they can really help us to anticipate and, if not avoid, then at least mitigate the next calamity. The answer is not much. The problem is that believers in such theories, or in any other form of insight that is not widely understood, invariably find themselves in the position of Cassandra. They see the future, or think they do, but cannot convince those around them. In that sense, many disasters are true tragedies, in the classical sense of the term. The prophet of doom cannot persuade the skeptical chorus. The king cannot be saved from his nemesis.

But there is a good reason why the Cassandras cannot persuade, and that is their inability to attach precision to their prophecies. When exactly will disaster strike? They generally cannot say. It is true that some disasters are "predictable surprises," like "gray rhinos" that we see rumbling toward us.[23] Yet sometimes, at the moment they strike, these gray rhinos metamorphose into "black swans"—seemingly bewildering events that "no one could have foreseen." This is partly because many black swan events—pandemics, earthquakes, wars, and financial crises—are governed by power laws, rather than a normal probability distribution of the sort that our brains more readily comprehend. There is no average pandemic or earthquake; there are a few very large ones and a great many quite small ones, and there is no reliable way of predicting when a very large one will come along.[24] In normal times, my family and I live not far from the San Andreas fault line. We know "the big one" could happen at any time, but how big and exactly when, no one can say. The same goes for man-made disasters such as wars and revolutions (which are more often disastrous than not) as well as financial crises—economic disasters that have lower death tolls but, often, comparably disruptive consequences. A defining feature of history, as chapter 3 shows, is that there are many more black swans—not to mention "dragon kings," events so large in scale that they lie beyond even a power-law distribution[25]—than a normally distributed world would lead us to expect. All such events lie in the realm of uncertainty, not of calculable risk. Moreover, the world we have built has, over time, become an increasingly complex system prone to all kinds of stochastic behavior, nonlinear relationships, and "fat-tailed" distributions. A disaster such as a pandemic is not a single, discrete event. It invariably leads to other forms of disaster—economic, social, and political. There can be, and often are, cascades or chain reactions of disaster. The more networked the world becomes, the more we see this (chapter 4).

Unfortunately, our brains have not evolved in ways that equip us to comprehend or tolerate a world of black swans, dragon kings, complexity, and chaos. It would be wonderful if the advance of science had liberated us from at least some of the irrational ways of thinking that characterized the ancient and medieval worlds. ("We have sinned. It is God's judgment.") But other forms of magical thinking have grown even as religious belief has diminished. "This disaster lays bare the conspiracy" is an increasingly common response to any adverse event. Then there is that vague deference to "the science," which proves, on close inspection, to be a new form of superstition. "We have a model; we understand this risk" is a phrase that has been uttered more than once before several recent calamities, as if gimcrack computer simulations with made-up variables constitute science. In succession to the Oxford historian Keith Thomas's seminal *Religion and the Decline of Magic,* chapter 5 suggests, we must prepare to write *Science and the Revival of Magic.*[26]

Disaster management is made still more difficult by the fact that our political systems increasingly promote into leading roles individuals who seem especially oblivious to the challenges described in the preceding paragraphs: subprime forecasters rather than superforecasters. The psychology of military incompetence has been the subject of an excellent study.[27] Less has been written at a general level about the psychology of political incompetence, the subject of chapter 6. We know that politicians seldom seek out expert knowledge without some ulterior motive.[28] We know, too, that inconvenient expert knowledge is quite easily sidelined. But can we identify general forms of political malpractice in the field of disaster preparedness and mitigation? Five categories come to mind:

1. Failure to learn from history
2. Failure of imagination
3. Tendency to fight the last war or crisis
4. Threat underestimation
5. Procrastination, or waiting for a certainty that never comes

Henry Kissinger's "problem of conjecture"—which he formulated in the context of nuclear strategy—captures the asymmetries of decision making under uncertainty, especially in a democracy:

> Each political leader has the choice between making the assessment which requires the least effort or making an assessment which requires more effort. If he makes the assessment that requires least effort, then as time goes on it may turn out that he was wrong and then he will have to pay a heavy price. If he acts on the basis of a guess, he will never be able to prove that his effort was necessary, but he may save himself a great deal of grief later on. . . . If he acts early, he cannot know whether it was necessary. If he waits, he may be lucky or he may be unlucky. It is a terrible dilemma.[29]

Leaders are rarely rewarded for what they did to avoid disasters—for the non-occurrence of a disaster is rarely a cause for celebration and gratitude—and more often are blamed for the pain of the prophylactic remedies they recommended. The contrast between today's style of leadership and the presidency of Dwight Eisenhower forms part of chapter 7.

Yet not all failures are failures of leadership. Often the real point of failure is further down the organizational hierarchy. As the physicist Richard Feynman proved in the aftermath of the space shuttle *Challenger*'s destruction, in January 1986, the fatal lapse was not the White House's impatience for a successful launch to coincide with a presidential address, but the insistence of midlevel bureaucrats at NASA that a risk of catastrophic failure their own engineers put at 1 in 100 was in fact 1 in 100,000.[30] This, as much as blunders at the top, turns out to be a feature of many modern disasters. There is, as the Republican congressman Tom Davis said after Hurricane Katrina, a "vast divide between policy creation and policy implementation."[31] Such disconnects can be found in disasters of any scale, from a sunken ship to a collapsed empire, suggesting that there is a "fractal geometry of disaster" (chapter 8).

The behavior of ordinary people—whether in decentralized networks or acephalous crowds—can matter even more than the decisions of leaders or orders issued by governments in the event of a disaster. What leads some people to adapt rationally to a new threat, others to act passively as bystanders, and others to go into denial or revolt? And why can a natural disaster end up triggering a political one as disgruntled people form themselves into a revolutionary crowd? What causes a crowd to flip from wisdom to madness? The answer, I suggest, lies in the changing structure of the public sphere. For a disaster is directly experienced by only a minority of people. Everyone else hears about it through some network of communication. Even in the seventeenth century, the nascent popular press could sow confusion in people's minds, as Daniel Defoe found when he researched the plague of 1665 in London. The advent of the internet has greatly magnified the potential for misinformation and disinformation to spread, to the extent that we may speak of twin plagues in 2020: one caused by a biological virus, the other by even more contagious viral misconceptions and falsehoods. This problem might have been less serious in 2020 had meaningful reforms of the laws and regulations governing the big technology companies been implemented. Despite ample evidence after 2016 that the status quo was untenable, almost nothing was done.

NOT THE END OF MEDICAL HISTORY

We tend to think of epidemics and pandemics narrowly, in terms of particular pathogens' impacts on human populations. However, it is as much the social networks and state capacities that the pathogen encounters that determine the magnitude of a pandemic's impact. Population fatality rates are not inscribed in the ribonucleic acid of a coronavirus. They vary from place to place and from time to time, for reasons that are as much social and political as genetic.

For most of history, ignorance of medical science left communities more or less defenseless against new strains of disease. And the bigger and more commercially integrated a society, the more likely it was to suffer a pandemic, as the Greeks and Romans found out to their detriment. It was precisely the existence of trans-Eurasian trade routes that enabled the bacterium *Yersinia pestis* to kill so many fourteenth-century Europeans. Likewise, European expansion overseas, beginning roughly a century and a half later, led to the so-called Columbian Exchange: pathogens brought by Europeans devastated indigenous American populations; Europeans then brought back syphilis from the New World; and by shipping enslaved Africans to the Caribbean and the Americas, Europeans also brought malaria and yellow fever to those places. By the late nineteenth century, the European empires could claim to be conquering contagious disease. Yet fin de siècle failures to cope with public health crises, such as the return of the bubonic plague, became sources of grievance for indigenous nationalists, just as outbreaks of cholera in ports and industrial cities were grist to the mills of progressives and social democrats at home. As late as the 1950s, pandemics were still seen as a recurrent feature of the global order.

The later twentieth century was a time of seeming progress. Even as they plotted to wage biological warfare against each other, the Soviet Union and the United States collaborated to eradicate smallpox and competed to contain malaria. From the 1950s to the 1980s, great strides were made in multiple fields of public health, from vaccination to sanitation. Indeed, by the late twentieth century it seemed to some as if the threat of a pandemic had receded. With the rise of the randomized controlled clinical trial as the standard for medical research, we had arrived, or so it seemed, at "the end of medical history."[32] We had not, of course. Beginning with the HIV/AIDS pandemic, a succession of new viruses exposed the vulnerability of an increasingly networked world.

We had countless warnings that humanity's most clear and present danger was a new pathogen and the global pandemic it could cause. Yet somehow these warnings did not translate into swift, effective action in a majority of countries when the gray rhino became a black swan in January 2020. In China, the one-party state responded to the outbreak of the novel coronavirus in much the same way that its Soviet counterpart had responded to the 1986 Chernobyl nuclear disaster: with lies. In the United States, a populist president, echoed by cable news, at first dismissed the threat as a mere seasonal flu, then erratically intervened in his administration's response. But a distinct scandal was the abject failure of the government agencies whose one job was biodefense. In Britain the pattern was similar. In Europe, federalist aspirations (and the Euroskeptic notion of a European superstate) were initially exposed as hollow as each country sought to save itself, reimposing national frontiers and seeking to hoard scarce medical equipment. Talk of a European "community of fate" (*Schicksalsgemeinschaft*) resumed only when it was clear that Germany would not suffer the fate of Italy. In each case, the disaster was a moment of revelation not just of the pathogen's virulence but of the defects of the polities concerned. For the same virus was far less devastating in Taiwan and South Korea, to name two East Asian democracies whose preparedness proved equal to the challenge. Chapter 9 seeks to explain why that was, and the harmful role that the parallel "infodemic" of fake news and conspiracy theories played. Chapter 10 considers the economic consequences of the pandemic and offers an explanation for the apparently paradoxical behavior of financial markets in the face of the biggest macroeconomic shock since 1929–32. Finally, chapter 11 considers the geopolitical consequences of the pandemic and casts tentative doubt on the popular view that China will be the principal beneficiary and the United States the principal loser from COVID-19.

ELON'S WAY

What general lessons can we learn from the historical study of catastrophes?

First, it may simply be impossible to predict or even attach probabilities to the majority of disasters. From earthquakes to wars to financial crises, the major disruptions in history have been characterized by random or by power-law distributions. They belong in the domain of uncertainty, not risk.

Second, disaster takes too many forms for us to process with conventional approaches to risk mitigation. No sooner have we focused our minds on the threat of Salafi jihad than we find ourselves in a financial crisis originating in subprime mortgages. No sooner have we relearned that such economic shocks often lead to populist political backlashes than a novel coronavirus is wreaking havoc. What will be next? We cannot know. For every potential calamity, there is at least one plausible Cassandra. Not all prophecies can be heeded. In recent years we may have allowed one risk—namely climate change—to draw our attention away from the others. In January, even as a global pandemic was getting under way—as flights laden with infected people were leaving Wuhan for destinations all over the world—the discussions at the World Economic Forum were focused almost entirely on questions of environmental responsibility, social justice, and governance (ESG), with the emphasis on the *E*. As will become clear, I see the dangers arising from climbing global temperatures as real and potentially catastrophic, but climate change cannot be the sole threat we prepare for. Recognition of the multiplicity of threats we confront, and the extreme uncertainty of their incidence, would encourage a more flexible response to disaster. Not coincidentally, the states that did best in 2020 included three—notably Taiwan and South Korea (and initially Israel)—that face multiple threats, including an existential threat from neighbors.

Third, not all disasters are global. However, the more networked human society becomes, the greater the potential for contagion, and not just of the biological variety. A networked society needs to have well-designed circuit breakers that can swiftly reduce the connectivity of the network in a crisis, without atomizing and paralyzing society completely. Moreover, any disaster is either amplified or dampened by flows of information. Disinformation in 2020—for example, viral fake news about bogus therapies—made COVID-19 worse in many places. By contrast, effective management of information flows about infected people and their contacts helped contain the pandemic in a few well-run countries. The global network of scientific research worked wonders.

Fourth, as chapter 9 shows, COVID-19 exposed a serious failure of the public health bureaucracy in the United States and a number of other countries. It was tempting—and many journalists succumbed to the temptation—to lay all the blame for the excess mortality caused by the pandemic on the president. This was the kind of error Tolstoy mocked in *War and Peace:* the tendency to attach too much importance in the historical process to individual leaders. In reality, there were multiple points of failure in 2020, from the assistant secretary for preparedness and response at the Department of Health and Human Services to the governor of New York and the mayor of New York City to traditional and social media. On paper, the United States was ready for a pandemic—better prepared and better resourced than any country in the world. Almost as well prepared—on paper—was the British government. Yet when, in January, reports from China made it clear that the new coronavirus now known as SARS-CoV-2 was both contagious and lethal, there was a disastrous failure to act, on both sides of the Atlantic. The American epidemiologist Larry Brilliant, a key figure in the campaign to eradicate smallpox, has said for many years that the formula for dealing with an infectious disease is "early detection, early response."[33] In Washington and London there was just the opposite. Would a different kind of threat produce an equally sluggish and ineffectual reaction? If the problems exposed by the pandemic are not specific to the public health bureaucracy but are general problems of the administrative state, then it probably would.

Finally, there is a tendency throughout history, at times of acute social stress, for religious or quasi-religious ideological impulses to impede rational responses. We had all previously contemplated the danger of a pandemic, but more as entertainment (*Contagion*) than as a potential reality. Even now, when other science fiction scenarios are being realized—not only rising temperatures and climatic instability but also the rise and expansion of the Chinese surveillance state, to name just two—we struggle to react coherently and consequently. In the summer of 2020, millions of Americans took to the streets of nearly three hundred cities to protest loudly and sometimes violently against police brutality and systemic racism. However shocking the incident that precipitated the protests, this was risky behavior amid a pandemic of a highly contagious respiratory disease. At the same time, the rudimentary precaution of wearing a mask became a symbol of partisan affiliation. The fact that, in some parts of the country, gun buying seemed more popular than mask wearing testified to the potential for a public-order as well as a public-health disaster.

COVID-19 is not the last disaster we shall confront in our lifetimes. It is just the latest, after a wave of Islamist terrorism, a global financial crisis, a rash of state failures, surges of unregulated migration, and a so-called democratic recession. Next up probably won't be a disaster attributable to climate change, as we rarely get the disaster we expect, but some other threat most of us are currently ignoring. Perhaps it will be a strain of antibiotic-resistant bubonic plague, or perhaps a massive Russian-Chinese cyberattack on the United States and its allies. Perhaps it will be a breakthrough in nanotechnology or in genetic engineering that has disastrous unintended consequences.[34] Or perhaps artificial intelligence will fulfill Elon Musk's forebodings, reducing an intellectually outclassed humanity to the status of "a biological boot loader for digital super intelligence." Musk was notable in 2020 for dismissing the threat posed by COVID-19. ("The coronavirus panic is dumb," he tweeted on March 6.) He has also argued that "humans will solve environmental sustainability" and that even death itself—the existential threat to every individual—can be overcome with some combination of DNA editing and neurological data storage. Yet Musk is in other respects pessimistic about our future as a civilized species on Earth:

> Civilization has been around for . . . 7,000 years or something like that. If you counted from the first time there was any writing, any recorded symbols, besides cave paintings, that's a very tiny amount of time considering the universe is 13.8 billion years old. . . . And it's been . . . kind of a roller coaster, on the civilization front. . . . There is a certain probability that is irreducible, that something may happen to us, despite our best intentions, despite everything we try to do. There's a probability at a certain point that some either external force or some internal unforced error causes civilization to be destroyed. Or sufficiently impaired such that it can no longer extend to another planet.[35]

For Musk, the choice is essentially between "the singularity," in the sense of unstoppable progress in AI, and the end of civilization ("Those are the two possibilities"). Hence his contrarian warning that "the biggest problem the world will face in 20 years is population collapse." Hence his proposal to colonize Mars.

We simply cannot know which of all the possible future disasters—discussed more fully in the conclusion—will strike and when. All we can do is learn from history how to build social and political structures that are at least resilient and at best antifragile; how to avoid the descent into self-flagellating chaos that so often characterizes societies overwhelmed by disaster; and how to resist the siren voices who propose totalitarian rule or world government as necessary for the protection of our hapless species and our vulnerable world.

1

THE MEANING OF DEATH

This fell sergeant, death, is strict in his arrest.

—Hamlet

WE ARE ALL DOOMED

"We're doomed." This line, uttered by the Caledonian Cassandra of the British television sitcom *Dad's Army,* Private James Frazer, was one of the running jokes of my youth. The trick was to say it at the most incongruous moment possible—when the milk had run out or you had missed the last bus home. There's a wonderful scene in one episode ("Uninvited Guests") when Frazer—played by the great John Laurie—tells the other members of his Home Guard platoon a bloodcurdling story of a curse. As a young man, he was anchored off a small island near Samoa, where—according to his friend Jethro—there was a ruined temple, inside which stood an idol decorated with a giant ruby "the size of a duck's egg." They set out to steal the ruby, hacking their way through dense forest. But just as Jethro laid his hands on it, they were confronted by a witch doctor, who cursed Jethro with the words "DEATH! THE RUBY WILL BRING YE DEATH! DE-E-ATH."

PRIVATE PIKE: Did the curse come true, Mr. Frazer?

PRIVATE FRAZER: Aye, son, it did. He died . . . last year—he was eighty-six.

We are all doomed, if not necessarily cursed. I shall be dead by 2056, at the latest. My additional life expectancy at the age of fifty-six years and two months is, according to the Social Security Administration, 26.2 years, which would get me to eighty-two, four years less than Frazer's cursed friend. Rather more encouragingly, the UK Office for National Statistics gives a man of my age an additional two years, with a 1 in 4 chance of making it to ninety-two. To see if I could improve on these numbers, I went to the Living to 100 Life Expectancy Calculator, which bases its estimate on a detailed questionnaire about one's lifestyle and family history. Living to 100 told me I probably wouldn't make a century, but I had a better-than-even chance of living thirty-six more years.[1] It might, of course, have been another story if I had caught COVID-19 back in January, as the disease then had a fatality rate of 6 percent for my age group, and perhaps slightly higher if we factor in my mild asthma.

To die at fifty-six would certainly be a disappointment, but it would be a good result by the standards of the majority of the 107 billion human beings who have ever lived. In the United Kingdom, where I was born, life expectancy at birth did not reach fifty-six until 1920, exactly a hundred years ago. The average for the entire period from 1543 until 1863 was just under forty. And the United Kingdom was notable for its longevity. Estimates for the world as a whole put life expectancy below thirty until 1900, when it reached thirty-two, and below fifty until 1960. Indian life expectancy was just twenty-three in 1911. Russian life expectancy fell to a nadir of twenty in 1920. There has been a sustained upward trend over the past century—life expectancy at birth roughly doubled between 1913 and 2006—but with numerous setbacks. Life expectancy in Somalia today is fifty-six: my age.[2] It is still low there partly because infant and child mortality is so high. Around 12.2 percent of children born in Somalia die before they reach the age of five; 2.5 percent die between the ages of five and fourteen.[3]

When I try to put my own experience of the human condition into perspective, I think of the Jacobean poet John Donne (1572–1631), who lived to the age of fifty-nine. In the space of sixteen years, Anne Donne bore her husband twelve children. Three of them—Francis, Nicholas, and Mary—died before they were ten. Anne herself died after giving birth to the twelfth child, who was stillborn. After his favorite daughter, Lucy, had died and he himself had very nearly followed her to the grave, Donne wrote his *Devotions upon Emergent Occasions* (1624), which contains the greatest of all exhortations to commiserate with the dead: "Any man's *death* diminishes *me,* because I am involved in *Mankinde;* And therefore never send to know for whom the *bell* tolls; It tolls for *thee.*"

The Neapolitan artist Salvator Rosa painted perhaps the most moving of all memento mori, entitled simply *L'umana fragilità* (*Human Frailty*). It was inspired by an outbreak of bubonic plague that had struck his native Naples in 1655, claiming the life of his infant son, Rosalvo, as well as carrying off Salvator's brother, his sister, her husband, and five of their children. Grinning hideously, a winged skeleton reaches out of the darkness behind Rosa's mistress, Lucrezia, to claim their son, even as he makes his first attempt to write. The mood of the heartbroken artist is immortally summed up in the eight Latin words the baby, guided by the skeletal figure, has inscribed on the canvas:

Conceptio culpa
Nasci pena
Labor vita
Necesse mori

"Conception is sin, birth is pain, life is toil, death is inevitable." I remember being thunderstruck when, on my first visit to the Fitzwilliam Museum, in Cambridge, I read those words. Here was the human condition, stripped down to its bleak essentials. By all accounts, Rosa was a lighthearted man, who also wrote and acted in satirical plays and masques. At around the time of his son's death, however, he wrote to a friend, "This time heaven has struck me in such a way that shows me that all human remedies are useless and the least pain I feel is when I tell you that I weep as I write."[4] He himself died of dropsy at the age of fifty-eight.

Death was ubiquitous in the medieval and early modern world in a way that we struggle to imagine. As Philippe Ariès argued in *The Hour of Our*

Death, death was "tamed" by being, like marriage and even childbirth, a social rite of passage, shared with family and community and followed by funerary and mourning rites that offered familiar consolations to the bereaved. Beginning in the seventeenth century, however, attitudes changed. As mortality became more perplexing, even while its causes became better understood, so Western societies began to create a certain distance between the living and the dead. While the Victorians excessively sentimentalized and romanticized death—creating in literature "beautiful deaths" that bore less and less relation to the real thing—the twentieth century went into denial about the "end of life." Dying became an increasingly solitary, antisocial, almost invisible act. What Ariès called "an absolutely new type of dying" arose, which removed the moribund to hospitals and hospices and ensured that the moment of expiration was discreetly hidden behind screens.[5] Americans eschew the verb "to die." People "pass." Evelyn Waugh cruelly satirized this American way of death in *The Loved One* (1948), inspired by an unhappy sojourn in Hollywood.

The British way of death is only slightly better, however. In Monty Python's *The Meaning of Life,* death is one enormous faux pas. The Grim Reaper—John Cleese, shrouded in a black cloak—arrives at a picturesque English country home where three couples are in the middle of a dinner party:

GRIM REAPER: I am death.

DEBBIE: Well, isn't that extraordinary? We were just talking about death only five minutes ago. . . .

GRIM REAPER: Silence! I have come for you.

ANGELA: You mean . . . to—

GRIM REAPER: Take you away. That is my purpose. I am death.

GEOFFREY: Well, that's cast rather a gloom over the evening, hasn't it? . . .

DEBBIE: Can I ask you a question?

GRIM REAPER: What?

DEBBIE: How can we all have died at the same time?

GRIM REAPER: (*After long pause, points finger at serving dish*) The salmon mousse.

GEOFFREY: Darling, you didn't use canned salmon, did you?

ANGELA: I'm most dreadfully embarrassed.

THE IMMINENT ESCHATON

Each year, around the world, around fifty-nine million people expire—roughly the entire population of the world at the time King David ruled over the Israelites. In other words, roughly 160,000 people die each day—the equivalent of one Oxford or three Palo Altos. Around 60 percent of those who die are sixty-five or older. In the first half of 2020, roughly 510,000 people worldwide died of the new disease COVID-19. Each death is a tragedy, as we shall see. But even if none of these people would have died then anyway—which is unlikely, given the age profile of the dead—that represents only a modest (1.8 percent) increase in total expected deaths for the first half of 2020. In 2018, 2.84 million Americans died, so around 236,000 died per month, and 7,800 a day. Three quarters of those who died were sixty-five or older. By far the biggest killers were heart disease and cancer, which accounted for 44 percent of the total. In the first half of 2020, according to the Centers for Disease Control and Prevention, there were 130,122 American deaths recorded as "involving COVID-19." However, total excess (above-normal) mortality from all causes was close to 170,000. If none of these people would have died anyway—again unlikely—that represented an 11 percent increase in deaths for that period above the baseline derived from recent averages.

We are all doomed, then, even if medical scientists are able to extend life expectancy still further—as some predict, beyond a century. Despite the ongoing quest for solutions to the problem that life is a terminal condition,[6] immortality remains a dream—or, as Jorge Luis Borges intimated in "The Immortal," a nightmare.[7] But are we also doomed, collectively, as a species? The answer is yes.

Life, as our physicist mother never tired of reminding my sister and me, is a cosmic accident—a view also held by better-known physicists such as Murray Gell-Mann.[8] Our universe began 13.7 billion years ago, in what we call the Big Bang. On our planet, with the help of ultraviolet rays and lightning, the chemical building blocks of life developed, leading to the first living cell 3.5 to 4 billion years ago. Starting around 2 billion years ago, sexual reproduction by simple multicellular organisms unleashed waves of evolutionary innovation. About 6 million years ago, a genetic mutation in chimpanzees led to the first humanlike apes. *Homo sapiens* appeared extremely recently, 200,000 to 100,000 years ago, dominated other human types around 30,000 years ago, and had spread to most of the planet by around 13,000 years ago.[9] A lot of things had to be just right for us to get to this point. But the "Goldilocks" conditions in which we flourish cannot endure indefinitely. To date, around 99.9 percent of all species ever to have inhabited Earth have become extinct.

In other words, to quote Nick Bostrom and Milan M. Ćirković, "extinction of intelligent species *has* already happened on Earth, suggesting that it would be naive to think it may not happen again."[10] Even if we avoid the fate of the dinosaurs and the dodos, "in about 3.5 billion years, the growing luminosity of the sun will essentially have sterilized the Earth's biosphere, but the end of complex life on Earth is scheduled to come sooner, maybe 0.9–1.5 billion years from now," since conditions will by then have become intolerable for anything resembling us. "This is the default fate for life on our planet."[11] We might conceivably be able to find another habitable planet if we solve the problem of intergalactic travel, which involves almost unimaginably vast distances. Even then, we shall eventually run out of time, as the last stars will die roughly a hundred trillion years from now, after which matter itself will disintegrate into its basic constituents.

The thought that, as a species, we may have around a billion years left on Earth should be reassuring. And yet many of us seem to yearn for doomsday to come much sooner than that. The "end time," or eschaton (from the Greek *eskhatos*), is a feature of most of the world's major religions, including the most ancient, Zoroastrianism. The Bahman Yasht envisages not only crop failures and a general moral decay but also "a dark cloud [that] makes the whole sky night" and a rain of "noxious creatures." Although Hindu eschatology assumes vast cycles of time, the one currently under way, Kali Yuga, is expected to end violently, when Kalki, the final incarnation of Vishnu, descends on a white horse at the head of an army to "establish righteousness upon the earth." In Buddhism, too, there are apocalyptic scenes. Gautama Buddha prophesied that, after five thousand years, his teachings would be forgotten, leading to the moral degeneration of mankind. A bodhisattva named Maitreya would then appear and rediscover the teaching of dharma, after which the world would be destroyed by the deadly rays of seven suns. Norse mythology, too, has its Ragnarök (twilight of the gods), in which a devastating great winter (Fimbulvetr) will plunge the world into darkness and despair. The gods will fight to the death with the forces of chaos, fire giants, and other magical creatures (*jötunn*). In the end, the ocean will completely submerge the world. (Devotees of Wagner have seen a version of this in his *Götterdämmerung*.)

In each of these religions, destruction is the prelude to rebirth. The Abrahamic religions, by contrast, have a linear cosmology: the end of days really is The End. Judaism foresees a Messianic Age with the return to Israel of the exiled Jewish Diaspora, the coming of the Messiah, and the resurrection of the dead. Christianity—the faith established by the followers of a man who claimed to be that Messiah—offers a much richer version of the eschaton. Prior to the Second Coming of Christ (*parousia*), as Jesus himself told his followers, there would be a time of "great tribulation" (Matthew 24:15–22), "affliction" (Mark 13:19), or "days of vengeance" (Luke 21:10–33 offers the most detail of the Gospels). The Revelation of Saint John offers perhaps the most striking of all visions of doom—of a war in heaven between Michael and his angels and Satan, an interlude when Satan would be cast down and bound for a thousand years, after which Christ would reign for a millennium with resurrected martyrs by his side, only for the Whore of Babylon, drunk with the blood of the saints, to appear atop a scarlet beast, and a great battle to be fought at Armageddon. After that, Satan would be unleashed, then thrown into a lake of burning sulfur, and, finally, the dead would be judged by Christ and the unworthy cast down into the fiery lake. The description of the four horsemen of the Apocalypse is astonishing:

> And I saw when the Lamb opened one of the seals, and I heard, as it were the noise of thunder, one of the four beasts saying, Come and see. And I saw, and behold a white horse: and he that sat on him had a bow; and a crown was given unto him: and he went forth conquering, and to conquer.
>
> And when he had opened the second seal, I heard the second beast say, Come and see. And there went out another horse that was red: and power was given to him that sat thereon to take peace from the earth, and that they should kill one another: and there was given unto him a great sword.
>
> And when he had opened the third seal, I heard the third beast say, Come and see. And I beheld, and lo a black horse; and he that sat on him had a pair of balances in his hand.
>
> And I heard a voice in the midst of the four beasts say, A measure of wheat for a penny, and three measures of barley for a penny; and see thou hurt not the oil and the wine.
>
> And when he had opened the fourth seal, I heard the voice of the fourth beast say, Come and see.
>
> And I looked, and behold a pale horse: and his name that sat on him was Death, and Hell followed with him. And power was given unto them over the fourth part of the earth, to kill with sword, and with hunger, and with death, and with the beasts of the earth. (Revelation 6:1–8)

The day of wrath is heralded by a great earthquake, an eclipse of the sun, and a blood moon. The stars fall to the earth, and the mountains and islands are "moved out of their places."

A clever feature of the Christian eschaton was the uncertainty Christ left in his disciples' minds about its timing: "But of that day and hour knoweth no man, no, not the angels of heaven, but my Father only" (Matthew 24:36).

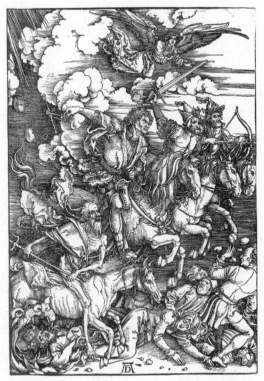

Albrecht Dürer, *The Four Horsemen of the Apocalypse* (1498).

The destruction of Jerusalem in AD 70 at the hands of Titus was interpreted by the early Christians as fulfillment of Jesus's prophecy that the Second Temple would be destroyed, but the subsequent spectacular events Christ had prophesied did not materialize.[12] By the time of Augustine of Hippo, it seemed prudent to downplay the millennium, as he did in *The City of God* (AD 426), consigning it to the realm of the unknowable and (implicitly) remote.

Perhaps the decline of Christian millennialism helps explain the revolutionary impact of Muhammad's new religion when it erupted from the Arabian Desert in the seventh century. In a number of respects, Islam simply dusted down the more exciting parts of Revelation. In Mecca, Muhammad taught his followers that the Day of Judgment would be preceded by the appearance of the one-eyed al-Masih ad-Dajjāl (the false messiah), with an entourage of seventy thousand Jews from Isfahan. Isa (Jesus) would then descend to triumph over the false messiah. In Sunni doctrine, the *ashrāṭ al-sā‘a*—the conditions of the hour—would include a huge black cloud of smoke (*dukhān*) covering the earth, a succession of sinkings of the earth, and the appearance of Ya‘jūj and Ma‘jūj (Gog and Magog) to ravage the earth and slaughter believers. After Allah had disposed of Gog and Magog, the sun would rise from the west, the Dābbat al-Ard (Beast of the Earth) would rise out of the ground, and, after the sounding of the divine trumpet, the dead would also rise (al-Qiyāmah) for the final judgment (Yawm al-Hisāb). When this prophecy failed to come true, however, Muhammad impatiently turned from redemption to imperialism. Allah, he argued in Medina, wanted Muslims to preserve his honor by punishing the unbelievers—to go from awaiting Judgment Day to expediting it with acts of jihad.[13] Shia eschatology is broadly similar to Sunni, but with the return of the Twelfth Imam, Muhammad al-Mahdi, foreseen after a period of declining morality and modesty.

For Christians, the Islamic conquests of the Near East and North Africa were just the biggest of a number of ghastly threats—Vikings, Magyars, and Mongols were also menacing Christendom. These and other disasters were interpreted by some as intimations of the end time; Christian eschatology never entirely receded. Joachim of Fiore (1135–1202) divided history into three ages, of which the third would be the final one. Likewise, in the wake of the Black Death of the 1340s—in terms of its mortality rate the biggest calamity ever suffered by Christians—there were those who inferred that the end was nigh. In 1356, a Franciscan monk named John of Roquetaillade wrote *Vademecum in tribulationibus,* prophesying a time of troubles in Europe that would feature social upheaval, tempests, floods, and more plagues.[14] Similar quasi-revolutionary visions inspired the Taborites in Bohemia in 1420 and the Franciscan Johann Hilten's 1485 prophecies of the twilight of the papacy.[15] And again, in the wake of Martin Luther's epoch-making challenge to the ecclesiastical hierarchy, millennialism gave sects as diverse as the Anabaptists, the Diggers, and the Levellers the confidence to defy established authority. Although the pursuit of the millennium abated in the eighteenth century, it revived again in the nineteenth and twentieth centuries, when some followers of the would-be prophet William Miller, later known as the Seventh-day Adventists, established a new church with a strongly millennialist doctrine that anticipated the end of the world in 1844. (The Millerites referred to mankind's survival that year as "the Great Disappointment.") Jehovah's Witnesses and members of the Church of Jesus Christ of Latter-day Saints (Mormons) both hold their own distinctive views of the imminence of the eschaton. Numerous modern cult leaders have persuaded their followers that the end was nigh. A number—notably Jim Jones, David Koresh, and Marshall Applewhite—achieved localized apocalypses in the form of mass suicides.

The end of the world, in short, has been a remarkably recurrent feature of recorded history.

DOOMSDAYS

It might be thought that the advance of science would ultimately liberate human beings from religious and pseudo-religious eschatology. Not necessarily. As the sociologist James Hughes has said, few of us are "immune to millennial biases, positive or negative, fatalist or messianic."[16] Just over a century ago, as the first truly industrialized war ground toward its conclusion—a war waged with tanks, planes, submarines, and poison gas—there were apparitions of the Virgin Mary in the Portuguese village of Fatima, a battle at Armageddon (Megiddo, in what was then Palestine), the proclamation of a Jewish home in the Holy Land, a German offensive named after the Archangel Michael, and a global pandemic more lethal than the war itself.[17] One of many intimations of impending apocalypse was the rise to power of Vladimir Ilyich Lenin, who unleashed a wave of anticlerical violence and iconoclasm across the Russian Empire.[18] As *The New York Times* reported on June 21, 1919, Lenin was widely seen by Russian peasants as "none other than the antichrist foretold in the Scriptures."[19]

To the Cologne-born political theorist Eric Voegelin, the reality was that Communism, like the Nazism he had to flee in 1938, was itself based on a flawed utopian interpretation of Christianity. Voegelin defined "gnosis" as "a purported direct, immediate apprehension or vision of truth without the need for critical reflection; the special gift of a spiritual and cognitive elite." Gnosticism, he argued, was a "type of thinking that claims absolute cognitive mastery of reality." When it took the form of a political religion, it harbored a dangerous and misguided ambition to "immanentize the eschaton"—in other words, to create a heaven on earth.[20] Voegelin's modern gnostics sought the "redivinization of society . . . substituting more massive modes of participation in divinity for faith in the Christian sense."[21] (Voegelin speculated that this shift to "massive participation" might be a response to the sheer difficulty of sustaining an authentic Christian faith.)[22] Writing more recently but in a similar spirit, the historian Richard Landes has detected the same urge in a wide range of historical and modern millennialist movements, up to and including Salafi jihadism and radical environmentalism.[23]

Far from displacing the eschaton, science seemed to bring it nearer. When J. Robert Oppenheimer witnessed the first atomic explosion at White Sands, New Mexico, he famously thought of Krishna's words from the Bhagavad Gita (the Hindu Song of the Lord): "I am become Death, the destroyer of worlds."[24] At the very beginning of the Cold War, the artist Martyl Langsdorf, whose husband was a key figure in the Manhattan Project, came up with the image of a "Doomsday Clock."[25] It first appeared in the *Bulletin of the Atomic Scientists* to illustrate the fear of many physicists—including some who had been involved in the creation of the atomic bomb—that a "technology-induced catastrophe" might be terrifyingly close. Midnight on the Doomsday Clock meant nuclear Armageddon. For many years, it was the *Bulletin*'s editor, Eugene Rabinowitch, who decided where the hands on the clock stood. After his death, a committee took over, meeting twice a year to adjust the clock. During the Cold War, the closest it came to midnight was in the years 1953–59, when the Doomsday Clock was moved to two minutes before midnight. The scientists also thought the years 1984–87 were fraught with peril: it was three minutes to midnight for four straight years. Popular literature reflected these anxieties. In Nevil Shute's *On the Beach* (1957), the year is 1963 and the people of Melbourne helplessly await a lethal cloud of radioactive fallout in the aftermath of World War III, which has been triggered, somewhat implausibly, by an Albanian nuclear attack on Italy. The choice is between heavy drinking and a government-issued suicide pill. In Raymond Briggs's graphic novel *When the Wind Blows* (1982), an elderly couple, Jim and Hilda Bloggs, dutifully build a fallout shelter, acting as if World War III will be as survivable as World War II had been.

Yet the reliability of the Doomsday Clock is open to question. Historians today agree that the most dangerous moment in the Cold War was the Cuban Missile Crisis. But the Doomsday Clock was at seven minutes to midnight throughout 1962, and it went back to 11:48 p.m. the following year, remaining there even as President Lyndon B. Johnson escalated the American involvement in the Vietnam War. Remarkably, the atomic scientists decided we were back to two minutes to Armageddon in January 2018,[26] and two years later they moved the clock forward to one hundred seconds to midnight, on the grounds that "humanity continues to face two simultaneous existential dangers—nuclear war and climate change—that are compounded by a threat multiplier, cyber-enabled information warfare, that undercuts society's ability to respond. The international security situation is dire, not just because these threats exist, but because world leaders have allowed the international political infrastructure for managing them to erode."[27] Somehow, today's doom is always better than last year's.

The nightmare of nuclear war was not the only apocalyptic vision to haunt the Cold War world. From the 1960s until the 1980s, a fear of global overpopulation led to a succession of mostly misguided and often downright harmful efforts to "control" reproduction in what was then called the Third World. Stephen Enke, of the RAND Corporation, argued that paying poor people to agree to sterilization or the insertion of intrauterine devices (IUDs) would be 250 times more effective in promoting development than other forms of aid. Paul Ehrlich's *The Population Bomb,* commissioned by the Sierra Club, predicted mass starvation in the 1970s, with devastating famines killing hundreds of millions of people. Lyndon Johnson was convinced, as were a majority of members of Congress, which increased the U.S. Agency for International Development's budget for family planning by a factor of twenty.

As president of the World Bank, former defense secretary Robert McNamara declared in 1969 that the bank would not finance healthcare "unless it was very strictly related to population control, because usually health facilities contributed to the decline of the death rate, and thereby to the population explosion." Some American institutions—including the Ford Foundation and the Population Council—toyed with the idea of mass involuntary sterilization of entire populations. The consequences provide yet another illustration that people convinced of an imagined impending apocalypse can do a great deal of real harm. Encouraging, if not quite forcing, Indian women to accept IUDs and Indian men to accept vasectomies led to much suffering. At the height of the Indian Emergency of the mid-seventies, the government of Indira Gandhi carried out more than eight million sterilizations. Nearly two thousand people died because of botched operations. The United Nations also supported the Chinese Communist Party's even more brutally administered "one-child policy."[28] With hindsight, we can see that the solution to the problem of rising population was not mass sterilization but the "Green Revolution" in agricultural technology, pioneered by agronomists such as Norman Borlaug.

Today's latter-day millennialists are the prophets of catastrophic climate change. "Around 2030," the Swedish environmentalist Greta Thunberg has written, "we will be in a position to set off an irreversible chain reaction beyond human control that will lead to the end of our civilization as we know it."[29] "The world is going to end in 12 years if we don't address climate change," the Democratic congresswoman Alexandria Ocasio-Cortez prophesied in 2019.[30] Thunberg's emergence as the personification of radical environmentalism recalls past forms of eschatology, not least in the severity of the sacrifices she demands. "We don't need a 'low carbon economy,'" she declared at the World Economic Forum in January 2020. "We don't need to 'lower emissions.' Our emissions have to stop if we are to have a chance to stay below the 1.5-degree target. . . . Any plan or policy of yours that doesn't include radical emission cuts at the source, starting today, is completely insufficient."[31] The new green revolution—or Green New Deal—proposed by Ocasio-Cortez, Thunberg, and others implies a drastic reduction in all CO_2 emissions, with little regard for the economic and social costs. We shall return to this subject below; suffice

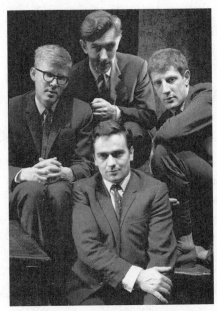

"Now is the end—perish the world!" The *Beyond the Fringe* cast prepares for the end time.

for now to say that warnings of the imminent end of the world risk becoming (like the cry of "wolf!" in the children's story) less credible through repetition.

The inescapable fact remains: millennialist prophets, gnostic pursuers of the eschaton, scientists warning of calamity, and authors imagining it—all of these groups together have succeeded in predicting no fewer than a hundred of the last zero ends of the world. In the theatrical comedy revue *Beyond the Fringe* (1961), Peter Cook plays Brother Enim, a prophet who has led his followers to a mountaintop to await the apocalypse:

JONATHAN MILLER: How will it be, this end of which you have spoken, Brother Enim?

ALL: Yes, how will it be?

PETER COOK: Well, it will be, as 'twere a mighty rending in the sky, you see, and the mountains shall sink, you see, and the valleys shall rise, you see, and great shall be the tumult thereof.

MILLER: Will the veil of the temple be rent in twain?

COOK: The veil of the temple *will* be rent in twain about two minutes before we see the sign of the manifest flying beast-head in the sky.

ALAN BENNETT: And will there be a mighty wind, Brother Enim?

COOK: Certainly there will be a mighty wind, if the word of God is anything to go by. . . .

DUDLEY MOORE: And will this wind be so mighty as to lay low the mountains of the earth?

COOK: No, it will not be quite as mighty as that—that's why we have come *up* on the mountain, you stupid nit. . . .

MILLER: When will it be, this end of which you have spoken?

ALL: Aye, when will it be, when will it be?

COOK: In about thirty seconds' time, according to the ancient pyramidic scrolls . . . and my Ingersoll watch.

The prophet and his followers compose themselves for the end of the world and count down:

COOK: Five, four, three, two, one—zero!

ALL: (*Chanting.*) Now is the end—perish the world!

A pause.

COOK: It *was* GMT, wasn't it?

MILLER: Yes.

COOK: Well, it's not quite the conflagration I'd been banking on. Never mind, lads, same time tomorrow . . . we must get a winner one day.

THE STATISTICS OF CALAMITY

What we really have to fear is big disasters that do not kill us all, but just a large number of us. The trouble is that we struggle to conceptualize both the potential scale of disasters and their likelihood. "One death is a tragedy; a million is a statistic." That aphorism is conventionally credited to Stalin, an attribution that can be traced back to a 1947 *Washington Post* column by Leonard Lyons:

> In the days when Stalin was Commissar of Munitions a meeting was held of the highest ranking Commissars, and the principal matter for discussion was the famine then prevalent in the Ukraine. One official arose and made a speech about this tragedy—the tragedy of having millions of people dying of hunger. He began to enumerate death figures. . . . Stalin interrupted him to say: "If only one man dies of hunger, that is a tragedy. If millions die, that's only statistics."[32]

Lyons didn't cite a source, but either he or Stalin almost certainly borrowed the phrase from the Berlin satirist Kurt Tucholsky, who in turn attributed it to a French diplomat: "War? I don't find that so terrible. The death of one human being, that's a catastrophe. A hundred thousand dead—that's a statistic."[33] We encounter a version of this mentality in our time, as Eliezer Yudkowsky has observed: "People who would never dream of hurting a child hear of an existential risk, and say, 'Well, maybe the human species doesn't really deserve to survive.' . . . The challenge of existential risks to rationality is that, the catastrophes being so huge, people snap into a different mode of thinking. Human deaths are suddenly no longer bad, and detailed predictions suddenly no longer require any expertise."[34]

We must at least try to make sense of the statistics. Making due allowance for the grave defects of historical sources, we may say that there have probably been in all of recorded history seven major pandemics with victims greater than 1 percent of the estimated world population, of which four killed

more than 3 percent and two—the Plague of Justinian and the Black Death—
more than 30 percent, though the toll of the former may well have been much
less.[35] Likewise, the available data on mortality resulting from warfare point
to the existence of a small number of very lethal conflicts. Data from the physicist L. F. Richardson and the social scientist Jack Levy, as well as other, more
recent studies, point to seven large-scale wars that killed in excess of 0.1 percent of the estimated world population at the time they broke out. The two
world wars were the deadliest conflicts in history in absolute terms. In Richardson's analysis of all "deadly conflicts" between 1820 and 1950, the world
wars were the only magnitude-7 wars, that is, the only ones with death tolls
in the tens of millions. They accounted for three fifths of all the deaths in his
sample, which included homicides, wars, and everything in between.[36] The
world wars killed around 1 and 3 percent, respectively, of the world population in 1914 and 1939. There may have been comparably devastating conflicts
in earlier periods, notably the wars of the Three Kingdoms era in third-century
China, between the Han and Jin dynasties.[37] In relative terms—that is, the proportions of combatant forces killed—the War of the Triple Alliance (1864–70)
is ranked among the deadliest of modern history, yet it is more or less unknown outside the countries that fought it: Argentina, Brazil, and Uruguay,
which combined against Paraguay. On the whole, then, pathogens have been
significantly more lethal than wars. Indeed, most of the people who lost their
lives in the War of the Triple Alliance died of disease, not enemy action. According to Pasquale Cirillo and Nassim Taleb's estimates, "no armed conflict
has ever killed more than 19 percent of the world population."[38] The conquistadors killed orders of magnitude fewer Central and South Americans than
did the diseases they brought with them from Europe, to which the indigenous peoples had no resistance.[39]

Similar exercises can be carried out for civil wars as well as genocides or
democides—mass murders of populations, as distinct from fatalities incurred
in interstate warfare. The total victims of Stalinism within the Soviet Union
may have exceeded twenty million—a "statistic" indeed. Mortality rates in excess of 10 percent have also been estimated for Pol Pot's reign of terror in Cambodia, as well as for the civil wars in Mexico (1910–20) and Equatorial Guinea

(1972–79). In Richardson's list of magnitude-6 deadly conflicts, six out of seven were civil wars: the Taiping Rebellion (1851–64), the American Civil War (1861–65), the Russian Civil War (1918–20), the Chinese Civil War (1927–36), the Spanish Civil War (1936–39), and the communal slaughter that accompanied Indian independence and partition (1946–48).

We are inclined to assume that no century was as bloody as the twentieth. Yet the exemplary violence meted out by the thirteenth-century Mongol leader Chingis (Genghis) Khan is said to have reduced the populations of Central Asia and China by more than thirty-seven million—a figure that, if correct, is equivalent to nearly 10 percent of the world's population at that time. Tamerlane's late-fourteenth-century conquests in Central Asia and northern India were also notably bloody, with an estimated death toll in excess of ten million. The Manchu conquest of China in the seventeenth century may have cost the lives of as many as twenty-five million people. In addition to the Taiping, several pre-1900 Chinese rebellions and their suppression caused human suffering on a scale that may have matched or exceeded that inflicted on the people of China by twentieth-century civil wars. The eighth-century An Lushan Rebellion is thought to have cost the lives of more than thirty million people. Also devastating to the provinces affected were the roughly contemporaneous Nien and Miao rebellions and the Muslim rebellions in Yunnan and northwestern China. In these cases, death tolls have to be inferred from provincial and local censuses taken before and after the rebellions. The declines seem to imply mortality rates ranging from 40 to 90 percent, though once again it is likely that disease and starvation caused as much death as organized violence, and probably much more.

Finally, there is reason to think that the mortality rates arising from some episodes of Western European conquest and colonization of the Americas and Africa were as high as those of the twentieth century. As noted above, the overwhelming majority of victims of the European conquest of the Americas succumbed to disease, not to violence, so those who speak of "genocide" debase the coinage of historical terminology just as much as those who call nineteenth-century famines in India "Victorian holocausts." However, the forcible enslavement of the Congolese people by the Belgian crown after 1886 and the suppression of the Herero uprising by the German colonial authorities in 1904 do bear comparison to twentieth-century acts of organized violence. The proportion of the population estimated to have been killed in the Congo under Belgian rule may have been as high as a fifth. The estimated mortality rate in the Herero War was higher still—more than 1 in 3, making it, by that measure, the bloodiest conflict of the entire twentieth century. The absolute number of dead, however, was 76,000, while an estimated 7 million were killed in the Congo between 1886 and 1908.[40] Though it is conventional to normalize data by calculating percentages, we should always remember that, *pace* Stalin, a million deaths are always a million tragedies—a million premature and painful deaths—whether the denominator is numbered in the tens of millions or the billions, or whether they are carried out by two warring superpowers or a million murderers. Richardson was surprised to find that, while the world wars accounted for some 36 million deaths—around 60 percent of all the "deadly quarrels" in his 130-year period—the next-largest category was the magnitude-0 events (conflicts in which 1 to 3 people died), which were responsible for 9.7 million deaths. The remainder of the 315 recorded wars, combined with all the thousands of quarrels of intermediate size, accounted for less than a quarter of the casualties of all the deadly quarrels.[41] We ought also to make some allowance for the fact that, thanks to rising life expectancy, a death in the twentieth century—especially in the rich countries of Europe and North America—nearly always implied a bigger loss in terms of quality-adjusted life years than a death in previous eras.

Many of the greatest economic disasters in history have, not surprisingly, coincided with the great pandemics and conflicts discussed above. Not all, however. The Great Depression, which is generally dated from the Wall Street Crash of October 1929, was a consequence of structural imbalances in the world economy, a rigid system of fixed exchange rates, beggar-thy-neighbor protectionism, and errors of monetary and fiscal policy. The economist Robert Barro has compiled the best available global list of twentieth-century economic disasters, ranked by their impact on real per capita gross domestic product (GDP) as well as their financial consequences. Out of sixty declines of 15 percent or more in real per capita GDP, thirty-eight were attributable to

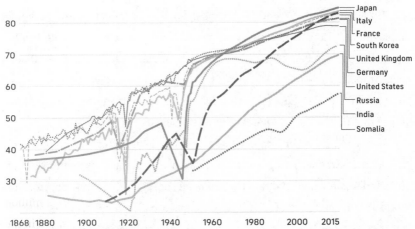

Life expectancy at birth, 1868–2015 (the average number of years a newborn would live if the pattern of mortality in the given year were to stay the same throughout its life).

war and its aftermath, while sixteen were a result of the Great Depression. Out of the thirty-five countries in his sample, the biggest declines (each of 64 percent) were in Greece from 1939 to 1945 and Germany from 1944 to 1946. The World War II experiences of the Philippines and South Korea were not much better: each suffered reductions of per capita GDP of 59 percent.[42] As the United Kingdom has uniquely long time series, allowing modern economic indicators to be estimated for at least the past three centuries—and for England back to the late thirteenth century—we can also identify years of severe economic hardship in earlier periods. According to the Bank of England, the worst year in English economic history was in fact 1629* (when the economy contracted by 25 percent), with 1349 (down 23 percent) a close second. The last annual contraction larger than 10 percent came in 1709, when economic activity was steeply reduced throughout Europe by the "Great Frost," the coldest winter in five hundred years, which has been attributed to the exceptionally low sunspot activity known as the Maunder Minimum, as well as to volcanic eruptions in the two preceding years at Mount Fuji, in Japan, and Santorini and Vesuvius, in Europe.[43] The worst year of the twentieth century

---

*The reason for the severity of the 1629 contraction is not immediately obvious: war with Spain was going badly, but the main theater of operations that year was the Caribbean. The year is best known to political historians as the beginning of Charles I's eleven-year "Personal Rule" without a parliament.

was 1921 (minus 10 percent), a time of steep postwar deflation and high unemployment.[44] However, no five-year period can compare with the late 1340s,
a period when the Black Death reduced the population by more than 40 percent. At its halfway point, the year 2020 seemed likely to witness the worst
contraction in British history since 1709—in late June the International Monetary Fund forecast a 10.2 percent reduction in GDP.[45]

There are, however, limits to what can be gleaned from economic data.
As I learned when writing a dissertation on the German hyperinflation of
1923 and again when studying the financial consequences of the outbreak of
World War I, the times of most intense crisis are also times when economic
statistics cease to be collected or are collected only erratically. The World
Bank has a comprehensive data collection that includes GDP per capita data
for nearly every country in the world since 1960. But if one looks at those
countries that have suffered the most economic and political disruption in the
past sixty years—Afghanistan, Cambodia, Eritrea, Iraq, Lebanon, Somalia,
Syria, Venezuela, and Yemen—in each case there are, unsurprisingly, gaps in
the data that coincide with the times of maximum disruption. Who can say
precisely how severe their economic disasters were?[46] All we know is that
these same countries can nearly all be found near the top of the Fragile States
Index, formerly a ranking of "failed" states.[47] A further challenge is the (at
first sight paradoxical) finding that the period 1914–50, a time of world war,
depression, and a collapse of globalization, was also a period when human
development—measured broadly in terms of life expectancy, education, the
percentage of national income spent on social projects, and the level of
democracy—advanced significantly across a broad front.[48]

Disaster, in short, is harder to quantify than might be assumed, even in
the modern era of statistics. Death tolls are often inaccurate. To understand
the significance of a disaster, we need to know not just the absolute number
of corpses but excess mortality—the number of deaths that would not otherwise have happened, relative to a baseline calculated as an average of recent
years. In trying to assess the scale of a disaster, the choice of denominator can
make a great deal of difference. What was a catastrophic famine for some
parts of Bengal in 1943, as we shall see in chapter 6, looks altogether smaller

if the death toll is expressed as a percentage of the entire Indian population, and scarcely registers relative to world population in the context of the world's worst war. My aim, in what follows, is to enable the reader to compare the different forms that doom takes, not to assert that all disasters are somehow the same. Up to September 2020, COVID-19 had killed an estimated 0.0114 percent of the world population, making it the twenty-sixth-most-disastrous pandemic in history. The Spanish flu of 1918–19 was roughly 150 times more deadly. But for those cities most affected, in the months when they were hardest hit, COVID-19 was as bad as the Spanish flu, if not worse. In terms of excess mortality, April 2020 in New York City was nearly 50 percent worse than October 1918 and three and a half times worse than September 2001, the month of the 9/11 terrorist attack on the World Trade Center.[49] In the first half of 2020, the population of London was struck as hard by COVID-19 as it had been by the German rocket attacks in the second half of 1944, confronting the government in each case with a comparable challenge: how to protect people from a lethal threat without paralyzing the city.[50] This is not to equate al-Qaeda or the Nazis with the virus SARS-CoV-2, but merely to show that disaster, in the sense of excess mortality, can take diverse forms and yet pose similar challenges.

Each premature death, as Stalin may have said, is in some sense a tragedy; the younger the victim, the more painful the death, the greater the tragedy. As the next chapter shows, however, some disasters are more authentically tragic than others.

2

CYCLES AND TRAGEDIES

> The vicissitudes of fortune, which spares neither man nor the proudest of his works, which buries empires and cities in a common grave.
>
> —Gibbon

IN SEARCH OF CYCLES

Are disasters predictable? In preliterate societies, they surely were not. Life was dominated by the effects of natural forces, only some of which—notably the seasons—were rhythmic and predictable. Disasters were intelligible only with reference to supernatural forces. In polytheistic religions, "the gods" were often merely the names given to conflicting natural forces. Indeed, the unsatisfactory nature of polytheism prompted the Epicureans' rejection of any kind of divine agency. Writing in the first century BC, the Roman philosopher Titus Lucretius Carus proposed the existence of an infinite universe composed of atoms with an essentially random dynamic.[1] It was only slowly that the idea developed of an ultimate and purposeful supernatural arbiter with the capacity to generate historical cycles. The Old Testament book of Ecclesiastes offers an early cyclical theory: "The thing that hath been, it is that which shall be; and that which is done is that which shall be done" (1:9). In the Old Testament, however, Yahweh's purpose unfolds itself in a complex historical narrative: the Creation, Abraham, the entrance into Egypt, the Exodus, Solomon, the captivity, the rededication of the Temple. To this, the early Christians' New

Testament added a revolutionary coda—the Incarnation, the Crucifixion, and the Resurrection—and the prospect of an ultimate apocalypse, ending the historical cycle.[2]

Early Roman historians sought to give meaning to history by invoking the role of a purposeful, if sometimes capricious, "Fortune." Polybius's *Rise of the Roman Empire* argued that the "vicissitudes" of Fortune in fact had a purpose: the triumph of Rome. A similar conception can be found in the work of Tacitus, though here it was Rome's destruction that was the divine objective. For Tacitus, as for Polybius, "the actual course of events" was "often dictated by chance," but events "also had their underlying logic and causes."[3] An additional superhuman factor that Polybius acknowledged was the Stoic notion of historical cycles, culminating in periodic natural catastrophes:

> When a deluge or a plague or a failure of crops . . . result[s] in the destruction of much of the human race . . . all the traditions and arts will simultaneously perish, but when in the course of time a new population has grown up again from the survivors left by the disaster, as a crop grows up from seed in the ground, a renewal of social life will begin.[4]

Imperial Chinese historiography also had its cyclical features from the earliest times, with the Mandate of Heaven being bestowed on dynasties and then withdrawn when no longer merited, giving rise to a dynastic cycle. Though the First Qin Emperor sought to challenge this Confucian notion, it ultimately proved ineradicable. As in the West, cyclical theories and millenarian theories competed, but the dynastic cycle became institutionalized under the Tang dynasty.[5] Though notionally supplanted by Marxism-Leninism since 1949, it remains a remarkably prevalent way of thinking about Chinese history, with the Communist Party as just the latest dynasty.

Cyclical theories of history have thus been a recurrent feature of Western and Eastern intellectual life. In *The New Science* (1725), Giambattista Vico argued that civilization went through a recurring cycle (*ricorso*) of three ages: the divine, the heroic, and the human. He considered his life's work to be "a rational civil theology of divine providence . . . a demonstration, so to speak, of the historical fact of providence, for it must be a history of the forms of order which, without human discernment or intent, and often against the designs of men, providence has given to this great city of the human race."[6] There is a close parallel between Vico's approach and that of the twentieth-century British sage Arnold Toynbee.[7] Adam Smith's *Wealth of Nations* (1776) laid the foundation for a strictly economic analysis of society that also implied a cyclical historical process. Here it was not blind fate but an "Invisible Hand" that led individuals to act, unwittingly, in the common interest, even while pursuing their own selfish ends, leading a society first to growth, then to "opulence," then to "the stationary state." In his much bleaker *Essay on the Principle of Population* (1798), Thomas Malthus proposed a demographic cycle, in which either starvation or "vice" was the inevitable consequence of the innate tendency of population to outgrow the supply of food. Karl Marx combined the Hegelian dialectic with the rudiments of Ricardian political economy. The result was a model of historical change through class struggle, culminating in the materialist apocalypse foretold in *Capital*:

> The monopoly of capital becomes a fetter upon the mode of production, which has sprung up and flourished along with and under it. Centralization of the means of production and socialization of labor at last reach a point where they become incompatible with their capitalist integument. This integument is burst asunder. The knell of capitalist private property sounds. The expropriators are expropriated.[8]

Like Peter Cook's followers on top of their hill, Marx's are still waiting.

CLIODYNAMICS

In recent years, proponents of "cliometrics" and "cliodynamics" have sought to revive the cyclical approach. For the premodern period, the Malthusian model would appear to offer the best fit.[9] However, variations on the Malthusian model have also been proposed for some modern crises.[10] A good illustration is the various attempts to explain the Arab revolutions of 2010–12 in terms of a "youth bulge." In one study of countries where youth population growth rates exceeded 45 percent over five years, "not a single one managed to avoid major political shocks. The risk of a particularly violent civil war was very high for these countries (about one chance out of two)." (This would suggest that trouble lies ahead for four sub-Saharan African countries: Niger, Kenya, Uganda, and Malawi.)[11] In and of itself, a youth bulge is not a predictor of upheaval; but in combination with low economic growth, a strongly autocratic state, and an expansion of higher education, it is.[12] The most ambitious project in this neo-Malthusian vein, led by the sociologist Jack Goldstone, looked at 141 instances of instability between 1955 and 2003, including crises of democracy, civil war, and state collapse. States with higher levels of infant mortality were nearly seven times more likely to suffer from internal instability than those with lower levels. Armed conflict in bordering states also increased the likelihood of instability, as did state-led discrimination against at least one minority group.[13]

Loosely related to the neo-Malthusians are the historians and social scientists who have sought the key to the cycles of history in generational conflicts, though here issues of political culture dominate demographics. In the 1920s, Karl Mannheim argued that the "critical period" of adolescence shaped the character of a generation for life. The Arthur Schlesingers *père et fils* both wrote about the "cycles of American history," positing a regular rotation between liberal and conservative consensus.[14] More recently, William Strauss and Neil Howe have proposed a cycle of generational realignment that unfolds every eighty to ninety years.[15] In each of these periods, there is supposedly a four-stage cycle of "turnings": a "High," an "Awakening," an "Unraveling," and finally a "Crisis." Like Oswald Spengler before them, Strauss and Howe associate each of these turnings with a season, beginning with spring and ending with winter. The last American Crisis, they suggest, was the period spanning the Great Depression and World War II. If the pattern holds steady, then we have entered a new fourth turning, which began with the global financial crisis of 2008–9 and will culminate in the 2020s as the baby boom generation surrenders power to the millennials.[16]

The defect of all such cyclical theories is that they leave relatively little room for the interplay of geographical, environmental, economic, cultural, technological, and political variables. The most ambitious ventures in cliodynamics attempt to remedy this in various ingenious ways.[17] The historian Ian Morris identifies "cycles of state growth and collapse . . . in Southwest Asia around 3100 BCE (the end of the Uruk Expansion), 2200 BCE (the fall of Egypt's Old Kingdom and the Akkadian Empire), and 1200 BCE (the end of the Bronze Age), and in South Asia around 1900 BCE (the fall of the Indus civilization)," suggesting that "in each case [there was a] feedback relationship between cultural evolution and the environment." For Morris, war was the key, and in particular the way the breeding of bigger horses transformed the arid steppes of central Eurasia from a wasteland into a zone for trade and warfare, not to mention the spread of disease.[18] Climatic variables have grown fashionable in recent years, not surprisingly. To give just one example, Qiang Chen has sought to relate episodes of drought to dynastic crises in the history of imperial China.[19] Other scholars have emphasized the role of floods.[20]

In *Historical Dynamics* (2003), the historian Peter Turchin proposed a novel model for the rise and fall of states. New states, he argued, tend to form at the contested frontiers of existing ones (the "meta-ethnic frontier"), for at such zones of recurrent conflict, the pressure is greatest for a people to develop what, in his *Muqaddimah,* the fourteenth-century Islamic scholar Ibn Khaldun called *asabiyyah*—social cohesion, implying a capacity for collective action. But when a state attains a certain level of civilization—with all the attendant luxuries and inequalities—the incentive for cooperation fades and *asabiyyah* declines.[21] In *War and Peace and War* (2006), Turchin added a new element: successful empire builders, like the Romans, incorporate rather than annihilate conquered peoples. However, success plants the seeds of decline: not only the depletion of *asabiyyah* but also the familiar Malthusian cycle. With peace and stability comes prosperity; with prosperity comes population growth; that leads to overpopulation; and overpopulation results in unemployment, low wages, high rents, and, in some cases, shortages of food. As living standards deteriorate, people become liable to revolt. Ultimately, the collapse of social order results in civil war; imperial decline is then inevitable.[22] *Secular Cycles* (coauthored with Sergey Nefedov) formalized this framework. Four variables interact to bring about social/political change:

1. Population numbers in relation to "carrying capacity"
2. State strength (i.e., fiscal balance)
3. Social structure (specifically the size of the social elite and its consumption levels)
4. Sociopolitical stability

In this "structural demographic theory," the cycle has four phases:

1. Expansion: Population is growing rapidly, prices are stable, and wages keep pace with prices.
2. Stagflation: Population density approaches the limits of carrying capacity; wages decrease and/or prices rise. Elites enjoy a period of prosperity, as they can command high rents from their tenants.
3. General crisis: Population declines; rents and prices fall, and wages rise. Life might improve for the peasantry, but the consequences of an enlarged elite sector begin to be felt in the form of intra-elite conflict.
4. Depression: This phase of endemic civil war ends only when the elite has shrunk to the point that a new secular cycle can begin.[23]

Turchin and Nefedov argue that "the dominant role in internal warfare appears to be played by elite overproduction leading to intra-elite competition, fragmentation, and conflict, and the rise of counter-elites who mobilize popular masses in their struggle against the existing order."[24] The moment of cyclical crisis also features rising inflation and state bankruptcy.[25] Turchin's most recent contention is that the theory can be applied to the contemporary United States. Like Neil Howe, he has for some time predicted a crisis in or close to the year 2020.[26]

Cliodynamics is an exciting new field, without question. Turchin and his collaborators' massive historical database, Seshat, has gathered data for hundreds of polities spanning six continents from the Neolithic to the middle of the last millennium. It sets a new standard for the systematic historical study of political structures.[27] A remarkable paper by the young Korean scholar Jaeweon Shin and coauthors proposes a refinement of Turchin's model that introduces information technology as a variable. "Sociopolitical development," they write, "is dominated first by growth in polity scale, then by improvements in information processing and economic systems, and then by further increases in scale." There may, they suggest, be a "Scale Threshold for societies, beyond which growth in information processing becomes paramount, and an Information Threshold, which once crossed facilitates additional growth in scale."[28] Looking especially at the failure of New World societies (with the possible exception of the one in Cuzco) to develop systems of written record, they ask, "Could some of the frequent collapses seen in societies be due to a polity's never developing sufficient information-processing capacities, so that it stumbles or even collapses through poor performance due to lack of external connectivity, internal coherence, or inability to compete with polities whose superior information-processing abilities have enabled more growth in size?"[29]

Yet, as Turchin and Nefedov acknowledge, any cyclical process must itself be subject to distinctly noncyclical forces: extreme climate fluctuations, pandemics, and technological discontinuities, as well as major conflicts, which, as we have seen, have an almost random incidence in terms of both timing and scale.[30] Turchin's identification of 2020 as the likely next "spike" of sociopolitical instability in the United States—the successor to 1870, 1920, and 1970—may prove prophetic.[31] Higher immigration since the 1970s has clearly coincided with stagnating real wages, though other factors—technological change and Chinese competition—played at least as important a role. Elite overproduction is nicely captured by the rising cost of Yale tuition expressed in terms of average annual manufacturing wages, as well as the increase in the number of MBAs and lawyers as a percentage of the population. Elite fragmentation is clearly visible in the paralyzing partisanship of Washington, D.C., as well as the heated competition for legislative positions and the rising cost of election campaigns. The United States also looks badly lacking in the *asabiyyah* needed to prosecute foreign wars to a successful conclusion.[32]

Nevertheless, despite the recent heated discussions of mass shootings and police forces' use of lethal violence, rates of violence remain much lower in 2020
than they were in 1870, 1920, or 1970, as Turchin's own data show. Americans may own more guns than ever, but they use them against one another
much less frequently than in past spikes of violence.[33] In any case, how much
of 2020's instability—most obviously the eruption of mass protests in support
of Black Lives Matter in late May and June—should be attributed to the impact of a pandemic that no cyclical theory of history could have predicted?

A similar objection can be made about other cyclical theories currently
in vogue. The hedge fund manager Ray Dalio has devised his own model of
the historical process, which revolves around debt dynamics rather than demographic dynamics. Rather like Turchin, Dalio discerns "big cycles . . . com-
prised of swings between 1) happy and prosperous periods in which wealth
is pursued and created productively and those with power work harmoniously
to facilitate this and 2) miserable, depressing periods in which there are fights
over wealth and power that disrupt harmony and productivity and sometimes
lead to revolutions/wars."[34] Dalio's philosophy of history is homespun, a little
like George Soros's autodidactic approach to behavioral psychology. "Most
things," Dalio writes, "happen repeatedly through time. . . . There are only
a limited number of personality types going down a limited number of paths
that lead them to encounter a limited number of situations to produce only a
limited number of stories that repeat over time." He proposes what he calls a
"formula for what makes the world's greatest empires and their markets rise
and fall," based on "the 17 forces . . . that have explained almost all of these
movements throughout time." Elsewhere he writes of a "single measure of
wealth and power . . . made up as a roughly equal average of eight measures
of strength. They are: 1) education, 2) competitiveness, 3) technology, 4) economic output, 5) share of world trade, 6) military strength, 7) financial center strength, and 8) reserve currency." He also talks of four interacting cycles
of debt, money and credit, wealth distribution, and geopolitics.[35] The conclusion Dalio draws from his four-cycle theory is that the United States' days of
prosperity and primacy are numbered, much as the United Kingdom's were in
the 1930s. As for the dollar, "cash is trash."[36]

The difficulty with this approach is that it cannot explain nonevents that the model, had it existed in the past, would have wrongly predicted. Why didn't Great Britain decline and fall in the years after 1815, for example? Its debt-to-GDP ratio reached a peak of 172 percent in 1822. After five years of deflation (from 1818 to 1822), economic inequalities were acute and led to a wave of political unrest. Following the suicide of the hated Viscount Castle-reagh, on August 12, 1822, the international order established at the Congress of Vienna began to crumble. Yet the British Empire went from strength to strength in the early nineteenth century, and the revolutions happened on the other side of the English Channel in 1830 and 1848. One might equally well ask why the United States didn't decline and fall in the 1970s. Inflation took a heavy toll on the savings of bondholders. After Richard Nixon broke the last remaining link between the dollar and gold, the inflation rate rose to double digits. Meanwhile, there were riots in inner cities and protests on college cam-puses. The president himself was forced to resign, and the country ignomini-ously lost the Vietnam War. Yet American power endured and recovered rapidly in the 1980s. In 1989, two years after the publication of Paul Kenne-dy's *The Rise and Fall of the Great Powers*—another work of cyclical history, which emphasized the vital importance of manufacturing capacity and fiscal balance, and on that basis foresaw American decline—the United States won the Cold War as the Soviet empire in Central and Eastern Europe was swept away in a wave of revolutions, while Japan's bid for great-power status evap-orated as the country's asset-price bubble burst.

The reality, as we shall see, is that history is a process too complex to be modeled, even in the informal ways favored by Turchin and Dalio. Moreover, the more systematic modeling is done of historical phenomena—notably pan-demics, but also climate change or environmental degradation—the easier it becomes to go "from being roughly right towards being precisely wrong."[37]

DIAMOND IN THE ROUGH

If economic, social, or political collapses could be foreseen, presumably at least some of them could be averted. In *Collapse* (2011), the American polymath

Jared Diamond offered something less rigid than a cyclical theory, more a kind of collapse-avoidance checklist for a world increasingly worried about man-made climate change. "Collapse" he defined as "a drastic decrease in human population size and/or political/economic/social complexity, over a considerable area, for an extended time." Its proximate cause could be inadvertent damage to a population's environment, natural climate change unrelated to human activity, or war (aggression by a hostile neighbor). But collapse was most likely to come about because the society in question failed to address the threat or threats it faced.[38] And unlike the protracted decline into old age that individuals experience, societal collapses could be swift:

> One of the main lessons to be learned from the collapses of the Maya, Anasazi, Easter Islanders, and those of other past societies (as well as from the recent collapse of the Soviet Union) is that a society's steep decline may begin only a decade or two after the society reaches its peak numbers, wealth, and power. In that respect, the trajectories of the societies that we have discussed are unlike the usual courses of individual human lives, which decline in a prolonged senescence. The reason is simple: maximum population, wealth, resource consumption, and waste production mean maximum environmental impact, approaching the limit where impact outstrips resources. On reflection, it's no surprise that declines of societies tend to follow swiftly on their peaks.[39]

Either society fails to anticipate the cause of its collapse, or it fails to perceive it when it strikes (the problem of "creeping normalcy"), or it fails to try to solve it because of political, ideological, or psychological barriers, or it tries to solve it but doesn't succeed.

Diamond's book analyzes seven collapses, two (Rwanda and Haiti) in the recent past, others more distant: the Greenland Norse, the inhabitants of Easter Island (Rapa Nui), the Polynesians of Pitcairn, Henderson, and Mangareva, the Anasazi of southwestern North America, and the Maya of Central America. He also considers three success stories: the Pacific island of Tikopia, central New Guinea, and Tokugawa-era Japan. The most important story he tells is an adult version of the Dr. Seuss story *The Lorax* (1971). The collapse of the population of Easter Island—from several tens of thousands in its heyday to between fifteen hundred and three thousand when Europeans first arrived, in the early eighteenth century—Diamond blames on "human environmental impacts, especially deforestation and destruction of bird populations; and the political, social, and religious factors behind the impacts, such as . . . a focus on status construction . . . and competition between clans and chiefs driving the erection of bigger statues requiring more wood, rope, and food."[40] With no trees to anchor the soil, Easter Island's fertile land suffered erosion, leading to poor crop yields, while the dwindling supply of wood meant islanders could no longer build canoes to fish. This led to internecine warfare and, ultimately, cannibalism. The moral is clear: despoil the planet and we shall all end up like the Easter Islanders.

There is, however, an alternative version of Easter Island's history. The counternarrative is that settlement of the island did not occur until AD 1200, that deforestation was mostly the work of rats who arrived with the settlers, that the tall stone statues were not transported horizontally on logs but were "walked" upright, that natives subsisted on seafood, rat meat, and vegetables they grew, and that the collapse of the island's society was the result of European impacts, notably the arrival of venereal disease, after 1722.[41] A further hypothesis is that the island's population was reduced by slavers from South America.[42] This is a far cry from the Lorax.

Still, perhaps Diamond's broader argument—that collapse is as much a social or political phenomenon as an environmental one—can be salvaged. "Nations undergo national crises," he writes in *Upheaval* (2019), "which . . . may or may not get resolved successfully through national changes. Successful coping with [crises caused by] either external or internal pressures requires selective change. That's as true of nations as of individuals."

One of the oldest ideas in Western political thought is the analogy between the individual human and the body politic—think of Abraham Bosse's frontispiece for Thomas Hobbes's *Leviathan,* which depicts a giant crowned figure towering over the landscape, his torso and arms made up of more than three hundred men. Diamond revives this idea with seven case studies of national crisis and recovery, in Finland, Japan, Chile, Indonesia, Germany, Australia, and the United States. The seven cases provide the basis for Diamond's twelve-step strategy for coping with a national crisis:

1. Acknowledge that you are in crisis, whether you are an individual or a nation.
2. Accept your personal/national responsibility to do something about the situation.
3. "Build a fence [not necessarily physical] to delineate one's individual/national problems needing to be solved."
4. Get material and emotional help from other individuals/nations.
5. Use other individuals/nations as models of how to solve problems.
6. You are more likely to succeed if you have "ego strength," which for states translates as a sense of national identity.
7. Diamond also recommends "honest self-appraisal" for both individuals and states.
8. It helps if you have experience of previous personal/national crises.
9. It also helps to have patience.
10. Flexibility is a good idea.
11. You will benefit from having "core values."
12. It also helps to have freedom from personal/geopolitical constraints.[43]

The problem with all this is that, in reality, nation-states are not that much like individual people. It would be much more accurate to say that, like any large-scale polity, they are complex systems. As such, they are not governed by the same broadly Gaussian rules as individual members of our species. For example, we human beings at adulthood are all roughly the same height. A histogram of human stature is a classic bell curve, with most of us somewhere between five and six feet tall and nobody shorter than about two feet or taller than about eight. There are no ant-size people and no human skyscrapers. This is not true of nation-states, a form of polity that became dominant only relatively recently in history. Two mega-states—China and India—account for 36 percent of the world's population. Then come eleven big states, from the United States down to the Philippines, each of which has more than one hundred million people, accounting for just over a quarter of the world's population. Seventy-five medium-size states have between ten million and a hundred million inhabitants: another third of the world's population. But then there are seventy-one with between one million and ten million (5 percent of humanity), forty-one states with between 100,000 and a million (0.2 percent), and a further thirty-three states with fewer than 100,000 residents.

Just as the sizes of states are not normally distributed, so, too, are the crises. The major upheavals—wars, revolutions, financial crises, coups—that historians love to study are low-frequency, high-impact events located in the tails of distributions that are anything but normal. The great revolutions of history—the English, the American, the French, the Russian, and the Chinese—did not happen everywhere. In the histories of most countries there are just a few forgettable revolts. Individual human histories are not like this. We may not all have adolescent and midlife crises, but enough of us do for the terms scarcely to need definition. We mostly have between one and four children. We nearly all have health crises of one sort or another. And, as we saw in chapter 1, we all die—mostly in a relatively narrow age range, again normally distributed. The life of an individual human is thus quite likely to follow a cyclical course. Some nation-states, by contrast, live a very long time. The United Kingdom is more than four hundred years old (its constituent parts are much older), and the United States is approaching 250. Others have been subject to tremendous institutional discontinuity. Chinese leaders love to claim that China is around five thousand years old, but this is a tall tale that originated with the Jesuits, who traced Chinese history as far back as 2952 BC, and was made official by Sun Yat-sen, who identified the mythical Yellow Emperor (Huangdi), whose reign is said to have begun in 2697 BC, as China's first ruler. In fact, the People's Republic of China celebrated its seventieth birthday in 2019, making it twelve years younger than Jared Diamond.

And the majority of the world's nation-states are not much older, having been formed, like Indonesia, in the period of decolonization that followed the end of the Second World War. What is the life expectancy at birth of a nation-state? No one can say.

In short, it is surely a category error to expect nation-states to behave like humans—like trying to extrapolate the incidence of pileups on highways from an understanding of the internal combustion engine. Precisely because complex polities are not subject to the same constraints as individual people, Diamond's metaphor is a misleading one. (It is even more misleading when he attempts to apply it to the entire human race.) In each of his seven cases, the nation in question successfully overcame the crisis or crises that afflicted it. Missing from the sample is one or more of the polities that irrevocably fell apart—such as the Soviet Union or Yugoslavia—or the former colonial pro-tectorates that didn't make it to independent statehood, or the innumerable ethnic groups who have never achieved self-government. If nation-states are scaled-up individuals, then what were these? There are options open to polities—for which dismemberment need not be fatal—that we humans just don't have.

CASSANDRA'S CURSE

"Can our current national emergency be viewed as perhaps a classical tragedy rather than as sordid drama?" asked the American playwright David Mamet in June 2020. "In our case, what brought about the plague of Thebes?"[44] It is a legitimate question. For if history is not cyclical, mimicking the life cycle of the individual human being, then perhaps it is dramatic, replicating on a much larger scale—on "the world's stage"—the classical human interactions of the theater.

Most celebrated disasters are tragedies and are routinely described as such by journalists. But some disasters are tragic in a strict sense—that is, they follow the conventions of classical tragedy. There is, as in Aeschylus's *Agamemnon,* a prophet, a chorus, and a king. The prophet foresees the disas-ter that lies ahead; the chorus is unconvinced; the king is doomed.

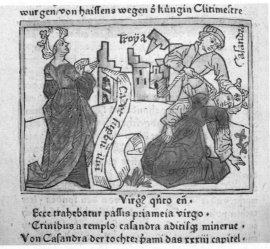

Woodcut illustration of Cassandra's prophecy of the fall of Troy (left) and her death (right), from Heinrich Steinhöwel's translation of Giovanni Boccaccio's *De mulieribus claris*, printed by Johann Zainer at Ulm, ca. 1474.

CHORUS MEMBER: If you don't know where you are, I'll tell you—you're at the house of the sons of Atreus. . . .

CASSANDRA: No . . . no . . . a house that hates the gods . . . house full of death, kinsmen butchered . . . heads chopped off . . . a human slaughterhouse awash in blood . . .

CHORUS MEMBER: This stranger's like a keen hound on the scent. She's on the trail of blood.

CASSANDRA: . . . I see evidence I trust—young children screaming as they're butchered—then their father eating his own infants' roasted flesh . . .

CHORUS MEMBER: We've heard about your fame in prophecy. But here in Argos no one wants a prophet.[45]

Cassandra has been brought back, a slave, from conquered Troy by the victorious Agamemnon. But the king's wife, Clytemnestra, plots his death, as revenge for her daughter Iphigenia, whom Agamemnon had sacrificed years before for the sake of a fair wind to the Trojan War. She also wants her lover, Aegisthus, to take Agamemnon's place. Cassandra sees all too clearly what is coming, but her curse is that she cannot convince any of her listeners:

> **CASSANDRA:** O evil woman, you're going to do it. Your own husband, the man who shares your bed—once you've washed him clean . . . there in the bath . . . How shall I describe how all this ends? It's coming soon. She's stretching out her hand . . . and now her other hand is reaching for him . . .

> **CHORUS MEMBER:** I still don't understand. What she's saying is just too confused. Her dark prophecies leave me bewildered. . . .

> **CHORUS:** What good ever comes to men from prophecies?[46] . . .

> **CASSANDRA:** But we'll not die without the gods' revenge. Another man will come and will avenge us, a son who'll kill his mother, then pay back his father's death, a wanderer in exile, a man this country's made a stranger. He'll come back and, like a coping stone, bring the ruin of his family to a close.[47]

When Agamemnon is indeed murdered, the members of the chorus are thrown into confusion and dissension. Aeschylus has them bickering indecisively about how to respond to the killing of their king.[48] Inexorably, the prophecy fulfills itself in the second and third parts of the *Oresteia* trilogy. In *Choephoroi* (*The Libation Bearers*), Agamemnon's son, Orestes, returns to Argos and, with his sister Electra, plots the murder of their mother and her lover. Having committed matricide, Orestes is then hounded by the Furies. In *The Eumenides* (*The Kindly Ones*), Orestes seeks justice from Athena—and is granted it, in the form of the first trial by jury.

In these ancient tragedies, the consequences of defying the gods are starkly represented. Orestes describes "the wrath of blood guilt"—the consequences of not avenging his father's death—in the most lurid terms: "From underneath the earth, infectious plagues, leprous sores which gnaw the flesh, fangs chewing living tissue, festering white rot in the sores."[49] By contrast, Athens is to be protected from such scourges by "the kindly ones" after they have been reconciled to Orestes's acquittal. As the chorus chants:

> Let no winds destroy the trees nor scorching desert heat move in to shrivel budding plants, no festering blight kill off the fruit. . . . I pray man-killing civil strife may never roar aloud within the city—may its dust not drink our citizen's dark blood, nor passions for revenge incite those wars which kill the state.[50]

Disaster was no unimaginable contingency in ancient Greece; it was never far away, held back only by the goodwill of the gods.

We see a similar tragic disaster in Sophocles's *Oedipus Rex,* where it is Thebes that is suffering divine retribution in the form of a plague:

> Our ship of State,
> Sore buffeted, can no more lift her head,
> Foundered beneath a weltering surge of blood.
> A blight is on our harvest in the ear,
> A blight upon the grazing flocks and herds,
> A blight on wives in travail; and withal
> Armed with his blazing torch the God of Plague
> Hath swooped upon our city.[51]

According to the oracle at Delphi, Oedipus must find the man who murdered his predecessor, Laius. But the prophet in this case, Tiresias, knows that Oedipus is himself the murderer, that he has committed not only patricide but also incest by marrying his own mother, Jocasta. When he sees the true nature of his predicament, Oedipus fulfills Tiresias's prophecy by blinding himself.

As Richard Clarke and R. P. Eddy have suggested, many modern disasters echo these classical tragedies.[52] Hurricane Katrina, the Fukushima nuclear disaster, the rise of ISIS, the financial crisis: in each case there was a Cassandra who was not heeded. Clarke and Eddy's "Cassandra Coefficient" has four components: the threat of disaster, the prophet of disaster, the decision maker, and the critics who disparage and reject the warning. In this framework, disasters are predictable, but a variety of cognitive biases conspire to prevent the necessary preemptive action. A disaster is hard to imagine if it has never happened before (or not recently), or because an erroneous consensus rules it out, or because its scale defies belief, or because it simply seems too outlandish.[53] The Cassandras may lack the skills of persuasion. The decision makers may be captives of diffuse responsibility, "agenda inertia," regulatory capture, intellectual inadequacy, ideological blinkers, downright cowardice, or bureaucratic pathologies such as "satisficing" (addressing a problem but not solving it) or withholding vital information.[54] And the "chorus"—not so much public opinion as expert opinion—can fall victim to a different set of biases: the craving for certainty (randomized controlled trials, peer-reviewed papers), the habit of debunking any novel theory, or the sunk cost of being invested in "settled science,"[55] not to mention the temptation to make countless false prophecies on opinion pages and talk shows.

Many experts crave calculable risk; they tend to dislike uncertainty. The distinction is an important one. As the Chicago economist Frank Knight argued in 1921, "Uncertainty must be taken in a sense radically distinct from the familiar notion of Risk. . . . A measurable uncertainty, or 'risk' proper . . . is so far different from an unmeasurable one that it is not in effect an uncertainty at all." Time and again an event will occur that is "so entirely unique that there are no others or not a sufficient number to make it possible to tabulate enough like it to form a basis for any inference of value about any real probability."[56] The same point was brilliantly expressed by John Maynard Keynes in 1937. "By 'uncertain' knowledge," he wrote in response to critics of his *General Theory,*

> I do not mean merely to distinguish what is known for certain from what
> is only probable. The game of roulette is not subject, in this sense, to
> uncertainty. . . . The expectation of life is only slightly uncertain. Even
> the weather is only moderately uncertain. The sense in which I am using

the term is that in which the prospect of a European war is uncertain, or . . . the rate of interest twenty years hence. . . . About these matters there is no scientific basis on which to form any calculable probability whatever. We simply do not know.[57]

To make matters worse, we struggle with even calculable risks because of a host of cognitive biases. In a famous article, Daniel Kahneman and Amos Tversky demonstrated, with a series of experiments, that people tend to miscalculate probabilities when confronted with simple financial choices. First, they gave their sample group 1,000 Israeli pounds each. Then they offered them a choice between (a) a 50 percent chance of winning an additional 1,000 pounds and (b) a 100 percent chance of winning an additional 500 pounds. Only 16 percent of people chose (a); everyone else (84 percent) chose (b). Next, they asked the same group to imagine having received 2,000 Israeli pounds each and confronted them with another choice: between (c) a 50 percent chance of losing 1,000 pounds and (d) a 100 percent chance of losing 500 pounds. This time the majority (69 percent) chose (c); only 31 percent chose (d). Yet, viewed in terms of their payoffs, the two problems are identical. In both cases you have a choice between a 50 percent chance of ending up with 1,000 pounds and an equal chance of ending up with 2,000 pounds (a and c) or a certainty of ending up with 1,500 pounds (b and d). In this and other experiments, Kahneman and Tversky identified a striking asymmetry: risk aversion for positive prospects, but risk seeking for negative ones.[58]

This "failure of invariance" is only one of many heuristic biases (evolved modes of thinking or learning) that distinguish real human beings from the *Homo oeconomicus* of neoclassical economic theory, who is supposed to make his decisions rationally, on the basis of all the available information and his expected utility. Other experiments show that we also succumb too readily to such cognitive traps as:

Availability bias, which causes us to base decisions on information that is readily available in our memories, rather than the data we really need

Hindsight bias, which causes us to attach higher probabilities to events after they have happened (*ex post*) than we did before they happened (*ex ante*)

The problem of induction, which leads us to formulate general rules on the basis of insufficient information

The fallacy of conjunction (or disjunction), which means we tend to overestimate the probability that seven events of 90 percent probability will all occur, while underestimating the probability that at least one of seven events of 10 percent probability will occur

Confirmation bias, which inclines us to look for confirming evidence of an initial hypothesis, rather than falsifying evidence that would disprove it

Contamination effects, whereby we allow irrelevant but proximate information to influence a decision

The affect heuristic, whereby preconceived value judgments interfere with our assessment of costs and benefits

Scope neglect, which prevents us from proportionately adjusting what we should be willing to sacrifice to avoid harms of different orders of magnitude

Overconfidence in calibration, which leads us to underestimate the confidence intervals within which our estimates will be robust (e.g., to conflate the "best-case" scenario with the "most probable"), and

Bystander apathy, which inclines us to abdicate individual responsibility when in a crowd.[59]

There are many other ways in which human beings can err. The term "cognitive dissonance" was coined by the American social psychologist Leon Festinger. In his seminal 1957 book on the subject, Festinger argued that "in the presence of an inconsistency there is psychological discomfort" and that therefore "the existence of [cognitive] dissonance . . . will motivate the [affected] person to try to reduce the dissonance and achieve consonance." Moreover, "when dissonance is present, in addition to trying to reduce it, the person will actively avoid situations and information which would likely increase the dissonance."[60] Yet there is considerable evidence that many people can learn to live with such dissonance for long periods of time. Cognitive dissonance often consists of saying one thing in public and another in private. This was once the basis of life in Communist systems all over the world. It turns out to be something people in capitalist societies can do just as easily—flying in private jets to conferences about the perils of climate change—with very little of the discomfort predicted by social psychology.

Or take the concept of "category error," a term coined by the Oxford philosopher Gilbert Ryle. In *The Concept of Mind* (1949), Ryle gave a very English example: "A foreigner watching his first game of cricket learns what are the functions of the bowlers, the batsmen, the fielders, the umpires and the scorers. He then says, 'But there is no one left on the field to contribute the famous element of team-spirit.'"[61] Ryle went on to make his most famous point, that René Descartes was wrong to represent the human mind as a "ghost in the machine"[62]—something distinct from the body. We no more have separate minds than a cricket team has a twelfth player with the job of boosting the others' morale. Yet similar category errors abound in modern discourse—for instance, the illusion that because nation-states are made up of millions of individual people, they should therefore experience crises in the same way individual people do.

THE BELLS OF HELL

It would be cheering to think that, in the late 1600s, mankind crossed a threshold from superstition to science, as suggested by the Welsh historian Keith Thomas in *Religion and the Decline of Magic*.[63] In reality, "the science" is a complex and contested realm, in which new paradigms only slowly overcome bad ones, as the American philosopher of science Thomas Kuhn argued long ago.[64] Moreover, scientific methods can be abused to produce any number of spurious correlations—for example, between the signs of the zodiac and the chances of survival of leukemia sufferers who receive a stem-cell transplant.[65] At the same time, the advance of science led to a decline not only of magical thinking but also of religious belief and observance. As G. K. Chesterton foresaw, this had the unintended consequence of creating spaces in people's minds for new forms of magical thinking.* Modern societies are highly susceptible to surrogate religions and magic, leading to new forms of irrational activity that, on close inspection, are quite similar to pre-1700 behaviors.

It would also be pleasing to believe that such wrongheadedness could be overcome by the methods of "superforecasting," as pioneered by Philip Tetlock, the political scientist who has sought to overcome individual biases by means of tournaments of skilled forecasters and various forms of accountability.[66] But Tetlock's finest forecasters in the Good Judgment Project said there was just a 23 percent chance that the British electorate would vote to leave the European Union just before they did exactly that. On February 20, 2020, Tetlock's superforecasters predicted only a 3 percent chance that there would be more than 200,000 coronavirus cases a month later. There were. Zeynep Tufekci was one of those writers who discerned the danger of COVID-19 relatively early. But in a 2014 article, she sounded an almost identical warning about the Ebola pandemic, predicting that there could be a million cases by the end of 2014; there were only about thirty thousand.[67]

Small wonder, in a world of seemingly random catastrophes that our minds are singularly ill equipped to anticipate, that the ordinary man has so often resorted to black humor. In the trenches of the Western Front in the middle of World War I, a song caught on among British soldiers that parodied a prewar Salvation Army anthem:

The Bells of Hell go ting-a-ling-a-ling
For you but not for me.

---

*Contrary to popular belief, Chesterton did not say, "When men stop believing in God, they don't believe in nothing. They believe in anything." The nearest thing is in his short story "The Miracle of Moon Crescent": "You hard-shelled materialists [are] all balanced on the very edge of belief—of belief in almost anything."

For me the angels sing-a-ling-a-ling
They've got the goods for me.
O Death, where is thy sting-a-ling-a-ling?
O Grave, thy victoree?
The Bells of Hell go ting-a-ling-a-ling
For you but not for me![68]

The Knightsbridge barrister who jotted down those words (transcribed from a letter he had been sent by his nephew, a second lieutenant who had heard his men singing them) understood very well their significance. They were not being directed at the Germans across no-man's-land, he suggested:

> I should guess that this odd triumphant credo . . . is not a defiance of the earthly foe, but merely one more manifestation of the courageous levity that this war has drawn forth. It is Tommy's light surface way of accepting death. To do even so tremendous a thing as that without a touch of humour would not be playing the game. We get therefore trench after trench filled with men who at any moment may be blown to atoms singing these astonishing words. . . . Isn't that wonderful? and incredible? It is not exactly religion, and yet it is religion. Fatalism with faith. Assurance with disdain.[69]

This was the eve of the Battle of the Somme, in terms of loss of life the greatest military disaster in British history (see chapter 6). In all, 13 percent (673,375) of the men who served in the British Army between 1914 and 1918 lost their lives and 32 percent were wounded.

In wars, as in plagues, we human beings have a strange propensity to believe that we, as individuals, will survive. Sometimes we are right about that: the survivors of the war did outnumber the fallen, after all. Toby Starr, the young officer who had heard his men sing "The Bells of Hell," was not only lucky but also brave: when he and two platoons under his command struck a German land mine, he was unscathed, and, "though much shaken, he at once organised a party with a machine gun to mow down the oncoming enemy, and having effectively repulsed them . . . was instrumental in rescuing, although under fire, a number of his own buried men." For this, Starr was awarded the Victoria Cross.[70] As a general rule, however, the bells of hell go ting-a-ling-a-ling with little regard for our personal qualities. And we tend to be rather bad at estimating the probability that they will go ting-a-ling-a-ling for us.

In proximity to sudden death, gallows humor may well be the right response. The American military has its own version of "The Bells of Hell," which takes the form of sardonic acronyms. "SOL" originated as an official abbreviation for "soldier," but as early as 1917 it had come to stand for "soldier out of luck" and later "shit out of luck" (applicable to everything from death to being late for dinner). In World War II, "SNAFU" stood for "situation normal: all fouled (or fucked) up"—"used acronymically," in the words of the *Oxford English Dictionary*, "as an expression conveying the common soldier's laconic acceptance of the disorder of war and the ineptitude of his superiors" or "to indicate that things are not going too well." In 1944, U.S. Air Force bomber crews came up with another acronym to describe a state of affairs even more extreme than SNAFU: "FUBAR"—"fouled (or fucked) up beyond all recognition." This could signify, again according to the dictionary, "bungled, ruined, messed up," but also "extremely intoxicated."

More recently, in the streets of San Francisco, a phrase originated that, like SOL, SNAFU, and FUBAR, has passed into general usage, to be uttered in the face of all kinds of adversity. "Shit happens" (rendered more politely as "Stuff happens" or "It happens") was first recorded in 1964 by a Berkeley master's student who was writing a thesis on "Gang Members and the Police." One of the gang members he interviewed—a sixteen-year-old African American youth—described how, as he and his friends were walking down San Francisco's Market Street after watching a movie, they were gratuitously stopped and threatened with arrest by two policemen. "That shit happens all the time," the young man observed. "There ain't a day we don't get roused like that."[71] In this particular incident, the police used racist language ("Now all you black Africans pick up your spears and go home! I don't want you guys walking up the street") but not violence. Yet it might have been otherwise. Like Toby Starr, though in quite different circumstances, the originator of "Shit happens" had survived a brush with disaster—doubtless one of many. For those who see disaster at close quarters on a regular basis, it is neither predictably cyclical nor ineffably tragic. It is just life.

3

GRAY RHINOS, BLACK SWANS, AND DRAGON KINGS

As flies to wanton boys, are we to the gods.
They kill us for their sport.

—*King Lear*

THE MENAGERIE OF CATASTROPHE

It became a commonplace among beleaguered leaders seeking to rally popular support in early 2020 to say that the COVID-19 pandemic was a war, albeit against an "invisible enemy."[1] A number of historians offered carefully qualified endorsements of this analogy.[2] For obvious reasons, a pandemic is very different from a war, of course. We think of a pandemic as a natural disaster, whereas a war is man-made—a distinction to which we shall return. In a pandemic it is a pathogen that kills people, whereas in a war people kill people. Nevertheless, the two kinds of disaster have much in common, besides the stark fact of excess mortality. Each belongs to that special class of rare, large-scale disaster that is the subject of this book.

Not all wars seem to come as a bolt from the blue. The outbreak of World War I in 1914 did. People in 1914 had long been aware that a large-scale European conflict was a possibility and understood how dire its consequences would be, and yet—even among the well educated and well informed—few grasped until late in July the imminence of Armageddon. The same might be said of those who in 2020 had been informed repeatedly of the threat posed by contagious new pathogens but opted to ignore or downplay the danger when the World Health Organization's "Disease X" actually appeared. In its initial phase, the pandemic therefore had more or less the same consequences as the opening few months of World War I: financial panic, economic dislocation, popular alarm, and a significant level of excess mortality, though among the elderly of both sexes, rather than prime-age males. One important difference was that the COVID-19 pandemic commenced without the offsetting boost to morale provided by patriotism. However, one similarity is that in each case there was a process of adjustment as it became clear that the crisis would not be "over by Christmas." Once they are over, disastrous events acquire a shape that was not discernible at the time to those whose lives were ruined by them. Nobody knew in August 1914 that the last shots of the war would be fired four and a quarter years later, just as nobody involved in the 1340 Anglo-French naval clash off Sluys knew that the two countries were embarking on a Hundred Years' War, as that phrase was not coined until 1823.[3]

Of course, some people know no history at all. "This is an incredibly unusual situation," one financial expert told the *Financial Times* in March 2020, "a kind of crisis we've never seen before."[4] This illustrates that people who use terms like "unprecedented" about a crisis are in general merely conveying their ignorance of history. Only slightly better were the many bad historical analogies deployed as people tried to understand the implications of the pandemic. In March the archbishop of Canterbury likened the impact to a nuclear explosion: "The initial impact is colossal," he said, "but the fallout last[s] for years and will shape us in ways we can't even begin to predict at the moment."[5] This is misleading. To see why, just reflect on what befell Hiroshima and Nagasaki when the first operational atomic bombs were detonated over them in August 1945. Roughly as many people were killed immediately by "Little Boy" in Hiroshima as had been killed in the Dresden firestorm six months before, which was around 35,000. But by the end of 1945 the Japanese death toll had risen much higher, to as many as 140,000 in Hiroshima and 70,000 in Nagasaki. In addition, there were large numbers of later deaths due to leukemia and cancer attributable to the radiation released by the two bombs.

At the time of writing (October 22, 2020), COVID-19 is estimated to have killed more than 1.1 million people worldwide over a period of roughly ten months. That is very probably an underestimate, judging by excess deaths relative to expected deaths in multiple countries.[6] And this figure will certainly rise in the months ahead, as this book is going to press. These are numbers that do indeed compare with the biggest battles of the world wars. Unlike the immediate shock wave and subsequent radiation from a nuclear explosion, however, SARS-CoV-2 is a virus that can be evaded if individuals and societies take the right precautions. The same "bomb" was dropped on Taiwan as on Italy and New York State. To date, seven people have died of COVID-19 in Taiwan, 33,523 in New York. This is not to say that geopolitical analogies are always invalid, or that only the study of other pandemics can help us understand this one. Rather, we need to think of COVID-19 as one of those rare catastrophes that befall humanity at irregular intervals in history. In addition to pandemics, these include major wars, violent revolutions, volcanic eruptions, earthquakes, and extreme weather-related events such as wildfires and floods. Historians tend to gravitate toward the study of such extreme disasters, with a preference for the man-made varieties. Yet they seldom reflect very deeply on their common properties.

A pandemic of the sort that swept the world in 2020 is about as frequent an event as a major war. One highly influential epidemiological model suggested that the pandemic of 2020, in the absence of non-pharmaceutical interventions, could kill up to forty million people worldwide.[7] Relative to a world population of 7.8 billion, that would approximate closely to the battlefield mortality in World War I. While it seems clear that the ultimate death toll from COVID-19 will not be so high—either because the Imperial College London model overestimated the infection fatality rate of the disease or because social distancing, economic lockdowns, and other measures really did avert mass death—there was no guarantee of this at the outset of the crisis.

If, as many contemporaries expected at its outset, World War I had lasted no longer than five months, it, too, would have been much less deadly.

A remarkable characteristic of these two disparate disasters is that each of them was repeatedly predicted by contemporaries for years before they occurred. In that sense they were both examples of what the American author Michele Wucker has called a "gray rhino"—something that is "dangerous, obvious, and highly probable"—along with "Hurricane Katrina, the 2008 financial crisis, the 2007 Minnesota bridge collapse, cyberattacks, wildfires [and] water shortages."[8] Yet when World War I and COVID-19 actually occurred, they were perceived to be very surprising events—"black swans." Nassim Taleb has defined a black swan as any event that "seems to us, on the basis of our limited experience, to be impossible."[9] Thanks to evolution and education, we have certain heuristic biases that lead us to expect most phenomena to be (like the heights of humans) normally distributed. But the statistical distributions of forest fires—to name just one example—obey a quite different set of rules: often, though not always, "power laws." There is no "typical" or average forest fire. Plotted on a graph, the distribution of fires is not the familiar bell curve, with most fires clustered around the mean. Rather, if you plot the size of fires against the frequency of their occurrence using logarithmic scales, you get a straight line.[10]

Power laws (or distributions that roughly resemble them) are surprisingly ubiquitous, though the steepness of that line varies.[11] They also characterize the distributions by size of meteorites and debris orbiting Earth, the craters on the moon, solar flares, and volcanic eruptions—to say nothing of the foraging patterns of various herbivores. In the human world, too, we encounter multiple power laws: daily stock market returns, box office revenues, the frequencies of words in most languages, the frequencies of family names, the sizes of power outages, the number of charges per criminal offender, individual annual health charges, and identity theft losses. The distribution of the 315 "deadly quarrels" identified by L. F. Richardson (see chapter 1) was not quite a power law: technically, it was a Poisson distribution, an essentially random pattern that applies not only to wars but also to radioactive decays, cancer clusters, tornado touchdowns, internet server hits, and, in a previous era, the deaths of cavalrymen caused by kicks from horses.

The precise mathematical distinction between power laws and Poisson distributions need not detain us here. For our purposes, it is enough to know that both distributions mean large events occur more frequently than in a normal distribution. In the case of war, Richardson strove to find patterns in his data for deadly conflict that might shed light on the timing and scale of wars. Was there a long-run trend toward less or more war? Was war related to the geographical proximity of states or to social, economic, and cultural factors? The answer in each case was no. The data indicated that wars were randomly distributed. (In Richardson's words, "The collection as a whole does not indicate any trend towards more, nor towards fewer, fatal quarrels.")[12] In this respect, wars do indeed resemble pandemics and earthquakes. We cannot know in advance when or where a specific event will strike, nor on what scale. While

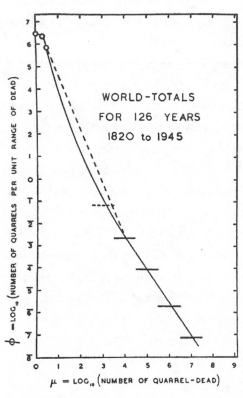

WORLD-TOTALS

FOR 126 YEARS

1820 to 1945

L. F. Richardson's representation of the number of conflicts of each magnitude compared with the number that died in each, from his *Statistics of Deadly Quarrels.* So far, the two world wars have been the only deadly quarrels of magnitude 7 (i.e., their death toll was in the tens of millions). So far, murders—deadly quarrels of magnitude 0 (i.e., a death toll of one)—have killed a quarter as many people as world wars have.

some modern researchers continue to discern in the data some more encouraging trend toward a more peaceable world,[13] the more persuasive view is that humanity remains prone to "conflict avalanches" or cascades of "randomly branching" armed conflict.[14]

There is one possible exception. The French geophysicist Didier Sornette has defined a "dragon king" as an event so extreme that it lies outside a power-law distribution. He finds examples in six domains: city sizes, acoustic emissions associated with material failure, velocity increments in hydrodynamic turbulence, financial drawdowns, the energies of epileptic seizures in humans and animals, and (possibly) earthquakes. Dragon kings, he argues, are "extreme events that are statistically and mechanistically different from the rest of their smaller siblings." They "exhibit a degree of predictability, because they are associated with mechanisms expressed differently than for the other events. Often, dragon-kings are associated with the occurrence of a phase transition, bifurcation, catastrophe, tipping point, whose emergent organization produces useful precursors."[15] It is not clear, however, how far such precursors can reliably be identified before the dragon king strikes.

How does an event go from being a gray rhino (eminently predictable) to being a black swan (hugely surprising) to being a dragon king (vast in magnitude)? To the historian, the transformation from gray rhino to black swan illustrates the problems of cognitive confusion discussed in the previous chapter. How else can an oft-predicted disaster be experienced, when it happens, as a bolt from the blue? However, the transformation from black swan to dragon king is the difference between a disaster that kills a great many people and one that has much wider and deeper consequences than the proximate body count. It is worth adding, even though it would be hard to prove statistically, that dragon kings would appear to exist outside the realm of catastrophe, too. There have been countless holy men and founders of religious cults; only three (Gautama Buddha, Jesus Christ, and Muhammad) founded world religions capable of attracting hundreds of millions of adherents and enduring for centuries. There have been and still are countless secular political theorists; none has matched Karl Marx in inspiring not only hundreds of millions of believers but also multiple political parties, revolutions, and states, including two of history's largest, the Soviet Union and the People's Republic of China. In the same way, there have been many periods of technological change in human history; only one, initially concentrated on the manufacture of textiles and iron and the application of steam power, constituted an industrial revolution. These extreme outliers seem more like dragon kings than black swans. Yet how predictable they are in practice is very far from clear.

If so many natural and man-made phenomena have power-law or Poisson distributions, how can history possibly be cyclical? If there is so much randomness in the world, how can tragedy be anything other than a rationalization of the bad luck that plague happened to strike Thebes during Oedipus's reign as king? As the atheist magician Penn Jillette has observed, "Luck is statistics taken personally."

LORENZ'S BUTTERFLY

Edward Lorenz, the pioneer of chaos theory, famously suggested that the flapping of a butterfly's wings in Brazil could set off a tornado in Texas. Even a tiny disturbance, he argued, can have huge effects in a complex system governed by nonlinear relationships. Lorenz discovered the butterfly effect in 1961, when he was experimenting at the Massachusetts Institute of Technology with a computer model he had designed to simulate weather patterns. (A mathematician by training, Lorenz had become a meteorologist during World War II.) He was repeating a simulation he had run before, but he had rounded off one variable from 0.506127 to 0.506. To his amazement, this tiny change drastically transformed the simulated weather generated by the computer.

Almost no one read Lorenz's pathbreaking paper on the subject when it was published in the *Journal of the Atmospheric Sciences* as "Deterministic Nonperiodic Flow."[16] It was not until nearly ten years later that he translated his insight into layman's language in a lecture with the title "Predictability: Does the Flap of a Butterfly's Wings in Brazil Set Off a Tornado in Texas?" "Two particular weather situations," he argued, "differing by as little as the immediate influence of a single butterfly, will generally after sufficient time evolve into two situations differing by as much as the presence of a tornado."

In his 1972 lecture, however, Lorenz added an important caveat: "If the flap of a butterfly's wings can be instrumental in generating a tornado, it can equally well be instrumental in preventing a tornado."[17] In Lorenz's view, this was what made long-range weather prediction so very difficult.

The same applies even more to economic forecasting. In 1966, the Nobel Prize–winning economist Paul Samuelson—like Lorenz, a professor at MIT—joked that declines in U.S. stock prices had correctly predicted "nine out of the last five recessions." Economic forecasters are in reality far worse at their jobs than weather forecasters. Of 469 downturns in national economies between 1988 and 2019, the International Monetary Fund had predicted only four by the spring of the year before they began.[18] As for the great financial crisis of 2008–9, only a handful of economists foresaw it with any real precision. Most, as Her Majesty the Queen pointed out, did not "see it coming."

The problem is that both the weather and the economy are complex systems—and, in the case of the economy, the system has been growing steadily more complex since the Industrial Revolution. A complex system is made up of very large numbers of interacting components, asymmetrically organized. Some such systems operate somewhere between order and disorder—"on the edge of chaos," in the phrase of the computer scientist Christopher Langton.[19] The system can operate for an extended period very nicely, apparently in equilibrium but in fact adapting all the time. However, there can come a moment when the system reaches a critical state. A very small catalyst (the butterfly that flaps its wings or the famous last grain of sand that causes the entire pile to collapse) can trigger a "phase transition" from one state or equilibrium to another.

Not long after some big phase transitions, historians arrive on the scene, because they tend to be attracted by events that inhabit the tails of the probability distribution. Unfortunately, these historians are generally no help at all. Misunderstanding complexity, they proceed to explain the huge calamity in terms of long-run causes, often dating back decades. A huge world war breaks out in the summer of 1914, to the avowed amazement of most contemporaries. Before long, the historians have devised a storyline commensurate with the disaster, involving power-hungry Germans and the navy they began building in 1898, the waning of Ottoman power in the Balkans dating back to the 1870s, and a treaty governing the neutrality of Belgium that was signed in 1839. This is what Nassim Taleb has rightly condemned as the "narrative fallacy"—the construction of psychologically satisfying stories on the principle of *post hoc, ergo propter hoc*.[20] Telling such stories is an age-old habit that is very hard to break. Recent versions of the retrospective fallacy trace the 9/11 terrorist attacks back to the execution of Sayyid Qutb, the Islamist writer who inspired the Muslim Brotherhood, in 1966;[21] or attribute the 2008 financial crisis to measures of financial deregulation dating back to the late 1970s.[22]

In reality, the proximate triggers of a crisis often suffice to explain the sudden phase transition. To understand why, we need to recognize that most of the "fat tail" phenomena historians like to study are essentially perturbations and sometimes complete breakdowns of complex systems. Complexity is a term now widely used by natural scientists as well as computer scientists to make sense of a wide range of different systems, such as the spontaneously organized behavior of half a million ants or termites, which allows them to construct complex hills and nests; the production of human intelligence from the interaction of a hundred billion neurons in the "enchanted loom" of the central nervous system; the action of the antibodies in the human immune system to combat alien bacteria and viruses; the "fractal geometry" whereby simple water molecules form themselves into intricate snowflakes, with myriad variants of sixfold symmetry, or plant cells form fern leaves; and the elaborate biological order that knits together multiple species of flora and fauna within a rain forest.[23]

There is every reason to think that man-made economies, societies, and polities share many of the features of complex adaptive systems. Indeed, economists such as W. Brian Arthur have been arguing along these lines for more than twenty years, going beyond Adam Smith's hallowed idea that an "Invisible Hand" caused markets to work through the interaction of profit-maximizing individuals, or Friedrich von Hayek's later critique of economic planning and demand management.[24] For Arthur, a complex economy is characterized by the dispersed interaction of multiple agents, a lack of any central control, multiple levels of organization, continual adaptation, the incessant creation of new niches, and an absence of general equilibrium. In this version of economics, Silicon Valley is a complex adaptive system. So is the internet itself.

Researchers at the Santa Fe Institute have for many years labored to see how such insights can be applied to other aspects of collective human activity.[25] This effort may recall Mr. Casaubon's effort in George Eliot's *Middlemarch* to find "the Key to all Mythologies,"[26] but the attempt is well worthwhile. Consider the following features that are characteristic of complex systems:

- "A small input can produce major . . . changes—an amplifier effect."[27]
- Causal relationships are often (though not always) nonlinear, so conventional methods of generalizing from observations to theory about their behavior, such as trend analysis and sampling, are of little use. Indeed, some theorists of complexity would go so far as to say that complex systems are wholly nondeterministic.
- When complex systems experience disruption, the scale of the disruption is therefore well-nigh impossible to predict.

What all this means is that a relatively minor shock can cause a disproportionate—and sometimes fatal—disruption to a complex system. As Taleb has argued, the global economy by 2007 had come to resemble an over-optimized electricity grid.[28] The relatively small surge represented by defaults on subprime mortgages in the United States sufficed to tip the entire world economy into the financial equivalent of a blackout.[29] Blaming such a crash on financial deregulation under Ronald Reagan is as illuminating as blaming the First World War on the naval plans of Admiral von Tirpitz.

EARTH-SHAKING EVENTS

History, broadly conceived, is the interaction of natural and man-made complexity. It would be very remarkable if this process resulted in predictable patterns. Even a relatively simple man-made edifice such as a bridge can fail "from deterioration of the bridge deck, corrosion or fatigue of structural elements, or an external loading such as floodwater. None of these failure modes is independent of the others in probability or consequence."[30] If it is hard for an engineer to foresee when a bridge may "go critical," then how much more difficult is it to anticipate the collapse of a large political structure?[31] The most that can be said is that historians these days are trying to relate more systematically the evolution of political structures to natural phenomena such as geological or climatic disruptions and pandemics.[32] The more such work is done, however, the more we realize how diverse and erratic is the incidence of disaster. We also begin to discern how artificial the distinction is between natural and man-made disasters. For there is a constant interaction between human societies and nature, so that even an endogenous shock such as a large earthquake is destructive of human life and health only in proportion to the proximity of large conurbations to the shifting fault line.

The history of disasters is a history of a poorly managed zoo full of gray rhinos, black swans, and dragon kings—as well as a great many unfortunate but inconsequential events and an infinity of nonevents. It is lucky for mankind that Earth has not so far been struck by any large extraterrestrial objects during our time of planetary predominance. The Vredefort Crater, in South Africa's Free State, was created around 2 billion years ago and has an estimated diameter of 190 miles. Sudbury Basin, in Ontario, dates back 1.8 billion years and has an estimated diameter of 81 miles. The Acraman Crater, in South Australia, was created 580 million years ago and is about 12 miles across. Finally, the Chicxulub Crater, on the Yucatán Peninsula, is more than 66 million years old and is 93 miles in diameter. Each of these bears witness to a devastating disaster that, for a protracted period, severely impaired Earth's viability as a habitat for organic life. As the estimated date of the Chicxulub impact coincides precisely with the Cretaceous-Paleogene boundary, it seems likely that it was the cause of the extinction of the dinosaurs. No comparable asteroid has struck Earth since the ascent of *Homo sapiens*—which is just as well. The 1490 Ch'ing-yang event seems to have been just an exceptionally large meteor shower. A quite different extraterrestrial shock—the 1859 Carrington Event, a "coronal mass ejection," or geomagnetic sun storm, that fired 100 million tons of charged particles at Earth's magnetosphere—had minimal impact, as electrification was still in its infancy.[33] Since the American astronomer John A. Eddy's seminal 1976 paper, exceptionally low solar activity has also been seen as the principal cause of the below-average temperatures between 1460 and 1550 (the "Spörer Minimum") and between 1645 and 1715 (the "Maunder Minimum").*[34] Thus far, humanity has been let off lightly by both outer space and our own solar system. The Chicxulub asteroid was between seven and fifty miles in diameter. If a similar object had struck Earth at any time in the past 300,000 years, it would have been "a species-destroying event," and not just because of the unimaginable impact of the initial blast. Oceans would have been acidified, land and sea ecologies would have collapsed, and the sky would have turned black, plunging any remnants of mankind into an extended cosmic winter.[35]

Earth has shown itself capable of generating its own geological disasters. The volcanic "super-eruption" at Yellowstone 630,000 years ago covered half the continental United States with ash. The eruption at what is now Lake Toba, in northern Sumatra, 75,000 years ago caused land temperatures to drop globally by between 5 and 15 degrees Celsius and the ocean surface to cool by 2 to 6 degrees Celsius, because of the huge quantity of ash and soot that was fired into the atmosphere. This catastrophe may even have brought the human race to the brink of extinction, reducing its total population to as few as four thousand individuals, with just five hundred females of childbearing age.[36] In 45 BC and again two years later, Alaska's Mount Okmok erupted. By analyzing the tephra (volcanic ash) found in six Arctic ice cores, researchers at the Desert Research Institute, in Reno, Nevada, and the Oeschger Centre for Climate Change Research, at the University of Bern, have posited a causal link between the Okmok eruptions and a decline in temperatures throughout the northern hemisphere at that time. The years 43 and 42 BC were the second- and eighth-coldest years on record, and the decade 43–34

---

*The "minima" are named after the British astronomers Edward Walter Maunder and his wife, Annie, who pioneered the study of sunspots, and the German Gustav Spörer, who first identified the low activity of the period after 1618.

BC was the fourth coldest. Temperatures in some Mediterranean regions were as much as 7 degrees Celsius below normal during the two years after the eruption. The weather in Europe was also unusually wet. This, the authors hypothesize, "probably resulted in crop failures, famine, and disease, exacerbating social unrest and contributing to political realignments throughout the Mediterranean region at this critical juncture of Western civilization."[37] Certainly, contemporary Roman sources testify to a period of abnormally cold weather in Italy, Greece, and Egypt. How far the resulting crop failures and food shortages explain the collapse of the Roman Republic is another question. Julius Caesar had already been appointed dictator for life in February of 44 BC, well before the larger second eruption of Okmok.

In any case, the Romans had a volcano much closer to home to worry about. Mount Vesuvius, on the shore of the Bay of Naples, had erupted on a massive scale in 1780 BC (the Avellino eruption)[38] and again around seven hundred years before its most famous eruption, in AD 79, during the reign of the emperor Titus. The Romans had some understanding of the dangers of earthquakes, having witnessed a severe one in Campania in AD 62 or 63. However, they did not know that the earth tremors felt near Vesuvius in the days before the eruption were intimations of catastrophe. Writing just a few years earlier, Seneca speculated that there might be a connection between earthquakes and the weather; he did not consider the connection to volcanoes. "There had been noticed for many days before a trembling of the earth," wrote Pliny the Younger to the historian Tacitus, "which did not alarm us much, as this is quite an ordinary occurrence in Campania."[39] The eruption on the morning of August 24 ejected a vast, tree-shaped cloud of stones, ashes, and volcanic gases to a height of twenty-one miles, raining molten rock, pulverized pumice, and ash onto the towns of Pompeii, Herculaneum, Oplontis, and Stabiae. As the huge cloud collapsed, it created a pyroclastic surge—a searingly hot blast of gas and debris that shot out sideways from the slopes of the volcano. The thermal energy released is estimated to have been 100,000 times greater than that of the atomic bombs dropped on Hiroshima and Nagasaki in 1945.[40]

Pliny the Younger's eyewitness account of the calamity illustrates how bewildering the eruption of Vesuvius was to even the best-educated Romans. Pliny's uncle and namesake was at Misenum, at the northwest end of the Bay of Naples, where he was in command of a naval fleet.

> On the 24th of August, about one in the afternoon, my mother desired him to observe a cloud which appeared of a very unusual size and shape. He had just taken a turn in the sun and, after bathing himself in cold water, and making a light luncheon, gone back to his books: he immediately arose and went out upon a rising ground from whence he might get a better sight of this very uncommon appearance.
>
> A cloud . . . was ascending, the appearance of which I cannot give you a more exact description of than by likening it to that of a [stone] pine tree, for it shot up to a great height in the form of a very tall trunk, which spread itself out at the top into a sort of branches. . . .
>
> This phenomenon seemed to a man of such learning and research as my uncle extraordinary and worth further looking into. He ordered a light vessel to be got ready. . . .
>
> Hastening then to the place from whence others fled with the utmost terror, he steered his course direct to the point of danger, and with so much calmness and presence of mind as to be able to make and dictate his observations upon the motion and all the phenomena of that dreadful scene. He was now so close to the mountain that the cinders, which grew thicker and hotter the nearer he approached, fell into the ships, together with pumice-stones, and black pieces of burning rock: they were in danger too not only of being aground by the sudden retreat of the sea, but also from the vast fragments which rolled down from the mountain, and obstructed all the shore.[41]

Incredibly, the elder Pliny then went ashore to visit his friend Pomponianus, dined with him, and went to bed, even as the eruption continued and the earth shook around them. Roused from sleep by his friend, Pliny sought to escape, using a pillow to protect himself from the falling stone and ash, but died from the toxic fumes (presumably from the pyroclastic surge) before he could board his vessel. The younger Pliny sought solace in the "miserable, though mighty, consolation that all mankind were involved in the same calamity, and that I was perishing with the world itself."[42] Though in the end he survived, it is, as we shall see, a common reaction: to feel, when confronted by a disaster, that one is facing the end of the world.

Pompeii and Herculaneum were destroyed and never rebuilt or resettled. Two millennia later, the tourist can visit their ruins and marvel, as I did as a boy, at the rude vitality of Roman life in the first century and the pathos of its devastating termination on that hellish summer's day. I shall never forget the perfectly preserved death agonies of the hundreds of fugitives who vainly sought refuge in the *fornici* (boathouses) along the beach at Herculaneum, which offered no protection whatever from the 500-Celsius-degree heat of the pyroclastic surge.[43] Yet the wider ramifications of the eruption of Vesuvius appear to have been minimal. The life and growth of the Roman Empire continued with barely a pause. And other settlements near Vesuvius recovered. Here is one of the stranger quirks of the politics of disaster: humans nearly always return to the scene, no matter how vast the disaster. Naples grew to be one of modern Italy's largest cities, despite another large eruption in 1631—smaller than Pliny's but bad enough to kill between three thousand and six thousand people.[44] Today Naples is the third-largest metropolitan area in Italy, with a population of 3.7 million. There is an evacuation plan for the eventuality of another eruption of Vesuvius, but it would be of little use if something on the scale of 1780 BC or AD 79 were to recur.[45]

Remarkably, Vesuvius did not produce the most destructive eruption of the Roman era: that was the Hatepe eruption of Mount Taupo, on New Zealand's North Island, in around 232. Major volcanic eruptions, such as Okmok, Taupo, and Paektu (on the China-Korea border, circa 946), differ from the other form of geological disaster, earthquakes, in that they have global impacts on the earth's climate. A huge Icelandic eruption in 536 lowered temperatures and shrank harvests across Eurasia. The period from around 1150 to 1300 was punctuated by five major volcanic events, each of which injected at least 55 million tons of sulfate aerosol into the stratosphere. The biggest, the eruption of Mount Samalas, on the Indonesian island of Lombok, in 1257, produced more than 275 million tons.[46] The fourteenth, fifteenth, and sixteenth centuries were much quieter, aside from the eruption of Kuwae, a submarine caldera between the Epi and Tongoa islands, in Vanuatu, in late 1452 or early 1453. The 1600s saw larger eruptions. The three biggest were at Huaynaputina, in Peru, in 1600; Mount Komagatake, in Japan, in 1640; and Mount Parker, in the Philippines, in 1641. However, these were dwarfed by Laki, in Iceland, in 1783–84, and Mount Tambora, in Indonesia, in 1815, each of which filled the stratosphere with around 110 million tons of sulfate aerosol. Since then, we have not had to deal with anything on such a scale. No subsequent volcanic eruption in the world—not even Krakatoa on August 26–27, 1883, though its eruption was loud enough to be heard in Western Australia[47]—has been even a quarter as large.

Death tolls are more or less unknown for the pre-1800 eruptions. The Dutch colonial authorities estimated that more than 71,000 people were killed by Tambora and 36,600 by Krakatoa. Modern estimates of the Krakatoa death toll, however, go as high as 120,000,[48] taking into account the numerous communities along the Sunda Strait that were wiped out by the tsunami the eruption caused.[49] The eruption of Laki killed between a fifth and a quarter of the population of Iceland and even larger proportions of livestock. But few people have ever lived in Iceland. Asia—and particularly Indonesia—is where volcanoes kill humans in the largest numbers. In the past ten thousand years, it has been estimated, Indonesia has accounted for only 17 percent of all volcanic eruptions, but 33 percent of the eruptions known to have produced human fatalities.[50] A more risk-averse species simply would not have settled there.

However, volcanic eruptions do more than kill those close to them. All these eruptions also had significant climatic consequences and hence agricultural and nutritional consequences. During the winter of 1601–2, Switzerland, Estonia, Latvia, and Sweden all experienced very low temperatures—ice remained in Riga harbor for much longer than usual—while in Russia, more than half a million people are thought to have died from starvation in the

1601–3 famine.[51] In the years that followed the eruptions of Komagatake and Parker, Japan, China, and Korea all saw cold summers, drought, poor harvests, and famine. Droughts were recorded in Ukraine, Russia, Java, parts of India, Vietnam, the Greek islands, and Egypt. France and England experienced a series of cold, wet summers. The five worst famines to hit Japan during the Tokugawa period—in 1638–43, 1731–33, 1755–56, 1783–88, and 1832–38—coincided with periods of significant volcanic activity.[52] After the eruption of Laki, Benjamin Franklin commented bemusedly on the presence of a "constant fog" over Europe and parts of North America. In Britain, the summer of 1783 was exceptionally warm because of the buildup of ash in the atmosphere, but then came a severe winter, caused by the high concentration of heat-absorbing sulfur dioxide in the atmosphere. Parish records in England and France indicate significant excess mortality owing to respiratory problems attributable to Laki's emissions. The 1783–84 winter was very harsh in North America, too: the Mississippi froze at New Orleans.[53] There was a similar pattern of unusual cold in the wake of Tambora's eruption from old England to New England, with associated bad harvests.[54] Krakatoa not only lowered northern hemisphere temperatures by around 0.4 degrees Celsius;[55] it also produced spectacular sunsets throughout the world for many months.[56] (One is believed to feature in the background of Edvard Munch's *The Scream*.)

Historians used to lump together all the evidence of lower-than-average temperatures from around 1500 to 1800 as evidence of a "Little Ice Age." A group of researchers recently advanced the bold claim that "the decline in global atmospheric CO_2 concentration by 7–10 ppm in the late 1500s and early 1600s which globally lowered surface air temperatures by 0.15°C [was] . . . a result of the large-scale depopulation of the Americas after European arrival [and] subsequent land use change," in particular the reversion of formerly cultivated land to natural forest.[57] On closer inspection, however, the Little Ice Age—whatever its causes—seems to fade from view. There were periods after 1600 when European temperatures were higher than the long-run average. Some regions of Europe were less cold and damp than others (there was not much of a Little Ice Age in Greece, for example). The largest negative

anomalies (temperatures lower than 0.8 degrees Celsius below average) were
in early-seventeenth-century northwestern Central Asia, a region ignored by
most Western historians.[58] One recent study finds no evidence of a change in
the distribution of summer temperatures in the Low Countries between the
fourteenth and twentieth centuries. If there had been a Little Ice Age, it would
surely have manifested itself in reduced crop yields and stagnating population, whereas no such trends are evident: indeed, by 1820 the population of
Europe was nearly two and a half times what it had been in 1500. English historians were for many years fascinated by paintings of the frozen Thames,
which seemed to testify to the existence of a Little Ice Age. This, however, resulted from the way that the wide piers of Old London Bridge acted like a dam,
creating a pool of still water that was liable to freeze over. Between 1660 and
1815, that happened a dozen times—to a thickness that permitted fairs to be
held on the ice in 1683–84, 1716, 1739–40, 1789, and 1814. It ceased after
the bridge was replaced in 1831.[59]

But can we also attribute major social and political upheavals to these
geological disruptions? A number have been suggested: the fall of Constantinople in 1453, Russia's Time of Troubles after the death of Tsar Boris Godu-
nov in 1605, the English colonization of North America,[60] and the outbreak
of the French Revolution,[61] not to mention the emergence of the deadly new
strain of cholera, *Vibrio cholerae,* in Bengal in 1817.[62] Some have even gone so
far as to link volcanically generated climate change to the rise of socialism
and nationalism. Yet, as with the Alaskan volcano's part in the downfall of the
Roman Republic, it seems a mistake to give geology too much of the credit for
history. A lot else was at work in each of these cases besides cold weather and
bad harvests. Rather, we should content ourselves by noting two points. First,
there is nothing remotely cyclical about the movements of the earth's tectonic plates. Second, despite our superior scientific knowledge, a very large
Tambora-like event would surprise us almost as much as Vesuvius astounded
the Romans, and for much the same reason: it has now been a very long time
since a really big volcanic eruption. It is precisely the erratic incidence of geological disaster—the long yet variable interludes—that explains the human
propensity to resettle in volcanic areas.

LIFE AND DEATH ON THE FAULT LINES

Earthquakes can rarely compete with volcanoes as world-historical events: their geographical reach is generally shorter, even when they generate tsunamis. Like volcanic eruptions, earthquakes follow a power law, making it extremely difficult to anticipate their timing and magnitude. All we can be sure of is their likely occurrence along the edges of the earth's tectonic plates. This is a terrible uncertainty to live with—or it would be if we thought about it too much. The difference is immense between a moment magnitude* 6.3 earthquake, such as the one that struck Christchurch, New Zealand, in February 2011, and a magnitude 9.0 one, such as the Tohoku quake, off Japan the following month. In terms of the shaking it caused, Tohoku was more than five hundred times larger; in terms of the energy it released, eleven thousand times larger.[63]

Probably the deadliest earthquake in history was the one that struck the Wei River valley, in China's Shaanxi Province, in January 1556. Although it was of magnitude 7.9–8.0, it affected a densely populated region, entirely destroying the cities of Huaxian, Weinan, and Huayin. The people living in the artificial caves carved into cliffs in the area of the Loess Plateau were especially vulnerable. The death toll was estimated to be above 800,000. Comparable disasters in more recent Chinese history were the 1920 Haiyuan earthquake (magnitude 7.8), which killed at least 200,000 people, and the 1976 Tangshan earthquake (magnitude 7.6), which killed around 242,000, exposing the shoddy quality of the buildings in the city as well as the absurdity of the Communist Party's earlier claims that it could predict earthquakes. (By comparison, the death toll of the 1906 San Francisco earthquake was at most three thousand, and the greater part of the destruction was in fact the result of fire—some of it deliberately started, for insurance purposes—rather than the earthquake itself.) There have been much larger earthquakes in modern

---

*Moment magnitude is nowadays the preferred measure of earthquake size and, so far as possible, is the measure of magnitude used here. It differs from the older and more familiar Richter scale of local magnitude. Moment is proportional to the slip on the fault multiplied by the area of the fault surface that slips. It is a better measure for very large earthquakes.

history, but most occurred in sparsely settled regions. The 1952 earthquake off Kamchatka, Russia, the 1960 earthquake that struck Valdivia, Chile, and the 1964 Good Friday earthquake in Prince William Sound, Alaska, were all magnitude 9.0 or higher, but they were far from major population centers.[64] Asian earthquakes have tended to be the most disastrous not because their size is exceptional, but because the populations close to Asian fault lines have been larger.

The Mediterranean world has had its disastrous earthquakes, too. In 526 and again in 528, the major Roman city of Antioch (today Antakya, in southern Turkey) was devastated by magnitude 7.0 earthquakes and tsunamis.[65] The chronicler John of Ephesus recorded that the disaster struck just after midday: the city wall, its churches, and most other buildings were destroyed.[66] The number of people killed has been put as high as 250,000 to 300,000[67]— the city was unusually crowded because of an influx of pilgrims to celebrate Ascension Day.[68] The earthquake was only one of multiple disasters that befell Antioch between 500 and 611, including the Plague of Justinian, suggesting a remarkable resilience on the part of the inhabitants—perhaps even antifragility.[69] Evidence of resilience, if not antifragility, also comes from southern Italy. Between December 5 and 30, 1456, the city of Naples—indeed, all of southern and central Italy[70]—was rocked by the biggest earthquake in the history of the Italian mainland (magnitude 6.9–7.3), exceeded only by the January 1693 Sicilian earthquake (7.4).[71] The same fault produced smaller quakes in 1688 and as recently as 2013.[72] The biggest Italian earthquake of modern times (magnitude 6.7–7.2) struck Messina on December 28, 1908, one of a succession to occur along the so-called Calabrian Arc (the others were in 1638, 1693, 1783, and 1905).[73] Around 90 percent of the city's buildings were destroyed, partly by the tremor, partly by the forty-foot tsunami that followed, and partly by fire, leaving sixty thousand to eighty thousand people dead.[74] Yet despite soubriquets such as "City of the Dead" and "City Without Memory,"[75] Messina has around 230,000 inhabitants today. People went back.[76] People nearly always go back.

Among the biggest earthquakes in European history, the one that struck Lisbon on November 1, 1755, repays study, not least because it so fascinated contemporaries. The earthquake of 1755 was not the first to hit the Portuguese capital—there had been others in 1321 and 1531—but it was the biggest. Seismologists today estimate that the 1755 earthquake had a magnitude of 8.4. Its epicenter was in the Atlantic Ocean, about 120 miles west-southwest of Cape St. Vincent. According to contemporary accounts, the quake lasted between three and a half and six minutes, opening sixteen-foot-wide fissures in the city center and toppling most buildings. Around forty minutes later, a tsunami hit the city, sweeping up the Tagus River, followed closely by two more huge waves. Candles lit for All Saints' Day were knocked over, starting a devastating fire. The best estimate is that between twenty and thirty thousand people were killed in Lisbon alone, a further fifteen hundred to three thousand people elsewhere in Portugal, and more than ten thousand in Spain and Morocco, for a total death toll (including deaths further afield) of thirty-five thousand to forty-five thousand. Before the earthquake, Lisbon had boasted seventy-five convents and monasteries and forty churches. Fully 86 percent of these buildings were destroyed. Of Lisbon's thirty-three thousand houses, approximately thirteen thousand were laid low; a further ten thousand sustained substantial damage. The Casa dos Contos—the Portuguese state treasury—was destroyed, as were the royal archives. The immediate cost was between 32 and 48 percent of Portugal's gross domestic product.[77]

The shocks from the earthquake were felt as far away as Finland and North Africa, and even in Greenland and the Caribbean. Tsunamis swept the coast of North Africa and struck Martinique and Barbados, across the Atlantic. Yet, unlike the particles released by a volcano, the shock waves released by an earthquake are short-lived. The historical significance of the 1755 earthquake lies principally in its political consequences for Portugal. Already an imperial power in decline relative to the Dutch, British, and French empires, Portugal was set further back by the costs of the disaster. The king, Joseph I, developed a phobia of all buildings, moving his court into a complex of tents and pavilions in the hills of Ajuda, then on the outskirts of Lisbon. However, his prime minister, Sebastião José de Carvalho e Melo, 1st Marquis of Pombal, seized the opportunity presented by the crisis: "Bury the dead and heal the living," he declared. He might have added: *And centralize power in my hands.* Pombal was not content with disposing of corpses, removing rubble, distributing food, establishing temporary hospitals for the injured, and preventing looting. He imposed price controls to combat the effects of shortages. He levied a 4 percent duty on all imports, in a mercantilist effort to improve the balance of trade. He persecuted the Jesuits and reduced the Church's political influence. And he sought to rebuild the city with structures that would be more resilient in a future earthquake.[78] The city the visitor sees today is still, to a remarkable extent, Pombal's Lisbon. The disaster was his opportunity.

Earthquakes often prompt such political as well as architectural reconstructions. This was also the case in Meiji-era Japan, after a huge earthquake struck Osaka and Tokyo on October 28, 1891. While many traditional Japanese structures survived—including wooden pagodas and the seventeenth-century keep of Nagoya Castle—newer iron railroad bridges and brick factories collapsed, calling into question the suitability of Western technology and engineering at a time when the government was wholeheartedly committing to remaking Japan on the basis of European and American models. Nationalist writers lost no time in condemning the injuries inflicted by falling bricks. In an earthquake, "Japanese-style building hurts people by breaking bones or arms," wrote one cultural conservative. "But brick buildings give the body harsher damage because bricks fall and cut people, and mortar gets deep into their cuts. The mortar can't be gotten out, so the cut festers. People can't be saved."[79] Such arguments did not halt the Meiji modernization program. However, the disaster led to the creation of the Imperial Earthquake Investigation Committee (IEIC), which rapidly established itself as the world's leading center for seismological research, in advance of Japan's Western role models. Nothing could illustrate better the extreme difficulty of predicting earthquakes than the subsequent history of Japanese seismology.

The full Japanese name of the IEIC translates as "the Board of Investigation for Preventing Earthquake Disasters." As an earthquake cannot be prevented, the board's job was therefore prediction. Fusakichi Omori believed he could foresee where the next earthquake was likely to occur along a known fault by first mapping the locations of all previous earthquakes along that line. The gaps left on the map—the areas that had been seismically quiet for the longest time—were likely to be the next sections of the fault to shift. However, Omori was skeptical when a junior seismologist, Akitsune Imamura, used this "gap theory" to predict that Sagami Bay, southwest of Tokyo, was the most probable epicenter of the next big earthquake. Imamura was vindicated on September 1, 1923, when the magnitude 7.9 Great Kanto earthquake leveled Tokyo and Yokohama, as it originated precisely in the gap he had located nearly twenty years before. The IEIC was duly replaced by a new Earthquake Research Institute, under the direction of a naval architect from Mitsubishi.[80] Yet the new institution was no more successful in predicting major earthquakes. Imamura now began to look for gaps in the Nankai Trough, the undersea fault line that runs from Kyushu to the center of Honshu. In 1944, a major earthquake and tsunami in the center of this fault convinced him that a second such event would occur at a gap at the southern end, opposite Shikoku, which indeed happened in 1946. This left only the "Tokai gap," which Imamura insisted would be the location of the next big quake. It has yet to happen. By contrast, the earthquake that struck Kobe in 1995—the Great Hanshin earthquake, which measured 6.9 on the moment magnitude scale and killed between 5,500 and 6,500 people—was not predicted by any leading seismologist. Indeed, the authorities had given such an earthquake a probability of between 1 and 8 percent, as compared with over 80 percent for a Tokai quake.[81]

An earthquake, to repeat, is only as deadly as there are centers of population (and frail buildings) near its epicenter. The advent of nuclear power after World War II created a new kind of risk, however. In the wake of the Kobe quake, the seismologist Katsuhiko Ishibashi coined the term *gempatsu-shinsai* (nuclear earthquake disaster) to describe the scenario of an earthquake and a tsunami hitting a nuclear power station. As a longtime proponent of the Tokai gap theory, Ishibashi worried about the Hamaoka nuclear plant, in Shizuoka Prefecture. However, his 2007 article "Why Worry?" looked prescient four years later. A "significant earthquake," he argued, "could take out reactors' external power [and] a tsunami could then overtop the seawalls, flood the EDGs [emergency diesel generators], disable cooling of the reactors and lead to meltdowns."[82] The Tokyo Electric Power Company (TEPCO) dismissed the warnings of Yukinobu Okamura that their plant at Fukushima might also be

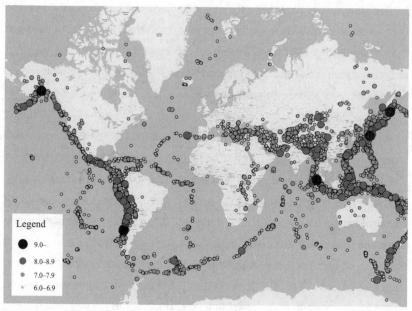

Earthquake locations and magnitudes, 1900–2017.

vulnerable to such a tsunami. The company took as its benchmark a modest quake that had happened in 1938. Okamura urged them to look back to the year 869 and a massive earthquake known as Jogan Jishin, which he believed had sent a tsunami two and a half miles inland, as far as the town of Sendai. Okamura and his team estimated that a magnitude 8.4 earthquake would unleash waves more than twenty feet high—enough to breach the nineteen-foot Fukushima seawall.[83] TEPCO dismissed these warnings—despite the fact that other power stations (notably the Onagawa nuclear plant) had much higher sea defenses—on the ground that raising the height of the seawall would only worry local residents. The government and the regulators essentially acquiesced in this.

The relative complacency of the Japanese authorities is all the more surprising in light of what happened on December 26, 2004, when a massive and protracted undersea earthquake with a magnitude of 9.1 to 9.3 occurred a hundred miles off the west coast of northern Sumatra. An estimated thousand miles of fault surface slipped about fifty feet along the subduction zone where the Indian Plate slides under the Burma Plate. This was followed by a major aftershock with magnitude 7.1 and multiple smaller aftershocks of up to 6.6 magnitude. The initial quake displaced around 7.2 cubic miles of water, creating devastating tsunamis that radiated outward—to the east and to the west—along the entire length of the slippage. These waves, which rose to heights of eighty to one hundred feet as they reached land, killed an estimated 227,898 people in fourteen countries, including Indonesia, Sri Lanka, India, and Thailand. The city of Banda Aceh suffered the most deaths, around 167,000, a large proportion of them children. But there were deaths as far away as Somalia and South Africa. The disaster exposed the poor quality of the tsunami warning systems, especially in Indonesia and Thailand.[84] In the latter, the role of Cassandra had been played by Samith Dhamasaroj, the former director general of the Thai Meteorological Department.[85]

Six years later, at 2:46 p.m. on March 11, 2011, a magnitude 9.0 earthquake struck eighty miles east of Sendai, about eighteen miles beneath the ocean surface. The relative movement between the two plates was about 260 feet, but the crucial feature of the quake was that an entire section of the subduction zone shifted in a massive block. "An area of seafloor the size of Connecticut jumped anywhere from 16 to 30 feet . . . shoving water toward Japan."[86] The quake lasted for three to five minutes, propelling a series of tsunami waves from the depths of the Pacific Ocean. Huge walls of water that formed as the waves neared land swept up to six miles inland, smashing everything in their path. More than nineteen thousand people were killed, drowned, or crushed to death.[87] Twenty-one-year-old Ryo Kanouya was told to return home to his village close to the shore at Fukushima to help elderly residents there. They were told to expect a ten-foot wave. He and his father ended up being swept out of their home:

> I was drained from my house into the soup of seawater, cars, houses, and everything the tsunami carried. To my surprise, I was able to reach the surface. My father and I recognized each other, [but] I watched him get washed away toward the mountainside. I was washed toward the ocean. . . .

Luckily a drawer for clothes came floating toward me and I climbed onto it. I felt relief. But I realized the incredible current was rapidly pulling me toward the ocean at high speed. When I was thinking what [I] should do next, I found a pile of debris sticking in a huge tree ahead of me. I held on with all of my remaining strength as I watched people being swept away around me.

Ryo was able to cling to the tree until the water level fell and finally was able to return to solid ground. Hiding next to a large rock, he nearly lost the will to keep moving, but the sight of a helicopter galvanized him. "If you don't move now, you're going to die," he thought. Stumbling through a wasteland of wreckage and corpses, he eventually saw a rescue vehicle. He and his father both survived, but the bodies of his grandmothers were never found.[88]

In addition to the human cost and the destruction of property, the Tohoku earthquake precipitated a grave crisis at the Fukushima Daiichi nuclear power plant. Although the active reactors shut down automatically when the earthquake was registered, the tsunami flooded the emergency generators powering the pumps that circulated coolant through the reactors' cores. As a result, there were nuclear meltdowns in three reactors, three hydrogen explosions, and the release of radioactive contamination, including large quantities of isotopes, into the air and sea. Considering how vulnerable the plant was to such a disaster, the most remarkable thing is that the consequences to date in terms of human health have been relatively modest.

Once again, the seismologists had failed. Kazuro Hirahara, the president of the Seismological Society of Japan, told the *Asahi Shimbun:* "There are many excuses we can make, but it amounted to a defeat for us. The only thing we can say is that it was beyond our expectations."[89] But this could equally well be said of all large earthquakes. Only the locations of earthquakes can be predicted—not their size and not their timing. Yet a map of the world, with the locations of the biggest earthquakes since 1500 plotted, reveals a puzzle. It is as if humanity took a collective decision to build as many as possible of its biggest cities on or close to fault lines. This illustrates the fatal interplay between the infrequency of disaster and the shortness of human memory. In

2011, those who recalled the 1938 earthquake off Fukushima made for old shelters that proved to be death traps as the much larger tsunamis struck.

AMERICAN DISASTER

Historically, the great American disaster has been, by Asian standards, not all that disastrous. As we have seen, the San Francisco earthquake of 1906 killed almost two orders of magnitude fewer people than the biggest Chinese earthquakes of modern times. But earthquakes are only one of the hazards that are more common in densely populated East Asia than in thinly populated North America. Consider two others that throughout history have intermittently wreaked havoc, again with little in the way of predictable periodicity: fires and floods, including those caused by hurricanes.

The biggest urban fire in modern Chinese history was the destruction of Changsha in 1938, when Kuomintang officials feared an imminent Japanese occupation. Whether an accident or a deliberate scorched-earth policy, the fire was disastrous: more than thirty thousand people lost their lives, and over 90 percent of the city's buildings were burned down. The biggest wildfire in modern Chinese history was the May 1987 Heilongjiang fire. Allegedly started by a forest worker who spilled gasoline from his brush cutter, the fire consumed three million acres of forest in the Greater Khingan Range, including one sixth of China's timber reserves. If one includes the forest across the border in Soviet territory, the area destroyed was close to eighteen million acres.[90] Prior to the 2020 California conflagrations, only one fire in American history came close in terms of casualties and destruction, and that was the Great Peshtigo fire, in northern Wisconsin and the Upper Peninsula of Michigan, which killed at least 1,152 people and burned altogether 1.2 million acres during the week of October 8–14, 1871. A further 2.3 million acres were partly damaged.[91]

Peshtigo, Wisconsin, was a logging town, supplying booming Chicago with timber from the forests close to Lake Michigan. The summer of 1871 had been one of the driest on record, and a reconstruction by the National Weather Service has shown that "after a long period of higher-than-usual temperatures and drought, a low-pressure front with cooler temperatures produced winds across the region. This whipped smaller fires into a giant conflagration. Hundred-mile-per-hour winds stoked the fire even more, with cool air fanning the flames and causing a gigantic column of hot air to rise. This produced even more wind—a vicious cycle that turned a routine wildfire into an inferno."[92] Yet the culprit was not the weather alone. Peshtigo's loggers had long been reckless in their practices, dumping waste from logging operations in large piles that acted as kindling. Railroad operations in the area were similarly cavalier. The town of Peshtigo itself was an all-wood tinderbox. Precautions taken after a smaller fire on September 27 proved woefully insufficient.[93] One who survived, the Reverend Peter Pernin, recalled a "dense cloud of smoke over-hanging the earth, a vivid red reflection of immense extent, and then [there] suddenly struck on my ear, strangely audible in the preternatural silence reigning around, a distant roaring, yet muffled sound, announcing that the elements were in commotion somewhere." As the situation intensified, "the wind heretofore violent rose suddenly to a hurricane, and quick as lightning opened the way for my egress from the yard by sweeping planks, gate, and fencing away into space."[94]

> The banks of the river as far as the eye could reach were covered with people standing there, motionless as statues, some with eyes staring, upturned towards heaven, and tongues protruded. The greater number seemed to have no idea of taking any steps to procure their safety, imagining, as many afterwards acknowledged to me, that the end of the world had arrived and that here was nothing for them but silent submission to their fate.[95]

At 10:00 p.m., Pernin and others opted to jump in the river, which offered only limited protection as flames flashed across its surface, and the cold temperature of the water ensured that many died from hypothermia or drowning. Pernin was able to emerge from the water at 3:30 a.m., chilled to the bone but alive.

Such fires were relatively common at the turn of the last century, wherever logging and railroad construction brought men close to large virgin forests: in northern Sweden, in Russia along the route of the Trans-Siberian Railway, on New Zealand's North Island, in Gippsland, Australia, as well as in British Columbia and Ontario. Comparable interactions between human settlements and natural waterways meant that the nineteenth century was also a time of great floods. In China, rapid population growth ultimately changed the course of the Yellow River. Forest clearance, drainage, and over-cultivation of marginal land led to soil erosion and elevated silting in the river itself, which, in turn, led to more flooding. When the river dams broke in 1853, a large part of northern China was "washed down."[96] Years of above-average precipitation put the entire waterway system connecting the Yellow and Yangtze rivers under stress. There were severe floods in 1887, 1911, 1931, 1935, 1938 (an intentional disaster intended to hamper the Japanese advance), and 1954, each causing significant loss of life. The 1887 flood is said to have caused at least 900,000 deaths; the 1931 flood, which began when the Yangtze River overflowed, may have claimed as many as 2 million; and the 1938 Yellow River flood killed between 400,000 and 500,000, though in each case more victims succumbed to starvation or disease than to drowning.

This pattern of catastrophic flooding explains the Communist regime's obsession with dam building. The high-circulation 5-jiao (half-yuan) banknote of the second series of the renminbi, first issued in 1955, features a dam on the back side. After swimming across the Yangtze River in 1958, Mao even wrote a poem about dams: "Great plans are being made / Walls of stone will stand upstream to the west." Yet not all the dams of the Mao era lived up to his heady rhetoric. The "Harness the Huai River" campaign to "give primacy to water accumulation for irrigation" was a typical 1950s initiative. The collapse of one of the dams built then—the Banqiao Dam—exposed the limits of Sino-Soviet collaboration. In August 1975, Typhoon Nina overwhelmed the dam by dumping a year's worth of rain (forty-two inches) in twelve hours,[97] causing one of the worst disasters in the history of the People's

Republic.[98] The breach unleashed the equivalent of a quarter of a million Olympic swimming pools of water, killing tens of thousands in a matter of hours. The secondary death toll from disease and starvation in the devastated area was in excess of 200,000 people.[99] The Cassandra figure in this disaster was the hydrologist Chen Xing, who had been purged during the Anti-Rightist Campaign for urging a halt to new dam construction but was now swiftly rehabilitated.[100] So horrific was the Banqiao Dam's failure that it remained a state secret until 1989. This did nothing to diminish the Communist Party's devotion to damming. In April 1992, the National People's Congress formally approved the Resolution on the Construction of the Yangtze River Three Gorges Project, the world's biggest-ever river dam development.*[101]

Though the United States is occasionally cursed as well as blessed in possessing numerous navigable rivers, the greatest being the Mississippi, the disasters they have caused pale in comparison with China's experience of flooding. The Johnstown Flood of 1889 remains the deadliest in American history. The catastrophic failure of the South Fork Dam on the Little Conemaugh River, fourteen miles upstream from the town of Johnstown, Pennsylvania, unleashed a torrent briefly equal to the average flow of the mighty Mississippi, killing more than 2,200 people. The Great Mississippi Flood of 1927 was vastly larger, inundating twenty-seven thousand square miles up to a depth of thirty feet, but it claimed no more than five hundred lives, though it rendered many more homeless. In 1965, after Hurricane Betsy swamped New Orleans, President Lyndon Johnson pledged federal protection for the city. But the work by the Army Corps of Engineers to reduce the risk of another such flood by building a Lake Pontchartrain Hurricane Barrier was halted by an environmental group's lawsuit.[102] The alternative option—a system of levees—proved inadequate.[103] When Katrina, a Category 4 hurricane with winds of up to 145 miles

---

*A catastrophic breach of the Three Gorges Dam—which became a distinct possibility following heavy rains in July 2020—would send ten billion cubic meters of water downstream toward the metropolises of Yichang (population 4.0 million), Wuhan (11.0 million), Nanjing (8.5 million), Changzhou (4.6 million), and Shanghai (24.3 million), threatening the lives and livelihoods of 350 million people, flooding a quarter of China's arable land, and potentially submerging nearly half the ground units of the People's Liberation Army.

per hour, struck the Mississippi delta not once but twice in the last week of August 2005, three of the levees failed, pouring millions of gallons of water into the city. In all, 1,836 Americans lost their lives as a result of Katrina, the overwhelming majority of whom were from Louisiana. Nearly three quarters of New Orleans's total housing stock was damaged.[104]

The impact of hurricanes on the United States illustrates the extreme difficulty of achieving and sustaining successful disaster preparedness. Unlike all the other forms of disaster discussed in this chapter, Atlantic hurricanes—all tropical cyclones officially recorded to have produced sustained winds of greater than seventy-four miles per hour—are not randomly or power-law distributed. Since 1851, a total of 296 North Atlantic hurricanes have made landfall in the United States. There is a reliable seasonality, the majority of hurricanes appearing between August and October, and there is relatively little variance: the decade with the most major hurricanes (the 1940s) had ten major hurricanes (measuring 3–5 on the Saffir-Simpson Hurricane Wind Scale), while the decade with the fewest (the 1860s) still had one. Nevertheless, *ex ante* estimates of the probability of a hurricane as large as Katrina varied from "once in 396 years" to "once in forty."[105] Ivor van Heerden, the South African scholar who served as assistant secretary of the Louisiana Department of Natural Resources in the 1990s, correctly anticipated the damage that a major hurricane would do to New Orleans, because of subsidence in the Mississippi delta and the loss of wetlands to oil and gas extraction.[106] But the Federal Emergency Management Agency (FEMA) failed to complete a credible disaster plan, even after conducting a disaster preparedness simulation in 2004 known as Hurricane Pam.[107] Not only did local officials and businessmen underestimate the dangers; the Army Corps of Engineers also failed to heed warnings (even when they came from the National Weather Service), and the administration of George W. Bush—preoccupied with the quite different threat of terrorism—subordinated FEMA to the new Department of Homeland Security, leaving FEMA officials "underfunded and entirely unprepared to handle any disaster."[108] The verdict of the bipartisan House committee that investigated the disaster was damning:

Too often during the immediate response to Katrina, sparse or conflicting information was used as an excuse for inaction rather than an imperative to step in and fill an obvious vacuum. Information passed through the maze of departmental operations centers and . . . "coordinating" committees, losing timeliness and relevance as it was massaged and interpreted for internal audiences.

As a result, leaders became detached from the changing minute-to-minute realities of Katrina. Information translated into pre-cast bureaucratic jargon put more than geographic distance between Washington and the Gulf coast. . . .

Critical time was wasted on issues of no importance to disaster response, such as winning the blame game [or] waging a public relations battle.[109]

This is not the last time we shall encounter such problems at both the local and federal levels of the U.S. government.

Yet the point still stands: Asian disasters tend to be worse than Western ones. Katrina was a national trauma in the United States, but the death toll was less than two thousand. The worst cyclones in South Asian history killed two orders of magnitude more people. The Backerganj Cyclone, which made landfall near present-day Barisal, Bangladesh, in October 1876, cost the lives of around 200,000 Bengalis, half lost to immediate drowning and half to subsequent famine and disease.[110] Less than a century later, in November 1970, the Great Bhola Cyclone struck East Pakistan (later Bangladesh), killing between 300,000 and 500,000 people, including 45 percent of the population of the city of Tazumuddin, forty miles southeast of Barisal.[111] Like Japan's earthquakes, Bangladesh's biggest cyclones are too far apart in time for living memory to provide sufficient awareness of the risk.[112] In the case of the Great Bhola Cyclone, the part of Cassandra had been played by an American: Dr. Gordon E. Dunn, whose 1961 report warning of just such a calamity, and recommending the construction of zones of artificial high ground, the Pakistani authorities had politely ignored.[113]

GREAT WAVES

Everyone knows *The Great Wave,* the most famous of all Japanese works of art, even if they do not know the name of the artist. He called himself Hokusai, and he published *Kanagawa oki nami ura (The Great Wave off Kanagawa)* at some point between 1829 and 1833. It is a woodblock print of the genre *ukiyo-e,* which translates, evocatively, as "picture of the floating world." Look closely at *The Great Wave,* which depicts not a tsunami but a so-called rogue wave, and you will see that it towers above the cowering oarsmen in three wooden fishing boats. They are on their way back to Kanagawa (now Yokohama). Mount Fuji is just visible in the distance. The artist is most certainly not implying that, after the great wave breaks, the sea will be a millpond.

There are waves in history, as we have seen, including some vast tsunamis. But the idea that those waves are like waves of light and sound is an illusion. In the 1920s, the Soviet economist Nikolai Kondratieff sought to show that there were such patterns in capitalism, inferring from British, French, and German economic statistics the existence of fifty-year cycles of expansion followed by depression.[114] For this contribution, which continues to be influential with many investors today, Stalin had Kondratieff arrested, imprisoned, and later shot. Unfortunately, modern research dispels the idea of such regularity in economic life. The economic historian Paul Schmelzing's meticulous reconstruction of interest rates back to the thirteenth century points instead to a long-run, "supra-secular" decline in nominal rates, driven mostly by the process of capital accumulation, punctuated periodically but randomly by inflationary episodes nearly always associated with wars.[115] Yet war is not the father of all and king of all, as Heraclitus claimed. Disaster takes many forms. Not all the dragon kings of history have been wars; no war has slain as many as the pandemic we call the Black Death.

It is tempting but misleading, then, to divide disasters into natural and man-made. Clearly, an earthquake is a geological event: aside from those caused by ill-designed nuclear tests in modern times, they are always exogenous to human society. Equally clearly, wars are started by human beings; they are endogenous to human society. Yet a natural disaster is a disaster in terms of human lives lost only to the extent of its direct or indirect impact on human settlements. The decisions to locate settlements near potential disaster zones—by a volcano, on a fault line, next to a river subject to severe flooding—are part of why most natural disasters are in some measure man-made. Still riskier decisions—building wooden towns next to logging operations or building nuclear power stations in tsunami danger zones—can further magnify the human cost of natural disasters.

In a similar way, wars can have their origins in natural events, for example if extreme weather or sustained climate change leads to an agrarian crisis, confronting a society with a choice between starvation and relocation. Humanity is a part of nature, and demographic ebbs and flows are a part of the integrated web of the world's ecological system. The disaster scenario that preoccupies so many people in our time is that "man-made climate change," in the form of rising average temperatures resulting from industrial and other emissions, will have catastrophic consequences. How far this can successfully be mitigated—that is, without unintended negative consequences—will be a function of the quality of decision making by democratic and undemocratic governments.

Despite our preoccupation with potential global disasters, in practice most disasters are local and relatively small in scale. As we shall see in chapter 8, there is a fractal geometry to catastrophe, in that a small disaster like a plane crash can, in a number of respects, closely resemble a large disaster such as a nuclear meltdown. The crucial distinction is between large disasters and colossal ones—the events in the furthest extremity of the right tail of the distribution: the dragon kings. Why do only a few disasters attain that status, killing not hundreds of thousands but millions or even tens of millions? Part of the answer is that there are limits to the geographical reach of most forms of disaster. Even the largest earthquake is not felt all over the world. Even the biggest wars are not in fact fought in every country. The world wars were notable for their compression in terms of space as well as time, with the bulk of casualties in World War II inflicted in two fatal triangles: one between the North Sea, the Black Sea, and the Balkans, the other from Manchuria to the Philippines to the Marshall Islands. Indeed, most of the world's landmass experienced little or no fighting at all. What matters is, first, whether or not a disaster strikes a densely populated part of the earth and, second, if the death and destruction in and around the epicenter have repercussions further afield. In the case of a large volcano, as we have seen, the smoke and ash emitted can spread very far and wide, profoundly affecting the climate on other continents. In the case of an earthquake or flood, too, there can be widespread ramifications if the initial shock disrupts the agricultural, commercial, or financial system of one, or more than one, country. In short, the most important feature of a disaster is whether or not there is contagion—that is, some way of propagating the initial shock through the biological networks of life or the social networks of humanity. Thus, no disaster can be understood without some appreciation of network science.

4

NETWORLD

Lest he should spread the contagion by bringing multitudes together, he erected his pulpit on the top of a gate: the infected stood within; the others without. And the preacher failed not, in such a situation, to take advantage of the immediate terrors of the people.

—David Hume, *History of England*

VOLTAIRE VS. POPE

Geneva is just over nine hundred miles from Lisbon as the crow flies. It is doubtful that anyone in the Swiss city felt even the slightest tremor on November 1, 1755, the day that the Portuguese capital was devastated by an earthquake and tsunami waves. And yet the news of the disaster spread much farther than the tremors of the earth, thanks to the network of publication and correspondence that had evolved in the Western world in the two centuries since the Reformation, when Geneva had been the capital of Calvinism. François-Marie Arouet, better known by his nom de plume, Voltaire, was already a long way down the path to religious skepticism by 1755. That was why he was in Geneva—Louis XIV had banned him from Paris. But the Lisbon earthquake crystallized Voltaire's revulsion against all those branches of philosophy that sought to reconcile humanity to such apparently arbitrary catastrophes.[1] In his uncharacteristically passionate "Poème sur le désastre de Lisbonne," Voltaire took issue—as bitterly as he and his publisher dared—with the optimistic theodicy of the German polymath Gottfried Wilhelm Leibniz ("We live in the best of all possible worlds") and the English poet Alexander Pope ("Whatever is, is right"), which struck him as intolerable complacency:

> "Heav'n, on our sufferings cast a pitying eye."
> All's right, you answer, the eternal cause
> Rules not by partial, but by general laws. . . .

> Yet in this direful chaos you'd compose
> A general bliss from individuals' woes?
> Oh worthless bliss! in injured reason's sight,
> With faltering voice you cry, "What is, is right"? . . .

> But how conceive a God, the source of love,
> Who on man lavished blessings from above,
> Then would the race with various plagues confound,
> Can mortals penetrate His views profound?[2]

The poem precipitated a heated response, not least from Jean-Jacques Rousseau.[3] This in turn prompted Voltaire to write his ironical masterpiece *Candide, or Optimism* (1759), in which the eponymous hero, accompanied by the Leibniz caricature Dr. Pangloss and an Anabaptist sailor, witnesses the destruction of Lisbon.[4]

The impact of the Lisbon earthquake on Voltaire and Rousseau—not to mention the Prussian philosopher Immanuel Kant, who wrote three separate texts on the subject—testifies to the power of social networks in the eighteenth century. Social networks, of course, long predated the Enlightenment. The Egyptian pharaohs had them in the fourteenth century BC. The "Silk Roads" had connected the Roman and Chinese empires. Christianity and later Islam, too, created enormous and enduring social networks that extended far beyond the Judaic and Arab societies where they had originated. The power structure of Renaissance Florence was based on complex familial networks. There was also a network of navigators, explorers, and conquistadors who often shared knowledge as Western Europe's warring kingdoms extended their commercial operations westward across the Atlantic and south around the Cape of Good Hope. And the Reformation was in many ways a networked revolution, made by interconnected groups of religious reformers all over northwestern Europe, whose capacity to spread their Protestant message had been decisively increased by the spread of the printing press beginning in the later fifteenth century. Still, the Enlightenment network stands out, not so much for its geographical range (70 percent of Voltaire's correspondents were French) as for the quality of the content that was shared on it.[5] In particular, the connections between the Continent and that "hotbed of genius" that was Scotland after the defeat of the Jacobites in 1746 were especially important for the development of some of the most important ideas of the modern age.[6]

Adam Smith is today better remembered for *The Wealth of Nations* (1776) than for his earlier *Theory of Moral Sentiments* (published the same year as *Candide*), but they are equally important works. "Let us suppose," wrote Smith in a remarkable passage in part 3 of *The Theory,*

> that the great empire of China, with all its myriads of inhabitants, was suddenly swallowed up by an earthquake, and let us consider how a man of humanity in Europe, who had no sort of connection with that part of the world, would be affected upon receiving intelligence of this dreadful calamity. He would, I imagine, first of all, express very strongly his sorrow for the misfortune of that unhappy people, he would make many melancholy reflections upon the precariousness of human life, and the vanity of all the labours of man, which could thus be annihilated in a moment. He would too, perhaps, if he was a man of speculation, enter into many reasonings concerning the effects which this disaster might produce upon the commerce of Europe, and the trade and business of the world in general. And when all this fine philosophy was over, when all these humane sentiments had been once fairly expressed, he would pursue his business or his pleasure, take his repose or his diversion, with the same ease and tranquillity, as if no such accident had happened.[7]

This was a profound insight, in some measure anticipating the Tucholsky-Stalin distinction between a tragedy and a mere statistic. "The most frivolous disaster which could befall himself would occasion a more real disturbance," argued Smith. "If he was to lose his little finger tomorrow, he would not sleep tonight; but, provided he never saw them, he will snore with the most profound security over the ruin of a hundred millions of his brethren, and the destruction of that immense multitude seems plainly an object less interesting to him, than this paltry misfortune of his own."

Smith then asked an important ethical question: "To prevent, therefore, this paltry misfortune to himself, would a man of humanity be willing to sacrifice the lives of a hundred millions of his brethren, provided he had never seen them? . . . When we are always so much more deeply affected by whatever concerns ourselves, than by whatever concerns other men; what is it which prompts the generous, upon all occasions, and the mean upon many, to sacrifice their own interests to the greater interests of others?" The answer he gave was not quite satisfactory:

> It is not the soft power of humanity, it is not that feeble spark of benevolence which Nature has lighted up in the human heart, that is thus capable of counteracting the strongest impulses of self-love. It is a stronger power, a more forcible motive, which exerts itself upon such occasions. It is reason, principle, conscience, the inhabitant of the breast, the man within, the great judge and arbiter of our conduct. . . . It is not the love of our neighbour, it is not the love of mankind, which upon many occasions prompts us to the practice of those divine virtues. It is a stronger love, a more powerful affection, which generally takes place upon such occasions; the love of what is honourable and noble, of the grandeur, and dignity, and superiority of our own characters.

A disaster such as Smith's hypothetical Chinese earthquake—perhaps he would have chosen the real Portuguese earthquake had Voltaire not been so upset by it—ought to elicit sympathy even in distant Edinburgh, for to be entirely unmoved would be a shaming kind of solipsism.

Yet the reality is that we struggle to live up to Smith's standard, that is, to concern ourselves with the fate of distant millions in order to placate our own consciences, if not out of genuine altruism. The British journalist (and card-carrying Communist) Claud Cockburn claimed that, during his spell as a copy editor on *The Times* in the late 1920s, he and colleagues had sometimes held a competition (with a small prize for the winner) to write the dullest printed headline. "I won it only once," he recalled, "with a headline which announced: 'Small Earthquake in Chile, Not Many Dead.'"[8] Sadly, no such headline was ever published in *The Times**—though "Earthquake in Chile" appeared in 1922 and 1928, and "Big Earthquake in Chile" in 1939.[9] Still, the initial, mostly nonchalant response of many people to the headline "Chinese City Admits Mystery 'Pneumonia' Virus Outbreak"—published in *The Times* on January 6, 2020—suggests that the moral Cockburns among us probably outnumber the Smiths.

AN INTRODUCTION TO NETWORKS

Networks matter. Indeed, they are arguably the single most important feature of both natural and man-made complexity. The natural world is to a bewildering extent made up of "optimized, space-filling, branching networks," in the words of the physicist Geoffrey West, which have evolved to distribute energy and materials between macroscopic reservoirs and microscopic sites over twenty-seven orders of magnitude.[10] The animal circulatory, respiratory, renal, and neural systems are all natural networks. So are plant vascular systems and the microtubial and mitochondrial networks inside cells.[11] The brain of the nematode worm *Caenorhabditis elegans* is the only neural network to have been comprehensively mapped, but more complex brains will in due course be given the same treatment.[12] From worms' brains to food chains (or "food webs"), modern biology finds networks at all levels of life on earth.[13] The sequencing of the genome has revealed a "gene regulatory network" in

---

*The headline did finally appear in 1979 in *Not the Times,* a spoof version of the newspaper produced during its yearlong absence due to strike action.

which "nodes are genes and links are chains of reactions."[14] Tumors, too, form networks.

In prehistory, *Homo sapiens* evolved as a cooperative ape, with a unique ability to network—to communicate and to act collectively—which sets us apart from all other animals. In the words of the evolutionary anthropologist Joseph Henrich, we are not simply bigger-brained, less hairy chimpanzees; the secret of our success as a species "resides . . . in the *collective brains* of our communities."[15] Like chimpanzees, but on a larger scale, we learn socially, by teaching and sharing. According to the evolutionary anthropologist Robin Dunbar, our larger brain, with its more developed neocortex, evolved to enable us to function in relatively large social groups of around 150 (as compared with around 50 for chimpanzees).[16] Indeed, our species should really be known as *Homo dictyous* ("network man").[17] The term coined by the ethnographer Edwin Hutchins is "distributed cognition." Our early ancestors were "obligate collaborative foragers" who became dependent on one another for food, shelter, and warmth.[18] It is likely that the development of spoken language, and the associated advances in brain capacity and structure, were parts of this same process, evolving out of apelike practices such as grooming.[19] In the words of the historians William H. McNeill and J. R. McNeill, the first "worldwide web" in fact emerged around twelve thousand years ago. Man, with his unrivaled neural network, was born *to* network.[20]

Social networks, then, are the structures that human beings naturally form, beginning with knowledge itself and the various kinds of representation we use to communicate it, as well as the family trees to which we all necessarily belong. Networks include the patterns of settlement, migration, and interbreeding that have distributed our species across the world's surface, as well as the myriad cults and crazes we periodically produce with minimal premeditation and leadership. Social networks come in all shapes and sizes, from exclusive secret societies to open-source mass movements. Some have a spontaneous, self-organizing character; others are more systematic and structured. All that has happened—beginning with the invention of written language—is that successive information and communication technologies have facilitated our innate, ancient urge to network.

In a previous work, I attempted to summarize the key insights of modern network science—a complex system of interdisciplinary research in its own right—under six headings.[21]

1. *No man is an island.* Conceived of as nodes in networks, individuals can be understood in terms of their relationships to other nodes: the edges that connect them. Not all nodes are equal. Located in a network, an individual can be assessed in terms not only of degree centrality (the number of her relationships) but also of betweenness centrality (the likelihood of her being a bridge between other nodes throughout the group), to give just two of a number of different measures. The individuals with the highest betweenness centrality are not necessarily the people with the most connections, but the ones with the most connections to others with many connections. A key measure of an individual's historical importance is the extent to which that person was a network bridge or broker. Sometimes, as in the case of the American Revolution, crucial roles turn out to have been played by people, such as Paul Revere, who were not leaders but connectors.[22] In their different ways, individuals who have high degree centrality or betweenness centrality act as network "hubs."

In 1967, the social psychologist Stanley Milgram sent out 156 letters to randomly chosen residents of Wichita, Kansas, and Omaha, Nebraska. The recipients were asked to forward the letter directly to the intended final recipient—a stockbroker in Boston—if he was known personally to them, or to forward it to someone they believed might know the final recipient, provided they knew that intermediary on a first-name basis; and also to send Milgram a postcard saying what they had done. In all, according to Milgram, forty-two of the letters ultimately got through. (A more recent study suggests it was just twenty-one.)[23] The completed chains allowed Milgram to calculate the number of people required to get the letter to its target: on average, 5.5.[24] This finding had been anticipated by the Hungarian author Frigyes Karinthy, in whose story "Láncszemek" ("Chains," published in 1929) a character bets his companions that he can link himself to any individual on earth they may name through no more than five acquaintances, only one of which he has to know personally. The phrase "six degrees of separation" was not coined until John Guare's 1990 play of that title, but it had a long prehistory.

2. *Birds of a feather flock together.* Because of homophily, social networks can be understood partly in terms of like attracting like. Homophily can be based on shared status (ascribed characteristics such as race, ethnicity, sex, or age, and acquired characteristics such as religion, education, occupation, or behavior patterns) or shared values, insofar as those can be distinguished from acquired traits.[25] An early illustration in the sociological literature was the tendency for American schoolchildren to self-segregate by race or ethnicity. However, it is not always self-evident which shared attribute or preference causes people to cluster together. Moreover, we must be clear about the nature of the network linkages. Are the links between nodes relationships of acquaintance or amity (or enmity)? Are we looking at a family tree—like the famous genealogies of the Saxe-Coburgs or the Rothschilds—or a circle of friends (the Bloomsbury Set) or a secret society (the Illuminati)? Does something other than knowledge—money, say, or some other resource—get exchanged within the network?

3. *Weak ties are strong.* It also matters how grouped a network is, and how connected it is to other clusters. The joke that we are all just six degrees away from Monica Lewinsky or Kevin Bacon is explained by what the Stanford sociologist Mark Granovetter called, paradoxically, "the strength of weak ties."[26] If all ties were like the strong ones between us and our close friends, the world would necessarily be fragmented. But weaker ties—to the acquaintances we do not so closely resemble—are the key to the "small world" phenomenon. Granovetter's initial focus was on the way people looking for jobs were helped more by acquaintances than by their close friends, but a later insight was that, in a society with relatively few weak ties, "new ideas will spread slowly, scientific endeavors will be handicapped, and subgroups separated by race, ethnicity, geography, or other characteristics will have difficulty reaching a *modus vivendi*."[27] Weak ties, in other words, are the vital bridges between disparate clusters that otherwise would not be connected at all.[28]

Granovetter's was a sociological observation. It was not until 1998 that the sociologist Duncan Watts and the mathematician Steven Strogatz formally demonstrated *why* a world characterized by homophilic clusters could simultaneously be a small world. Watts and Strogatz classified networks in terms of two relatively independent properties: the average closeness centrality of each node and the network's general clustering coefficient. Beginning with a circular lattice in which each node was connected only to its first- and second-nearest neighbors, they showed that the random addition of just a few extra edges across the center of the circle drastically increased the closeness of all nodes, without significantly raising the overall clustering coefficient.[29] Watts had begun his work by studying the synchronized chirping of crickets, but the implications of his and Strogatz's findings for human populations were obvious. In Watts's words, "the difference between a big- and a small-world graph can be a matter of only a few randomly required edges—a change that is effectively undetectable at the level of individual vertices. . . . The highly clustered nature of small-world graphs can lead to the intuition that a given disease is 'far away' when, on the contrary, it is effectively very close."[30]

Network size also matters because of Metcalfe's law—named after the inventor of Ethernet, Robert Metcalfe—which (in its original form) stated that the value of a telecommunications network was proportional to the square of the number of connected and compatible communicating devices. This is in fact true of networks generally: put simply, the greater the number of nodes in a network, the more valuable the network to the nodes collectively and therefore to its owners.

4. *Structure determines virality.* The speed with which an infectious disease spreads has as much to do with the network structure of the exposed population as with the virulence of the disease itself.[31] The existence of a few highly connected hubs causes the spread of the disease to increase exponentially after an initial phase of slow growth.[32] Put differently, if the reproduction number (how many other people are newly infected by a typical infected individual) is above 1, then a disease spreads rapidly; if it is below 1, the disease tends to die out. That reproduction number is determined as much by the structure of the network it infects as by the innate infectiousness of the disease.[33]

Many historians still assume that the spread of an idea or an ideology is a function of its inherent content in relation to some vaguely specified context. We must now acknowledge, however, that some ideas go viral, like some pathogens, because of structural features of the network through which they spread. (A good illustration is the way the abolitionist movement successfully spread its message through the British political establishment in the early nineteenth century.) New ideas are least likely to advance in a hierarchical, top-down network, where peer-to-peer links are restricted or prohibited. More recent research has shown that even emotional states can be transmitted through a network.[34] Though distinguishing between endogenous and exogenous network effects is far from easy,[35] the evidence of this kind of contagion is clear: "Students with studious roommates become more studious. Diners sitting next to heavy eaters eat more food."[36] However, we cannot transmit ideas and behaviors much beyond our friends' friends' friends (in other words, beyond three degrees of separation). This is because the transmission and reception of an idea or a behavior requires a stronger connection than the unwitting transmission of an infectious pathogen. Merely knowing people is not the same as being able to influence them to study more or to overeat. Imitation is indeed the sincerest form of flattery, even when it is unconscious.

The key point, as with epidemic disease, is that network structure can be as important as the idea itself in determining the speed and extent of diffusion.[37] In the process of a meme's going viral, a key role is played by nodes that are not merely hubs or brokers but "gatekeepers"—people who decide whether or not to pass information to their part of the network.[38] Their decision will be based partly on how they think that information will reflect back on them. Acceptance of an idea, in turn, can require it to be received from more than one or two sources. A complex cultural contagion, unlike a simple disease epidemic, first needs to attain a critical mass of early adopters with high degree centrality (relatively large numbers of influential friends).[39] In the words of Duncan Watts, the key to assessing the likelihood of a contagion-like cascade is "to focus *not* on the stimulus itself but on the structure of the network the stimulus hits."[40] This helps explain why, for every idea that goes viral, there are countless others that fizzle out in obscurity because they began with the wrong node, cluster, or network. The same often goes for infectious microbes, only a very few of which succeed in generating pandemics.

If all social network structures were the same, we would inhabit a very different world. For example, a world in which nodes were randomly connected to one another—so that the numbers of edges per node were normally distributed along a bell curve—would have some "small world" properties, but it would not be like our world. That is because the nodes in so many real-world networks follow Pareto-like distributions, that is, there are more nodes with a very large number of edges, and more nodes with very few, than would be the case in a random network. This is a version of what the sociologist Robert K. Merton called "the Matthew effect," after the Gospel of Saint Matthew: "For unto every one that hath shall be given, and he shall have abundance: but from him that hath not shall be taken away even that which he hath" (25:29). In science, success breeds success: to him who already has prizes, more prizes shall be given. Something similar can be seen in "the economics of superstars."[41] In the same way, as many large networks expand, nodes gain new edges in proportion to the number that they already have (their degree or "fitness"). There is, in short, "preferential attachment." We owe this insight to the physicists Albert-László Barabási and Réka Albert, who were the first to suggest that most real-world networks might follow a power-law distribution or be "scale-free."* As such networks evolve, a few nodes will become hubs with many more edges than other nodes.[42] Examples of such networks abound, ranging from the directorships of Fortune 1000 companies to citations in physics journals and links to and from webpages.[43] In Barabási's words:

> There is a hierarchy of hubs that keep these networks together, a heavily connected node closely followed by several less connected ones, trailed by dozens of even smaller nodes. No central node sits in the middle

---

*A scale-free network has a power-law character, in that the relative likelihoods of very high degree and very low degree are higher than if links were formed at random. In a scale-free network there is no typical node, and yet the "scale" of difference between nodes appears the same everywhere. Put differently, the scale-free world is characterized by fractal geometry: the town is a large family, the city is a large town, and the kingdom is a large city.

of the spider web, controlling and monitoring every link and node. There is no single node whose removal could break the web. A scale-free network is a web without a spider.[44]

In the extreme case (the winner-takes-all model), the fittest node gets all or nearly all the links.[45] An example of a scale-free network is the air transportation system, in which a large number of small airports are connected to medium-size airports, which in turn connect to a few huge and busy hubs.[46] By contrast, the U.S. National Highway System is more like a random network, in which each major city has roughly the same number of highways connecting it to others. Intermediate network structures can also be found: for example, the friendship networks of American adolescents are neither random nor scale-free.[47] As we shall see, scale-free networks have played a key role in the spread of some infectious diseases.[48] A network can be modular—that is, it can consist of a number of separate clusters nonetheless tied together by a few bridging edges. Some networks are both modular and hierarchical, such as the complex genetic systems that regulate metabolism, which put certain subsystems under the control of others.[49]

5. *Networks never sleep*. Networks are rarely frozen in time. Large networks are complex systems, which, as we saw in chapter 3, have emergent properties—the tendency of novel structures, patterns, and properties to manifest themselves in phase transitions that are far from predictable. A seemingly random network can evolve with astounding speed into a hierarchy. The number of steps between the revolutionary crowd and the totalitarian state has more than once proved to be surprisingly small. The seemingly rigid structures of a hierarchical order can disintegrate with equal rapidity.[50]

6. *Networks network*. When networks interact, the result can be innovation and invention. When a network disrupts an ossified hierarchy, it can overthrow it with breathtaking speed. But when a hierarchy attacks a fragile network, the result can be the network's collapse. Social networks can meet and fuse amicably, but they may also attack one another, as happened when Soviet intelligence successfully penetrated the elite networks of Cambridge graduates in the 1930s. In such contests, the outcome will be determined by

the relative strengths and weaknesses of the rival networks. How adaptable and resilient are they? How vulnerable to a disruptive contagion? How reliant on one or more "superhubs," the destruction or capture of which would significantly reduce the stability of the whole network? Barabási and his colleagues simulated attacks on scale-free networks and found that they could withstand the loss of a significant fraction of nodes, and even of a single hub. But a targeted attack on multiple hubs could break the network up altogether.[51] Even more dramatically, a scale-free network could quite easily fall victim to a contagious, node-killing virus.[52]

As we have seen, the death tolls from natural and man-made disasters are not normally distributed; many forms of disaster follow power laws or are randomly distributed, which makes it impossible to attach probabilities to the scale and timing of really large disasters. This is why the endeavor to find cyclical patterns in history is likely doomed to fail. Now comes a further complication. Disasters are mediated, interpreted, and in some cases (those involving contagion) literally transmitted by networks—and networks themselves have structures that are complex and subject to phase transitions. If not exactly scale-free, many social networks are closer to a scale-free than to a lattice-like structure, meaning that a few nodes have much higher centrality than most. If Cassandras had higher centrality, they might be more often heeded. If erroneous doctrines spread virally through a large social network, effective mitigation of disaster becomes much harder. Finally, and crucially, hierarchical structures such as states exist principally because, while inferior to distributed networks when it comes to innovation, they are superior when it comes to defense. In the face of contagion, much depends on the quality of governance: not just strategic decision making at the top but also the speed and accuracy of information flows up and down the command-and-control structure, and the effectiveness of operational execution.

BUGS AND NETWORKS

The history of mankind's changing susceptibility to infectious disease tends to be written as a history of pathogens—as one damned bug after another—with medical science as the ultimately triumphant hero.[53] Eventually the "epidemiological transition" is achieved, in which infectious disease dwindles and chronic conditions like cancer and heart disease become the principal causes of human mortality.[54] It might make as much sense to tell this history as the story of our evolving social networks. For the first 300,000 years of our existence as a species, we lived in tribal groups too small to sustain large-scale infectious diseases. That changed with the Neolithic or Agricultural Revolution. As Edward Jenner observed in the 1790s, "The deviation of man from the state in which he was originally placed by nature seems to have proved to him a prolific source of disease."[55]

Bacteria were the first life form to inhabit Earth. Most are harmless to humans; many are beneficial. Bacteria reproduce by binary fission: they replicate their chromosomal DNA, then split in two. That means they essentially clone themselves. However, many bacteria contain plasmids: circular DNA molecules inside the bacterial cell, but separate from the chromosome, that divide independently, allowing some evolutionary variation. The viruses known as bacteriophages ("phages" for short) are another source of modification. Without their phages, the bacteria that cause cholera and diphtheria would be harmless. Phages use the bacteria's protein-making machinery to reproduce. If they pick up an extra piece of DNA, either from the bacterial chromosome or from a resident plasmid, mutation occurs. After bacteria came single-celled protozoa, such as the plasmodium that causes malaria, and viruses.[56] Because of the different ways they reproduce, we can distinguish between bacteria, DNA viruses (e.g., hepatitis B, herpes, and smallpox), RNA viruses (e.g., influenza, measles, and polio), retroviruses (e.g., HIV and human T-lymphotropic virus), and prion diseases (e.g., BSE, or mad cow disease). Viruses are very small: some nucleic acid in a coat of protein molecules. The viruses that cause yellow fever, Lassa fever, Ebola, measles, and poliomyelitis all have fewer than ten genes; those that cause smallpox and herpes have between two hundred and four hundred genes. (The smallest bacteria have between five thousand and ten thousand.)[57] Viruses can enter all cellular forms of life, from protozoa to humans; once viruses are inside a cell, having evaded the immune system's response, their mission is to replicate, often with the assistance of the host cell's protein-manufacturing equipment, and then to spread, either destroying the cell or modifying it.[58] A critical point is that the ability of viruses to mutate makes them especially dangerous antagonists for us naked apes.[59]

The history of disease is a protracted interaction between evolving pathogens, insect or animal carriers, and human social networks. We have evidence of malaria infection in three-thousand-year-old Egyptian mummies and almost as ancient Chinese books, but it seems clear that *Plasmodium falciparum* began infecting and killing humans long before then.[60] *P. falciparum* is the most dangerous of five species of plasmodium; all are spread by mosquitoes, most commonly the female *Anopheles* mosquito. The deadliest bacillus in history, *Yersinia pestis*—a mutation of *Y. pseudotuberculosis,* which first emerged in China at least two and a half thousand years ago[61]—also requires intermediaries to infect humans, but two instead of one: fleas (specifically *Xenopsylla cheopis,* though the human flea, *Pulex irritans,* may also have played a role in the Black Death) and rodents such as rats, because only in rodents does the quantity of the bacillus reach a sufficient concentration to block the flea's stomach. When this happens, the flea is unable to ingest blood but continues to "feed" as it tries to sate its hunger, regurgitating the blood along with the parasite. A bite from an infected flea introduces *Y. pestis,* which then targets the lymph glands in the neck, armpit, or groin. Because *Y. pestis* doubles in number every two hours, the bubonic plague that it causes rapidly overwhelms the immune system, spreads into the bloodstream, and causes internal and skin hemorrhages.[62] Relatively small genetic changes could (and can) increase or decrease the virulence of the plague.[63] The three main biotypes, or "biovars," of bubonic plague are Antiqua, Medievalis, and Orientalis, which appear to be able to interbreed, exchanging genetic information and so varying their virulence over time.[64] Crucially, *Y. pestis* kills fleas relatively slowly. Moreover, infected fleas can hibernate for up to fifty days in linens and other porous materials. The bacillus kills rodents faster, but a colony of rapidly reproducing rats takes six to ten years to be annihilated. In a large enough rodent population, such as the tarbagan marmots of Qinghai, *Y. pestis* becomes endemic.

Two microbes that do not require insects to spread them are the ones that cause tuberculosis and leprosy, *Mycobacterium tuberculosis* and *Mycobacterium leprae,* respectively. The former is one of the slowest bacteria to reproduce, doubling its numbers in around twenty-four hours, but the more human beings crowd together, the more people it can infect. Many infected people do not go beyond the latent stage; those who do are killed by the destructive effect of the disease on the lungs, unforgettably depicted in the last act of Verdi's *La traviata* (1853). TB is spread through the air when an infected person coughs, sneezes, speaks, or spits. Leprosy spreads in a similar way, but the principal symptoms are patches of discolored skin with reduced sensation due to nerve damage. By contrast, syphilis is a sexually transmitted infection caused by the bacterium *Treponema pallidum.* Its progression is protracted. The first stage sees the appearance of chancres (small non-itchy patches of skin ulceration). In the secondary stage, treponemes spread to every organ in the body, including the central nervous system. There is then a multiyear latent phase, without symptoms. The tertiary stage is associated with symptoms of chronic neurodegeneration. Far more rapid is the progression of typhus, also known as typhus fever, the most epidemic version of which is caused by the bacterium *Rickettsia prowazekii,* carried by body lice. Last but not the least of the bacterial diseases that will feature in this book is the *Vibrio cholerae* bacillus, which can replicate every thirteen minutes and is spread in contaminated water. It is not the bacillus itself that causes cholera, but the toxin the bacillus produces (choleragen), which damages the cell membranes that regulate the absorption of fluids. Death does not occur from dehydration, technically, but from "untreated hypovolemic shock with metabolic acidosis."[65]

Three viral diseases in particular may be said to have played a historic role, in the sense that their impacts were disastrous. Smallpox is—or was—an infectious disease caused by one of two virus variants, *Variola major* and *Variola minor,* which emerged around ten thousand years ago in northeastern Africa. Chinese texts from as early as 1122 BC report cases of smallpox. Egyptian mummies, notably Ramses V (reigned 1149–1145 BC), also seem to have smallpox-like lesions. Initial symptoms of the disease included fever and vomiting; then came the sores in the mouth and the hideous skin rash. The disease required no intermediary: a carrier became infectious as soon as the first sores appeared and spread the virus by coughing or sneezing viruses in droplets. The pustules themselves were infectious: to touch the clothing or bedding of a smallpox sufferer was dangerous. The risk of death, as measured by the infection fatality rate (IFR), was high—around 30 percent, and even higher for babies. Survivors were left scarred for life—like Esther Summerson in Dickens's *Bleak House* (1853)—or blind. Smallpox was less contagious than chickenpox: its basic reproduction number (R_0) was close to 5, as compared with nearly 10 for chickenpox and 16–18 for measles. But it was much deadlier and is estimated to have killed three hundred million people in the twentieth century alone, until its eradication in the 1970s—the most successful vaccination campaign in history, but also the most sustained one.[66]

Yellow fever, by contrast, may never be eradicated. Transmitted by the *Aedes aegypti* mosquito, the virus can infect monkeys as well as people. Its symptoms are fever, headaches, and muscle aches, sensitivity to light, nausea, and dizziness, as well as redness in the face, eyes, or tongue. Smallpox may be gone, but yellow fever is endemic in forty-four countries around the world and infects about 200,000 people each year, of whom 30,000 die (IFR 15 percent), principally through organ failure.[67] Finally, there is influenza, the shape-shifting killer. A form of orthomyxovirus, influenza has three types (A, B, and C) according to differences in its matrix protein and nucleoprotein. Influenza A virus is further classified into subtypes based upon the characteristics of the two major surface glycoproteins, hemagglutinin (HA) and neuraminidase (NA). Three HA subtypes (H1, H2, and H3) and two NA subtypes (N1 and N2) have caused influenza epidemics. A respiratory disease that is spread when an infected person coughs or sneezes, influenza has a distinctive ability to reassort its genetic material—single-stranded RNA that is present in the virion as separate small pieces. As the genome reassorts, minor changes in the configuration of the surface antigens occurs ("antigenic drift"); in the case of influenza A, the changes can be bigger ("antigenic shift"). The possibility also exists of gene reassortment following coinfection with another human strain or an avian or swine virus.[68]

Three things, beginning in the Neolithic, have increased mankind's vulnerability to these and many other infectious diseases: ever larger human settlements, increased proximity to insects and animals, and exponentially rising human mobility—to be more succinct, urbanization, agriculture, and globalization. Towns and cities, and the crowded living quarters associated with them, have been fundamental to contagion for the diseases that spread directly between humans. For many others, however, the presence of insects and animals is crucial. At least eight common diseases originated in domestic animals (diphtheria, influenza A, measles, mumps, pertussis, rotavirus, small-pox, and tuberculosis), and three more in apes (hepatitis B) or rodents (plague and typhus). We have chimpanzees to thank for malaria and HIV; cows for measles; cows (probably) for smallpox and tuberculosis; rodents for typhus and bubonic plague; monkeys for dengue and yellow fever; birds and pigs for influenza. Long-distance travel, whether for trade or war, has ensured that any novel pathogen eventually crosses continents and seas, spreading origi-nally tropical diseases to temperate climes and vice versa.[69]

In other words, no matter how ingeniously they evolve, microbes are only as successful at infecting human beings as human networks allow, including the networks we share with animals. And, crucially, no matter how ingenious we are in devising prophylactics and remedies against disease, our efforts can be undercut by our networks. The more we live in cities, the more vulnerable to contagion we make ourselves. The more we live close to animals, the more vulnerable to new zoonoses we make ourselves. We intended to domesticate sheep, cows, chickens, dogs, and cats. We unintentionally shared and often still share our homes with lice, fleas, mice, and rats. Bats—of which there are more than a thousand species, and whose vast and crowded communities are espe-cially well suited to the evolution of new viruses—may not live in our houses, but their ability to fly often brings them close to human habitation. Cultures in which they are sold live for their meat, as we shall see, put themselves and their trading partners at grave risk.[70] And of course, the more we travel, the more vulnerable to plagues we make ourselves.

Microbes do not mean to kill us; they have evolved only to replicate them-selves. Rapidly lethal viruses such as the coronaviruses that caused severe acute respiratory syndrome (SARS) or Middle East respiratory syndrome (MERS) fail to proliferate because their victims become visibly ill and then often die before they can infect many other people. As a group of scientists observed presciently in 2007, "If pathogen transmission is inherently damaging to the host, selective pressure will act on the pathogen to balance the benefit of higher transmission against the loss of host viability as a result of higher virulence. . . . Virulence will be tempered to ensure that the host population does not go into decline."[71]

ANCIENT PLAGUES

The history of pandemics is therefore as much a history of social networks as a history of pathogenic evolution. Moreover, before the medical scientific breakthroughs of the later twentieth century, there was remarkably little we could do in the face of contagious diseases other than modify our social networks to limit spread. This proved remarkably difficult, not just because of misunderstandings about the nature of infectious diseases but also because human beings seem incapable of sufficiently modifying their patterns of interaction even when, as in the modern era, they grasp the risk posed by an invisible microbe. As a result, pandemics in the past have more often led to the involuntary disintegration of social networks—and sometimes of political structures—than to conscious and effective adaptation of collective behavior.

We owe the earliest account we have of an epidemic to the father of historiography, the Athenian Thucydides. The war between Athens and Sparta, Thucydides wrote in the opening chapter of his *History of the Peloponnesian War*, "was prolonged to an immense length, and . . . was . . . without parallel for the misfortunes that it brought upon Hellas." But the war was only one of a number of disasters to befall Greece:

> Never had so many cities been taken and laid desolate. . . . Never was
> there so much banishing and blood-shedding, now on the field of battle,

now in the strife of faction. . . . There were earthquakes of unparal-
leled extent and violence; eclipses of the sun occurred with a frequency
unrecorded in previous history; there were great droughts in sundry
places and consequent famines, and that most calamitous and awfully
fatal visitation, the plague.[72]

Note that of all the calamities that befell Thucydides and his city, the plague—
which struck in the war's second year (430 BC)—was the one he regarded as
the "most calamitous." According to his account, it originated in Ethiopia, spread
through Egypt to the port of Piraeus, and from there to Athens. The city was
vulnerable because, under Pericles's leadership, the Athenians had retreated
behind their city walls, intending to wage a largely naval war. However, the
arrival of the plague turned Athens into a death trap. Around a quarter of
the population died, including Pericles, his wife, and his two sons. Thucydides
himself also contracted the disease but survived. He recalled its symptoms
with harrowing precision:

> People in good health were all of a sudden attacked by violent heats
> in the head, and redness and inflammation in the eyes, the inward parts,
> such as the throat or tongue, becoming bloody and emitting an unnatu-
> ral and fetid breath. These symptoms were followed by sneezing and
> hoarseness, after which the pain soon reached the chest, and produced
> a hard cough. When it fixed in the stomach, it upset it; and discharges of
> bile of every kind . . . ensued, accompanied by very great distress. In
> most cases also an ineffectual retching followed, producing violent
> spasms. . . . Externally the body was not very hot to the touch, nor pale
> in its appearance, but reddish, livid, and breaking out into small pustules
> and ulcers. But internally it burned so that the patient could not bear to
> have on him clothing or linen even of the very lightest description; or in-
> deed to be otherwise than stark naked. What they would have liked best
> would have been to throw themselves into cold water; as indeed was
> done by some of the neglected sick, who plunged into the rain-tanks
> in their agonies of unquenchable thirst; though it made no difference

whether they drank little or much. Besides this, the miserable feeling of not being able to rest or sleep never ceased to torment them. The body meanwhile did not waste away so long as the distemper was at its height, but held out to a marvel against its ravages; so that when they succumbed, as in most cases, on the seventh or eighth day to the internal inflammation, they had still some strength in them. But if they passed this stage, and the disease descended further into the bowels, inducing a violent ulceration there accompanied by severe diarrhea, this brought on a weakness which was generally fatal. For the disorder first settled in the head, ran its course from thence through the whole of the body, and, even where it did not prove mortal, it still left its mark on the extremities; for it settled in the privy parts, the fingers and the toes, and many escaped with the loss of these, some too with that of their eyes. Others again were seized with an entire loss of memory on their first recovery, and did not know either themselves or their friends.

Birds and animals generally eschewed unburied corpses; those that ate the dead perished.

What exactly the Athenian plague was has long been debated. It used to be regarded as an outbreak of the bubonic plague, but other candidates have included typhus, smallpox, and measles—even Ebola or a related viral hemorrhagic fever. A 1994–95 excavation revealed a mass grave, along with nearly a thousand tombs, dated between 430 and 426 BC, just outside Athens's ancient Kerameikos cemetery. Some of the remains appeared to include DNA sequences similar to those of *Salmonella enterica*, the organism that causes typhoid fever. In any case, for the Athenians there was no remedy. "Neither were the physicians at first of any service, ignorant as they were of the proper way to treat it," wrote Thucydides, "but they died themselves the most thickly, as they visited the sick most often; nor did any human art succeed any better. Supplications in the temples, divinations, and so forth were found equally futile, till the overwhelming nature of the disaster at last put a stop to them altogether. . . . No remedy was found that could be used as a specific; for what did good in one case, did harm in another. . . . Men [died] like sheep, through having caught the infection in nursing each other. This caused the greatest mortality." The sole meaningful discovery was that those who survived were subsequently immune, "for the same man was never attacked twice—never at least fatally."

We see here the first example of what will become a familiar pattern. One of the world's most advanced and densely populated societies was brought low by a new pathogen. The plague returned twice more, in 429 and in the winter of 427–26. In the face of mass death, the social and cultural order unraveled:

> As the disaster passed all bounds, men, not knowing what was to become of them, became utterly careless of everything, whether sacred or profane. All the burial rites before in use were entirely upset. . . . Men now coolly ventured on what they had formerly done in a corner, . . . seeing the rapid transitions produced by persons in prosperity suddenly dying and those who before had nothing succeeding to their property. So they resolved to spend quickly and enjoy themselves, regarding their lives and riches as alike things of a day. Perseverance in what men called honor was popular with none, it was so uncertain whether they would be spared to attain the object; but it was settled that present enjoyment, and all that contributed to it, was both honorable and useful. Fear of gods or law of man there was none to restrain them. As for the first, they judged it to be just the same whether they worshipped them or not, as they saw all alike perishing; and for the last, no one expected to live to be brought to trial for his offences, but each felt that a far severer sentence had been already passed upon them all and hung ever over their heads, and before this fell it was only reasonable to enjoy life a little.

Disregard for both religion and law also undermined the city's famous democracy, leading to a reduction of noncitizen residents and ultimately to a period of oligarchy in 411, though democracy was soon after restored, albeit with some new judicial constraints. And, perhaps inevitably, Athens lost the Peloponnesian War. Knowing this history makes the dark tragedy of *Oedipus Rex* more intelligible.

By comparison with the Athens of Pericles, the Rome of the second century AD was a vastly larger and more complex society—and consequently still more vulnerable to a new pathogen. At its height, the Roman Empire encompassed around seventy million people, perhaps a quarter of all the humans alive at the time. Already highly susceptible to gastrointestinal infections and malaria, the Romans appear to have suffered the first major smallpox epidemic in the winter of 165–66, during the reign of the philosopher-emperor Marcus Aurelius (from 161 to 180).[73] The Romans believed they had brought the plague upon themselves by sacking the temple of Apollo at Seleucia during their war against the Parthians; in reality, returning soldiers may have brought the disease with them, or it may have accompanied slaves imported from Africa. According to Galen, the disease afflicted young and old, rich and poor alike, but slaves were disproportionately affected (all of Galen's died); the symptoms were fever, thirst, vomiting, diarrhea, and a black rash. The plague persisted until around 192, drastically reducing populations from Egypt to Athens, leaving towns and villages desolate, and encouraging attacks by Germanic tribes, especially along the Danube. "During some time," Edward Gibbon noted, "five thousand persons died daily in Rome; and many towns, that had escaped the hands of the Barbarians, were entirely depopulated."[74] Modern scholars estimate the death toll at between 10 and 30 percent of the imperial population.[75] There is evidence of a significant slowdown in economic activity (indicated by a steep decline in tree felling) as a consequence. The Roman army was reduced "almost . . . to extinction" in 172, according to one contemporary source.[76] The epidemic may also have stimulated the spread of Christianity through the empire, because Christianity not only offered an explanation for the catastrophes—as God's punishment of a sinful society—but also encouraged some behaviors that led to the disproportionate survival of believers.[77]

Yet the Roman Empire withstood this shock, just as it withstood the Plague of Cyprian (249–70), an outbreak of hemorrhagic fever that may have killed between 15 and 25 percent of the population of the empire. It was another, later pandemic that has tended to be seen as the death blow to the empire: the Plague of Justinian, a bubonic plague outbreak that began in the Egyptian city of Pelusium, near modern-day Port Said, in 541, reached Constantinople the following year, arrived in Rome in 543, and struck Britain in 544. It broke out again in Constantinople in 558, a third time in 573, and yet again in 586. Indeed, like the Black Death of the fourteenth century, the Plague of Justinian recurred again and again for the better part of two centuries. We can be sure it was bubonic plague from the detailed descriptions of the historian Procopius (here in Gibbon's paraphrasing):

> The greater number, in their beds, in the streets, in their usual occupation, were surprised by a slight fever; so slight, indeed, that neither the pulse nor the color of the patient gave any signs of the approaching danger. The same, the next, or the succeeding day, it was declared by the swelling of the glands, particularly those of the groin, of the armpits, and under the ear; and when these buboes or tumors were opened, they were found to contain a coal, or black substance, of the size of a lentil. If they came to a just swelling and suppuration, the patient was saved by this kind and natural discharge of the morbid humor. But if they continued hard and dry, a mortification quickly ensued, and the fifth day was commonly the term of his life. The fever was often accompanied with lethargy or delirium; the bodies of the sick were covered with black pustules or carbuncles, the symptoms of immediate death; and in the constitutions too feeble to produce an irruption, the vomiting of blood was followed by a mortification of the bowels. . . . Many of those who escaped were deprived of the use of their speech, without being secure from a return of the disorder.

Like the Athens of Thucydides, the Constantinople of Justinian was thrown into confusion. Physicians were helpless, funeral rites abandoned; bodies lay on the streets until mass graves could be dug. During the emperor's own illness, as Gibbon noted, "idleness and despondence occasioned a general scarcity in the capital of the East."[78] Yet "no restraints were imposed on the free and frequent intercourse of the Roman provinces: from Persia to France, the nations were mingled and infected by wars and emigrations; and the pestilential odor which lurks for years in a bale of cotton was imported, by the abuse of trade, into the most distant regions. . . . It always spread from the sea-coast to the inland country: the most sequestered islands and mountains were successively visited; the places which had escaped the fury of its first passage were alone exposed to the contagion of the ensuing year."[79]

How lethal was the Plague of Justinian? Gibbon offered no body count, noting only "that during three months, five, and at length ten, thousand persons died each day at Constantinople; that many cities of the East were left vacant, and that in several districts of Italy the harvest and the vintage withered on the ground." It has long been asserted that the plague resulted in the deaths of between a quarter and half of the population of the Mediterranean region, though a recent survey of non-textual sources (e.g., papyri, coins, inscriptions, and pollen archaeology) has cast doubt on this huge death toll.[80] Nevertheless, the plague put a stop to Justinian's campaign to restore the Western Roman Empire, which had been overrun by Germanic tribes a century before, leaving the way clear for the Lombards to invade northern Italy and establish a new kingdom there. It is too much to attribute Rome's ultimate decline to this pandemic, as we shall see.[81] Nevertheless, the extent of the disruption to the empire's finances and defenses seems to have been profound. And, as Gibbon noted, the lack of any barriers to social and commercial intercourse ensured that the plague did maximum damage:

> The fellow-citizens of Procopius were satisfied, by some short and partial experience, that the infection could not be gained by the closest conversation: and this persuasion might support the assiduity of friends or physicians in the care of the sick, whom inhuman prudence would have condemned to solitude and despair. But the fatal security . . . must have aided the progress of the contagion.[82]

THE DANCE OF DEATH

How, then, are we to explain the worst pandemic in human history—the Black
Death of the mid-fourteenth century—a catastrophic recurrence of the bubonic plague that had devastated the Roman Empire eight centuries before?
There seems an obvious paradox: the Europe that it struck was no longer integrated into a single empire (albeit one with barbarians at the gates) but was
more politically fragmented than at any time in its recorded history. Europe
in 1340 was a patchwork of kingdoms, principalities, duchies, bishoprics, and
numerous autonomous or semiautonomous city-states. To look at a map of
the continent on the eve of the Black Death is to be struck by a simple question: If pandemics need large networks to spread a contagious pathogen, how
was the Black Death even possible?

The answer is that the political geography of a continent is a poor guide
to its social network structure. First, the population of the world was probably around one and a half times what it had been in the time of the emperor
Justinian (329 million in 1300, as compared with 210 million in 500). The European population had doubled rather rapidly, to around 80 or 100 million,
between 1000 and 1300. The population of England had surged from around

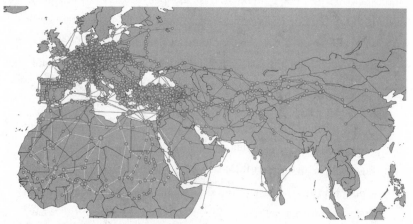

The network of pilgrimage and trade routes that connected European, African, and Asian cities in the fourteenth century. Bubble size is proportional to the centrality value of the cities.
Dark links indicate commercial routes and white links indicate pilgrimage routes.

2 million in 1000 to above 7 million in 1300, though there is evidence of some decline in the three decades before the Black Death, most likely because of climatic factors, harvest failures, and a Malthusian check. Second, there were significantly more towns in Western Europe in the fourteenth century than there had been in the sixth century. Each town can be thought of as a cluster in the network. The "weak ties" between the clusters were provided by trade and by war. These help to explain why the bubonic plague spread so much faster and was so much deadlier in Europe than in East Asia, where it originated. So sparse were social networks in much of Asia—so few were the ties between the clusters of settlement there—that this highly infectious disease took four years to travel across Asia, at a pace of just over six hundred miles per year.[83] The impact was very different in Europe, where the plague spread throughout England in the space of a year.[84] Tests on DNA evidence from plague sites in Belgium, England, France, and Germany show that different strains of plague spread along different routes.[85] Moreover, the plague came in multiple waves: in England, after the initial and biggest outbreak, a second wave came in 1361–62, followed by a third in 1369 and a fourth in 1375.

Between one third and three fifths of the population of Europe died. In Italy, around a hundred towns were altogether depopulated, including Arezzo (population in 1300, 18,000) and Salerno (13,000). The population of Genoa (60,000 residents in 1300) fell by 17 percent; those of Venice and Florence (each around 110,000) fell by, respectively, 23 and 66 percent, that of Milan (150,000) by 33 percent.[86] The population of England had already begun to decline in the early 1300s; after reaching 7 million in 1300, by 1450, after successive waves of plague, it was back down to 2 million.[87] The historian Mark Bailey estimates that half of peasant landowners and a quarter of magnate landowners died, either as a result of the Black Death or from the hardships that followed from it. Manorial court rolls reveal that unfree tenants were the social group hit hardest.[88]

Other influences explain the exceptionally lethal impact of the Black Death in Europe. The weather certainly played a part.[89] Deaths in all the multiple waves of plague in Europe peaked in the warmest months of the year, as summer temperatures suit the flea *Xenopsylla cheopis* better.[90] Wetter weather also increased the prevalence of *Yersinia pestis*.[91] On the other hand, the five major volcanic events between around 1150 and 1300 (see chapter 3) may have contributed to the lower-than-average temperatures and bad harvests that had left the population vulnerable. In England, for example, a severe cold snap and abnormally heavy rainfall contributed to four consecutive harvest failures after 1347. In addition to bubonic plague, pneumonic plague and septicemic plague—which have a higher (close to 100 percent) infection fatality rate—almost certainly contributed to the huge death toll.[92]

Yet of equal importance were the network connections from Asia to Europe and between Europe's commercial centers. The Tuscan town of Siena's golden age, from around 1260 until 1348, coincided with the rise and fall of the Mongol Empire. It was a time when Sienese merchants traveled as far as Tabriz to buy silks from Central Asia; a time when the pope received emissaries from the Yuan emperor Toghon Temür. Long ago lost, the artist Ambrogio Lorenzetti's huge, rotatable *Mappamondo* showed Siena at the center of a commercial network extending across Eurasia. Precisely this trade network provided the conduits along which the Black Death was transmitted.[93] Within Italy, bigger towns had higher mortality.[94] Bigger towns tended to be those, especially ports, with access to water transport.[95] This seems to have been true all across Europe.[96] In the terminology of network science, cities with the highest centrality in the network of trade (and of religious pilgrimage) were hit hardest by the plague.[97] Finally, social historians need occasional reminding that wars matter. The Hundred Years' War began on June 24, 1340, with the destruction of the French fleet at the Battle of Sluys by Edward III's naval expedition. Six years later Edward launched a cross-Channel invasion, capturing Caen and marching to Flanders, inflicting a heavy defeat on Philip VI's army at Crécy, and proceeding to conquer Calais. The French king's ally David II of Scotland then invaded England, only to be defeated at Neville's Cross (October 17, 1346). In 1355, Edward III's son the "Black Prince" led another force into France, winning another major English victory at Poitiers (September 19, 1356). A third English invasion went less well, leading to a temporary peace (the Treaty of Brétigny, May 8, 1360). The war resumed in 1369 and continued intermittently until 1453. A similar story can be told about Italy. In the 1340s and '50s, to give just one example, the Republic of Venice fought a succession of battles in Dalmatia against Louis I of Hungary and his allies, as well as against the rival republic of Genoa. Just as in Roman times—and as would continue to be true for the next six centuries of European history—armies marched on their stomachs, causing hunger wherever they went; but pestilence rode on their backs.

Historians have long debated the economic, social, and political consequences of the Black Death. A recent survey makes the argument that, unlike major wars, pandemics have tended to depress real interest rates and increase real wages (by killing people but leaving capital intact).[98] The picture is murkier than that implies, not least because war and plague so often coincided. It seems obvious from economic theory—and is borne out by at least some historical data for England and northern Italy—that such a drastic reduction in population must have created shortages of labor, roughly doubling real wages and lowering rates of return on land from above 10 to around 5 percent.[99] However, the most recent research on the English experience suggests some important crosscurrents, undermining the old view that the laboring peasantry—those who survived—were beneficiaries of the calamity. The post-plague spike in commodity prices—especially for salt, the price of which rose sevenfold from 1347 to 1352—meant that survivors' real wages were not initially improved much by the "greatest supply-side labor shock in history." For example, the price of grain in England jumped 230 percent above the long-term average in 1370, thanks to bad weather and bad harvests. An unidentified "pox" was also killing sheep, pigs, and cattle, which drove up livestock prices. All this, combined with chronic shortages of agricultural equipment (hoes and plows), meant misery for those the plague did not kill. The cost of living for laborers remained high for twenty years after the plague, coming down only during the late 1380s.[100]

Yet in the medium term there were significant improvements in the lot of ordinary Englishmen and -women who survived the Black Death. Competition for labor between landlords and other employers weakened government efforts to regulate wages. An increasing monetization of the English economy and a shift toward fixed, per annum, yearly rents began to break down the feudal association between land tenure and bondage. After the Black Death, a rising share of the people working the land were freemen—those yeoman farmers who were to become the backbone of the preindustrial English social structure. There was a shift in grain production toward wheat and barley and a significant increase in livestock farming, which required less labor than crop production. Per capita ale consumption soared after the plague, concentrating production in increasingly efficient large-scale breweries. There was increased manufacturing of woolen and leather goods. More people moved from the countryside to towns as former serfs sought employment in manufacturing, while single young women got jobs as domestics. After the Black Death, too, we see the emergence of the distinctive northwest European marriage pattern of delayed first marriages, lower fertility, and a larger unmarried female population. All of this (which also went on in Flanders and the Low Countries) stood in marked contrast to trends in Southern and Eastern Europe, where the Black Death was followed by a consolidation of feudalism, ensuring that serfdom, de facto if not de jure, would persist for another five centuries.

A surprising consequence of the Black Death in England was that it strengthened rather than weakened the English state. In the face of chronic shortages of both food and labor, the Crown instituted wage and price controls in 1351. To compensate for lost rents from the royal lands, it raised the per capita tax burden to triple what it had been in the early 1340s. At the same time, the 1351 Statute of Labourers compelled every able-bodied man to work and imposed novel forms of punishment (such as pillories and stocks) for "vagrancy," in an effort not so much to maintain order as to reduce labor mobility.[101] Taken together, this proved to be overreach and culminated in the 1381 Peasants' Revolt, which saw not only peasants but also villeins, burghers, and merchants take up arms. Yet the principal target of the rebels was not royal authority, in the person of Richard II, but the intermediate seignorial and ecclesiastical courts of local lords and clerics, the records of which were often singled out for destruction. In the words of Bailey, this was "a cleansing of the stables rather than a revolutionary overthrow of the system," revealing "the touching faith of the lower classes in royal justice."[102] Like most medieval rebellions, the Peasants' Revolt failed. The 1388 Statute of Cambridge imposed yet more restrictions on the mobility and activity of much of the peasantry.[103] On the other hand, there were meaningful improvements to the English rule of law. The Statute of Labourers created the office of justice of the peace, local magistrates whose role would endure until the legal reforms of the 1970s. Though restrictive in its content, the common law of villeinage promoted the idea of written precedence, established the importance of legal proofs, created the norms of due process, and reduced the scope of arbitrary behavior by lords, affording significantly greater legal protections to peasants.[104]

An earlier generation of medievalists, such as Michael Postan—who had himself been born in tsarist Bessarabia (now Moldova)—tended to see medieval England as a precursor of Alexander II's Russia, but with the demise of serfdom having a happier sequel. Their successors today are more inclined to look for deep continuities of English individualism and institutions. This may be to understate the contingent nature of political events in the three centuries between the Black Death and the Glorious Revolution, which repeatedly came close to changing the course of English history. Viewed through the lens of network science, the English authorities were wise to try to restrict mobility in the 1350s. As we have seen, it was precisely the relatively high geographical mobility of the English that had ensured the rapid spread of the plague. In Italy, too, the city-states sought to limit movement, paying out doles to those unable to work and imposing quarantines.[105] Yet making such measures effective was another matter. The wealthy were not easily dissuaded from fleeing to their rural retreats, like the seven young women and three young men in the Florentine writer Giovanni Boccaccio's *Decameron*. According to Baldassarre Bonaiuti, the Florentine diplomat also known as Marchionne di Coppo Stefani, "Many laws were passed that no citizens could leave [Florence] because of the said plague. For they feared that the *minuti* [literally, the little people] would not leave, and would rise, and the malcontents would unite with them . . . [But] it was impossible to keep the citizens in the city . . . for it is always so that large and powerful beasts jump and break fences."[106] More problematically, the crisis of religious faith and social trust elicited by the pandemic led to a parallel pandemic of the mind—and this in turn produced new and dangerous forms of mobility.

We should not underestimate the religious ferment generated by the Black Death. Heretical movements sprang up or were revived, as in the case of Lollardy in England. The most spectacular were the flagellant orders, men who sought to ward off the divine retribution of the plague with acts of penance and self-immolation. Beginning in Hungary in late 1348, the movement spread into Germany and then into Brabant, Hainaut, and Flanders. The flagellants moved in groups ranging in size from fifty to five hundred. "At Tournai a new band arrived every few days from mid-August to the beginning of October," wrote Norman Cohn, this extraordinary movement's historian. "In the first two weeks of the period bands arrived there from Bruges, Ghent, Sluys, Dordrecht and Liège; then Tournai itself joined in and sent off a band in the direction of Soissons."[107] When the burghers of Erfurt refused to open their gates to the flagellants, three thousand camped outside. Calling themselves Cross-bearers, Flagellant Brethren, or Brethren of the Cross, they wore white robes with a red cross on the front and back and similar headgear. Each band had a "master" or "father"—a layman, but one who heard confessions and imposed penances. Each procession lasted thirty-three and a half days, during which time the flagellants did not bathe, shave, change their clothes, or sleep in beds. All contact with women was prohibited. On arriving in a town, the brethren would proceed to its church, form a circle, and prostrate themselves, arms outstretched as if on a cross. On the master's command—"Arise, by the honor of pure martyrdom"—they would stand up and beat themselves with leather scourges tipped with iron spikes, chanting hymns as they did so, periodically falling back to the ground "as though struck by lightning." This ritual was carried out each day, twice in public and once in private. Crowds formed wherever the flagellants scourged themselves; their efforts to ward off further divine punishment were mostly welcomed.

We see here the way a pandemic of infectious disease can easily precipitate a pandemic of extreme behavior, which in turn further destabilizes the social order. For the flagellants were a millenarian movement with a potentially revolutionary agenda that increasingly flouted the authority of the clergy and directed popular wrath against Jewish communities, who were accused of willfully spreading the plague or of inviting divine retribution by their repudiation of Christ. Jewish communities were brutally massacred in numerous towns, notably Frankfurt (July 1349) and Mainz and Cologne (August). (An earlier pogrom in Strasbourg, where the Jews were burned to death in a hideous auto-da-fé, does not seem to have involved flagellants.)[108] Similar massacres of Jews occurred in Spain, France, and the Low Countries, too.[109] The wave of violence ended only after October 1349, when Pope Clement VI issued a bull condemning the flagellants.[110] All this testifies to the social and cultural upheaval created by the Black Death. Historians, however, have tended to miss that the most fundamental danger the flagellants posed was precisely their mobility, and therefore their ability to spread the plague.

The bug became a feature. To an extent that we find difficult to imagine, outbreaks of bubonic plague recurred in Europe from the mid-fourteenth to the early eighteenth century. In 1629, Venice lost around 48 percent of its population after the plague made its way through Mantua and Milan and into the city.[111] Manzoni's *I promessi sposi* (*The Betrothed*, first published in 1827) draws on the last great plague in Milan, in 1630. Plague features in Shakespeare's plays, but mostly as a familiar context, necessitating only allusions ("A plague on both your houses!" "Even so quickly may one catch the plague?"), not explanations. Only in *Romeo and Juliet* does it contribute to the plot: Romeo does not receive the crucial message about the drug that will simulate Juliet's death because the Franciscan friar charged with delivering it is forcibly quarantined. During Shakespeare's lifetime, London was afflicted with plague in 1582, 1592–93, 1603–4, 1606, and 1608–9, frequently closing the theaters where his plays were performed.[112]

In 1665, less than fifty years after Shakespeare's death, the plague struck London again, an epidemic famously reimagined, half a century after the fact, by Daniel Defoe.[113] Defoe's interest in the events of 1665 was more than historical: just two years before the publication of his *Journal of the Plague Year* (1722), a third of the population of Marseille had died in yet another plague outbreak. Defoe was in fact contributing to a live debate on how best to avoid another epidemic in England, which also produced Richard Mead's *Short Discourse Concerning Pestilential Contagion, and the Methods to Be Used to Prevent It* (1720). It was on the basis of Mead's advice that the Privy Council recommended, and Parliament passed, the 1721 Quarantine Act, which considerably extended the powers of the government beyond the previous 1710 Quarantine Act.[114]

Defoe's *Journal* describes the now familiar impact of bubonic plague on popular sentiment:

> The Apprehensions of the People, were likewise strangely encreas'd by the Error of the Times; in which, I think, the People, from what Principle I cannot imagine, were more adicted to Prophesies, and Astrological Conjurations, Dreams, and old Wives Tales, than ever they were before or since: Whether this unhappy Temper was originally raised by the Follies of some People who got Money by it; that is to say, by printing Predictions, and Prognostications I know not; but certain it is, Book's frighted them terribly.[115]

The examples he provides make it clear that seventeenth-century Londoners were as ready as sixth-century Romans or fourteenth-century Germans to infer supernatural causes and therefore remedies for the plague. Defoe makes his skepticism clear:

> I am speaking of the Plague, as a Distemper arising from natural Causes . . . propagated by natural Means. . . . 'Tis evident, that in the Case of an Infection, there is no apparent extraordinary occasion for supernatural Operation, but the ordinary Course of Things appears sufficiently arm'd, and made capable of all the Effects that Heaven usually directs by a Contagion. Among these Causes and Effects this of the secret Conveyance of Infection imperceptible, and unavoidable, is more than sufficient to execute the Fierceness of divine Vengeance, without putting it upon Supernaturals and Miracle.[116]

Notice here the phenomenon, which we shall encounter again, of the dual pandemic: the biological and the informational. Yet it is also clear from Defoe's text, as well as from the more reliable authorities he cited, that he had no real understanding of the epidemiology of the bubonic plague, believing that "the Calamity was spread by Infection, that is to say, by some certain Steams, or Fumes, which the Physicians call Effluvia, by the Breath, or by the Sweat, or by the Stench of the Sores of the sick Persons."[117]

Sometimes—often—we are right for the wrong reasons. The historian Edward Gibbon was born in 1737, six years after Defoe's death. Reading Gibbon's commentary on the Plague of Justinian more than a millennium earlier, we are startled to realize that Gibbon understands the causes of the bubonic plague only slightly better than Procopius.

> The winds might diffuse that subtile venom; but . . . such was the universal corruption of the air, that the pestilence which burst forth in the fifteenth year of Justinian was not checked or alleviated by any difference of the seasons. In time, its first malignity was abated and dispersed; the disease alternately languished and revived; but it was not till the end of a calamitous period of fifty-two years, that mankind recovered their health, or the air resumed its pure and salubrious quality.[118]

The salutary precautions to which Gibbon referred so condescendingly were quarantines and other restrictions on people's movement at a time of contagion. Defoe, too, understood the importance of such measures. "Had most of the People that travelled [not] done so," he wrote of the 1665 outbreak, "the Plague had not been carried into so many Country-Towns and Houses, as it was, to the great Damage, and indeed to the Ruin of abundance of People."[119] He also noted, approvingly, among the orders published by the lord mayor and aldermen of the city of London during the plague, the attempt to regulate the "multitude of Rogues and wandring Beggars, that swarm in every place about the City, being a great cause of the spreading of the Infection," and the prohibitions on "all Plays, Bear-Baitings, Games, singing of Ballads, Buckler-play, or such like Causes of Assemblies of People," as well as "publick Feasting" and "disorderly Tipling in Taverns."[120]

It is still frequently asserted that it was the progress of scientific understanding that helped mankind to dispel, or at least to hold in check, the threat of lethal infections. A closer look at the historical record reveals that, beginning in the Renaissance, men worked out the efficacy of quarantines, social distancing, and other measures now referred to as "non-pharmaceutical interventions" long before they properly understood the true nature of the diseases they sought to counter. It was enough to disrupt, however imperfectly, the social networks of the time—global, national, and local—to slow the spread of the still unknown and unguessed-at microbes.

5

THE SCIENCE DELUSION

So cometh now
My Lady Influenza . . .

—Rupert Brooke

MOSQUITO OR MAN

Sir Rubert William Boyce, one of the founders of the Liverpool School of Tropical Medicine, put it succinctly. The title of his 1909 book was *Mosquito or Man;* the subtitle, *The Conquest of the Tropical World.* "The Tropical Medicine Movement," he wrote, "has now spread all over the civilised world. . . . It can be said without exaggeration that the tropical world is today being steadily and surely conquered. The three great insect-carried scourges of the tropics—the greatest enemies mankind has ever had to contend with, namely Malaria, Yellow Fever and Sleeping Sickness—are now fully in hand and giving way. . . . The tropical world is unfolding once again to the pioneers of commerce. . . . This practical conquest . . . is destined to add a vast slice of the globe, of undreamt-of productiveness to [the British public's] dominions and activities." Such views were commonplace just over a century ago, at the confident zenith of the European empires. "The future of imperialism," wrote John L. Todd, a colleague of Boyce's at Liverpool, in 1903, "lay with the microscope."[1]

The idea of a scientific "conquest" of the natural world—of a hard-fought but ultimately conclusive victory of man (and microscope) over mosquito—is an almost irresistible one, even if we no longer think of imperialism as the beneficiary. In a previous work, I myself did not hesitate to describe modern medicine as one of the "six killer applications" of Western civilization.[2] It is nevertheless possible to recast this familiar story rather differently: not as a series of straightforward medical triumphs, but as something more like a cat-and-mouse feud between science, on the one side, and human behavior on the other. For every two steps forward that the men and women with the micro-scopes were able to take, the human race proved capable of taking at least one step back—by constantly, albeit unwittingly, optimizing networks and behav-ior to expedite the transmission of contagious pathogens. As a result, trium-phalist narratives about the end of medical history have repeatedly been given the lie: by the 1918–19 "Spanish" influenza, by HIV/AIDS, and most recently by COVID-19.

EMPIRES OF INFECTION

It might be thought that, when they began to sail beyond Europe's shores in pursuit of commercial opportunities in the fifteenth century, Europeans brought with them an understanding of science superior to that of the peoples they encountered in Africa, Asia, and the Americas. No doubt their skill at navigation was superior. But they can hardly be said to have excelled in med-ical science.

The overseas expansion of Europe was in some ways a consequence of the inability of any one power to dominate the continent. Several made the at-tempt, but time and again it proved impossible. This was not only because of a relative parity between the major kingdoms in terms of resources and mili-tary technology; it was also because armies on the brink of victory were re-peatedly defeated by a disease, typhus, the causes of which were not properly understood until 1916. Beginning at the Ottoman siege of Belgrade in 1456, the bacillus *Rickettsia prowazekii*—excreted by lice and scratched into their bites by dirty and hungry soldiers—repeatedly dashed the hopes of victorious generals, laying waste to their troops as no human foe could. Typhus ("El Tabardillo") killed a third of the Spanish army laying siege to Granada in 1489. Forty years later, the same disease devastated the French army at the gates of Naples. When the forces of the emperor Charles V besieged Metz in 1552–53, typhus delivered victory to its defenders.[3] In 1556, when Charles's nephew, the future emperor Maximilian II, marched eastward to assist the Hungarians against the forces of the Ottoman sultan Suleiman the Magnificent, the disease struck with such force that "the entire army scattered in all directions to escape the sickness." Typhus was among the deadliest combatants of the Thirty Years' War: in 1632 the disease so depleted the Swedish and imperial armies that a planned battle between the two sides at Nuremberg had to be abandoned.[4] Likewise, archaeological evidence confirms the presence of typhus at the siege of Douai, in northern France (1710–12), during the War of the Spanish Succession.[5] Thirty years later, during the War of the Austrian Succession, typhus killed 30,000 Prussians at the siege of Prague. In 1812, more than 80,000 French soldiers died during the first month of a typhus epidemic in Poland. By the time it reached Moscow, Napoleon Bonaparte's Grande Armée had been reduced from 600,000 men to just 85,000; perhaps as many as 300,000 had died of typhus and dysentery (though disease also took a heavy toll on the Russian side).[6] Again, evidence from a mass grave in Vilnius confirms that "General Typhus" capably assisted "General Winter" on the tsar's behalf.[7] Typhus also claimed many soldiers' lives during the Crimean War (1854–56), though cholera was the bigger killer in that conflict.

When Europeans crossed the Atlantic in what the historian Alfred W. Crosby called "the Columbian Exchange," they brought with them not only knowledge but pathogens of which they were entirely ignorant.[8] As Jared Diamond argued, what proved catastrophic for the Native Americans was not so much the conquistadors' guns and steel, but the germs they brought with them from across the sea: smallpox, typhus, diphtheria, hemorrhagic fever. Like the rats and fleas of the Black Death, the white men were the carriers of the fatal microbes, spreading them from Hispaniola to Puerto Rico to the Aztec capital, Tenochtitlán, to the Inca Empire of the Andes. The Aztecs lamented the devastating impact of the *cocoliztli* ("pestilence" in the Nahuatl language). In truth, they succumbed to a cocktail of different microbes, including *Salmonella enterica,* to which they had no resistance. European settlers understood that they had taken possession of a vast charnel house. The Franciscan missionary and historian Juan de Torquemada recorded that, "in the year 1576, a great mortality and pestilence that lasted for more than a year overcame the Indians [so that] the place we know as New Spain was left almost empty."[9] One of the things the Pilgrims gave thanks for at Plymouth at the end of 1621 was the fact that 90 percent of the indigenous peoples of New England had died of disease in the decade before their arrival, having first—considerately—tilled the land and buried stores of corn for the winter.[10] In 1500, in what was to become British North America, there had been roughly 560,000 American Indians; by 1700 the number had more than halved. This was just the beginning of a drastic decline that was to affect the entire North American continent as the area of white settlement spread westward. There were probably around 2 million indigenous people in the territory of the modern United States in 1500. By 1700 the number was 750,000; by 1820 there were just 325,000.

This was, however, an exchange. There is reason to believe that some of the explorers and conquerors who returned to Europe brought with them syphilis.* The modern view, based on skeletal evidence, is that the *Treponema pallidum* bacterium did indeed come to Europe from the New World after 1492, but that the venereal disease syphilis was the result of a novel mutation.[11] (If Henry VIII and Ivan the Terrible were indeed sufferers, as has sometimes been suggested,† the political consequences were profound.)[12] Meanwhile, the European transportation of enslaved Africans to the Americas—to compensate for the lack of local labor—made the exchange triangular, for they brought with them the flavivirus that causes yellow fever, the plasmodium that causes malaria, and the species of mosquito that is so well adapted to spreading both. Malaria and yellow fever flourished on the plantations of the Caribbean and the southern states of British America.[13] In the mid-seventeenth

---

*Modern research has debunked an earlier theory that there was treponeme infection in Europe before Columbus, but that it took the form of yaws, which is transmitted from skin to skin, and that syphilis spread in Europe only once hygiene improved and yaws declined, and with it cross-immunity to syphilis.
†The evidence is too flimsy to withstand scrutiny. Leg ulcers and obesity were Henry VIII's principal medical problems.

century, epidemics of yellow fever in Saint Kitts, Guadeloupe, and Cuba and along the east coast of Central America killed between 20 and 30 percent of the local population. The earliest definitive outbreaks in North America occurred in 1668 (New York) and 1669 (the Mississippi Valley).[14] This meant that later settlers in the Americas faced dauntingly high mortality rates in their first years after crossing the Atlantic. To survive was to be "seasoned." It also meant that armies recruited in Europe to fight in the New World were at a disadvantage—witness the disastrous losses to yellow fever suffered by Admiral Edward Vernon's force of 25,000 in 1740 and 1742, during the War of Jenkins' Ear, when he tried and failed to take Cartagena and Santiago de Cuba.[15] The same fate befell the French soldiers sent by Napoleon to retake Saint-Domingue from the Haitian revolutionary Toussaint L'Ouverture in 1802. "Yellow Jack" may even have played a part—along with the French navy—in tipping the military balance against George III's army at the Battle of Yorktown (1781).

The French historian Emmanuel Le Roy Ladurie called it "the unification of the globe by disease," the creation of a "common market of microbes."[16] Consequently, the European empires had to be built and sustained in spite of disease. A British soldier had a one-in-two chance of dying if he was posted to Sierra Leone; a one-in-eight chance in Jamaica; one-in-twelve in the Windwards and Leewards; one-in-fourteen in Bengal or Ceylon. Only if he had the luck to be sent to New Zealand was he better off than he would have been at home. A royal commission reported in 1863 that the mortality rate for enlisted men in India between 1800 and 1856 was sixty-nine per thousand, compared with a death rate for the equivalent age group in British civilian life of around ten per thousand. Troops in India also had a much higher incidence of sickness. With quintessentially Victorian precision, another royal commission calculated that, out of an army of 70,000 British soldiers, 4,830 would die each year and 5,880 hospital beds would be occupied by those incapacitated by illness.[17] Tropical diseases also took a heavy toll on the French colonial civil service throughout its existence. Between 1887 and 1912, a total of 135 out of 984 appointees (14 percent) died in the colonies. On average, retired colonial officials expired seventeen years earlier than their counterparts in the metropolitan service. As late as 1929, nearly a third of the sixteen thousand Europeans living in French West Africa were hospitalized for an average of fourteen days a year.[18] Céline's Grand Guignol depiction of French Equatorial Africa in 1916–17—he went there as a representative of the Forestry Company of Sangha-Oubangui—makes it clear that illness was a way of life, and life was expected to be shortened by service in the tropics: "Men, days, things—they passed before you knew it in this hotbed of vegetation, heat, humidity, and mosquitoes. Everything passed, disgustingly, in little pieces, in phrases, particles of flesh and bone, in regrets and corpuscles. . . ."[19]

The problem was that the empires grew much faster than the medical knowledge of those administering them. In 1860 the territorial extent of the British Empire had been some 9.5 million square miles; by 1909 the total had risen to 12.7 million. It now covered around 22 percent of the world's land surface—making it three times the size of the French empire and ten times the size of the German—and controlled roughly the same proportion of the world's population: some 444 million people in all lived under some form of British rule. According to the *St. James's Gazette,* the Queen Empress Victoria held sway over "one continent, a hundred peninsulas, five hundred promontories, a thousand lakes, two thousand rivers, ten thousand islands." A postage stamp was produced showing a map of the world and bearing the legend WE HOLD A VASTER EMPIRE THAN HAS BEEN. All this was joined together by three communications networks. There were barracks and naval coaling stations—thirty-three of them in all—dotted across the world, from Ascension Island to Zanzibar. New technology drew each node in the network closer together. In the days of sail it had taken between four and six weeks to cross the Atlantic; with the introduction of the steamship, that was reduced to two weeks in the mid-1830s and just ten days in the 1880s. Between the 1850s and the 1890s, the journey time from England to Cape Town was cut from forty-two days to nineteen. Moreover, steamships got bigger—in the same period, average gross tonnage roughly doubled—as well as more numerous, leading to proportionate increases in traffic volumes. The second network was the railway. The first in India—linking Bombay to Tanna, twenty-one miles away—was formally opened in 1853; within less than fifty years, track covering nearly 25,000 miles had been laid. In the space of a generation, the "te-rain" transformed Indian economic and social life: for the first time, thanks to the standard third-class fare of seven annas, long-distance travel became a possibility for millions of Indians. As the historian J. R. Seeley put it, the Victorian revolution in global communications had achieved "the annihilation of distance." Finally, there was the information network of the telegraph. By 1880 there were altogether 97,568 miles of cable across the world's oceans, linking Britain to India, Canada, Australia, Africa, and Australia. Now a message could be relayed from Bombay to London at the cost of four shillings a word, with the reasonable expectation that it would be seen the next day. In the words of Charles Bright, one of the apostles of the new technology, the telegraph was "the world's system of electrical nerves."[20]

All this did indeed help to project British power over greater distances than any previous empire had achieved. But the Victorian transport networks were also the fastest transmission mechanism for disease there had ever been. Even as pioneers of medical science peered into their microscopes, seeking a truly effective countermeasure against the mosquito, two great pandemics spread through the imperial transportation network. Cholera was a disease endemic to the Ganges River and its delta; its export to the world was one of the unintended crimes of the British East India Company.[21] There were no fewer than six cholera pandemics in the period from 1817 to 1923: 1817–23, 1829–51, 1852–59, 1863–79, 1881–96, and 1899–1923.[22] The first broke out near Calcutta, then moved overland to Siam (Thailand) and from there by ship to Oman and south to Zanzibar. By 1822 it had reached Japan, as well as Mesopotamia (Iraq), Persia (Iran), and Russia.[23] The second cholera pandemic began in 1829, again in India, then moved across the Eurasian landmass to Russia and Europe, and from there to the United States. The rapid growth of ports and manufacturing centers in the industrial world had created the perfect breeding grounds for the disease: crowded accommodation with abysmal sanitation. When cholera struck Hamburg in 1892, devastating the slum-dwelling *Lumpenproletariat* of the inner city, where the mortality rate was thirteen times higher than in the city's wealthy West End, the pioneering German bacteriologist Robert Koch commented, "Gentlemen, I forget

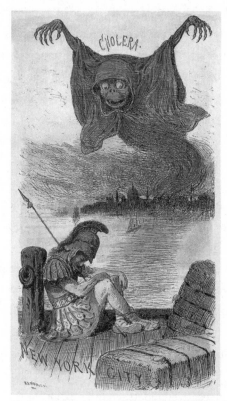

Cholera comes to New York while Science sleeps.
"Is This a Time for Sleep?" by Charles Kendrick,
1883.

that I am in Europe."[24] While modern social historians see the Hamburg epidemic as a parable of the class structure, in reality cholera's reign of terror in Europe's port cities was more a consequence of imperialism than of
capitalism.

The revival of bubonic plague followed the same pattern. The bacterium
reemerged from its reservoir among the Himalayan marmots in the 1850s and
spread down through China to Hong Kong, which it reached in 1894. From
there, multiple steamships transported infected fleas and rats to every continent. By the time it was brought under control in the mid-twentieth century,
the third plague pandemic had caused around fifteen million deaths, the vast
majority in India, China, and Indonesia. In Central and South America, around

thirty thousand died; in Europe, about seven thousand people; in North America, just five hundred, all of them in San Francisco, Los Angeles, and New Orleans, as well as a few unlucky communities in Arizona and New Mexico.[25] The first outbreak in San Francisco began in Chinatown in March 1900. The second followed the great earthquake and fire of 1906; the rat population exploded, creating a perfect breeding ground for *Y. pestis*. In all, 191 people died.[26]

QUACKS

More than half a millennium separated San Francisco in 1900 from Florence in 1350—and yet understanding of the causes of bubonic plague had barely advanced in that time. Fourteenth-century scholars at the University of Paris noted a hostile conjunction between Jupiter, Mars, and Saturn: "Warm and humid Jupiter was argued to have drawn up evil vapors from the earth and water, while Mars, hot and dry, set fire to the vapors, igniting the plague as well as other natural disasters. Saturn, for its part, was to add evil wherever it went and, when in conjunction with Jupiter, to cause death and depopulation."[27] In his *Consilio contro la pestilentia* (1481), the philosopher Marsilio Ficino likewise attributed the Black Death partly to "malignant constellations . . . conjunctions of Mars with Saturn [and] eclipses." However, the consensus view that emerged in the medieval period was atmospheric rather than astrological. The plague, it was argued, must be spread by a "poisonous vapor" (*vapore velenoso*) that lingered longest in "heavy, warm, damp, and fetid air," which could spread "from place to place . . . more rapidly than burning sulfur." The reason the disease killed some but not others had to do with "sympathy." If the body was in sympathy with the poisonous vapor—if someone was already inclined toward heat and dampness—susceptibility would be greater. By the late fifteenth century, nevertheless, doctors were testing urine, opening abscesses, and bleeding patients, as well as dispensing prophylactics and therapies. In 1479, for example, Machiavelli's uncle Bernardo was given a variety of experimental remedies based on rue and honey.[28]

Renaissance scholars, like earlier Muslim writers, revived the ideas of

Hippocrates and Galen, who identified six influences on human health: climate, motion and rest, diet, sleeping patterns, evacuation and sexuality, and afflictions of the soul.[29] This was worthless against the plague. But so, too, was "miasmatism." The "plague costume" devised by Venetian physicians—which combined a wax-covered gown with a long beak containing herbs—was as useless as the burning of sulfur in the streets of London in 1665. As for the attempts to fend off the plague with religious services, these—like the flagellants' processions—were worse than useless. As a member of the Observant branch of the Franciscan order told the Doge of Venice, "If God wishes it, it will not suffice to close the churches. It will need a remedy for the causes of the plague, which are the horrendous sins which are committed, the blaspheming of God and the saints, the schools of sodomy, the infinite usury contracts made at Rialto."[30] In 1625, the archbishop of Canterbury told the English ambassador to the Ottoman Empire, "Wee have here, with better knowledge, taken a course to appease God's wrathe in the pestilence, and therefore in parliament decreed solemne fasts and publicke praters throughout the whole kingdome, the king himself, at Westminster churche joyning with the lords and the rest of the commons."[31] In 1630, Pope Urban VIII excommunicated the Florentine sanitary commission for banning processions. The following year, the priest of Montelupo Fiorentino, a walled village twelve miles from Florence, defied Florentine rules against processions.[32] It cannot have done his flock much good.

Like their counterparts in England, the Florentine authorities understood that, whether or not the plague spread through miasma, the free movement of people did not help. In the Venetian empire, the Black Death prompted the innovation of isolating arriving sailors in a *lazaretto* for a mandatory period, though initially—in the seaport of Ragusa (present-day Dubrovnik) in 1377—it was for only thirty days.[33] In 1383, the authorities in Marseille extended the isolation period to forty days, giving the quarantine its name. (The duration was a biblical touch, inspired by the forty days and forty nights of the flood in Genesis, the forty years the Israelites spent wandering in the wilderness, and the forty days of Lent.)[34] Recurrent plague outbreaks led to the gradual development of five policies designed to limit contagion: controllable borders with marine or land quarantines to keep the disease out, as well as sanitary cordons to keep the infected in; social distancing in the form of bans on gatherings; burying of the dead in special pits, and destruction of the personal belongings and houses of the dead; lockdowns (the isolation and separation of the sick from the healthy), which included confinement to pesthouses and *lazaretti,* as well as infected people's homes; and health status tracking in the form of bills of health—certificates that testified that a ship or caravan did not carry the plague. Florence also experimented with the provision of free food and medical care to those whose livelihoods had been disrupted by plague, as much to discourage vagrancy as to reduce hardship.[35] The case of Ferrara illustrates how these measures came to be used together. In time of plague, the city closed all but two city gates and posted at them surveillance teams "composed of wealthy noblemen, city officials, physicians and apothecaries." Health status was tracked by bills of health (*fedi di sanità*), which certified that people were arriving from plague-free zones. If new arrivals had symptoms, they would be confined to *lazaretti* outside the city walls.[36] The enforcement of these and other public hygiene measures created a need for heavier policing. The head of Palermo's board of health noted in 1576 that his motto was "gold, fire, and the gallows"—gold to pay taxes, fire to burn infected goods, and the gallows for those who defied the board's orders.

None of this could be said to be based on science. It was more the product of intelligent general observation and a growing reluctance to leave one's fate in God's hands. Consequently, it was never wholly effective. In 1374, the ruler of Milan, Bernabò Visconti, ordered that the subordinate town of Reggio Emilia be cordoned off by armed troops. It did not stop the plague from reaching Milan. In 1710, the Habsburg emperor Joseph I decided to block the spread of diseases from the Balkans by creating a continuous "sanitary cordon" along his realm's southern frontier with the Ottoman Empire. By the middle of the eighteenth century, the border was policed by two thousand fortified watchtowers, positioned a half mile apart. The restriction to just nineteen border crossings ensured that anyone arriving on Habsburg territory was registered, housed, and isolated for at least twenty-one days. Their quarters were disinfected daily with sulfur or vinegar. As the English traveler Alexander Kinglake noted on crossing the border at Zemun, near Belgrade, in 1835:

> It is the Plague, and the dread of the Plague, that divide the one people from the other. . . . If you dare to break the laws of the quarantine, you will be tried with military haste; the court will scream out your sentence to you from a tribunal some fifty yards off; the priest, instead of gently whispering to you the sweet hopes of religion, will console you a[t] dueling distance, and after that you will find yourself carefully shot, and carelessly buried in the ground of the Lazaretto.[37]

All of this was established too late to save its progenitor: Joseph I died of smallpox in April 1711, having caught the disease from his prime minister, whose daughter was infected.[38] In 1720, when plague was ravaging Marseille, the French regent, Philippe of Orleans, sent Charles Claude Andrault de Langeron to take command. A new council of health severed communications between Marseille and Aix, Arles, and Montpellier, where plague walls were built. The crew of the ship thought to be infected were confined to an offshore *lazaretto*. For good measure, there was a general massacre of cats and dogs, which must have been welcomed by the rats of Provence.[39]

Science lagged far behind such experiments, which, for all their imperfections, did at least something to disrupt networks of contagion. To be sure, Girolamo Fracastoro had published a treatise in 1546 arguing that epidemic diseases such as smallpox and measles were caused by seeds (*seminaria*) and transmitted by direct contact, through the air, or from contaminated objects. However, Fracastoro's work was not influential.[40] George Watson's *The Cures of the Diseased in Remote Regions* (1598) was the first English textbook on that subject, but it did not help much, as the prescribed treatments were either bleeding or changes of diet.[41] It was not until the eighteenth century that a true advance in Western medical science occurred, with James Lind's first clinical trial, in 1747, which established the efficacy of citrus fruits as a remedy for scurvy; with William Withering's discovery that digitalis (foxglove) was, in the right dose, a remedy for dropsy (edema); and with the import to Europe of the Oriental practice of variolation against smallpox, which can in fact be traced back as far as tenth-century China. In 1714, two physicians— Emmanuel Timoni and Jacob Pylarini—wrote separate letters to the Royal Society in London, describing the "engrafting" of healthy people with infectious matter from smallpox pustules, which they had observed in Istanbul. Lady Mary Wortley Montague, the formidable wife of the British ambassador to the Ottoman capital—who had herself survived smallpox in 1715 and lost a brother to the disease—championed the procedure, having her five-year-old son inoculated in 1718, followed by her daughter in 1721. On returning to London, she convinced the eminent physician Sir Hans Sloane to conduct some trial inoculations on ten orphans and six condemned men. The procedure was risky, as children were in effect being given mild doses of the disease, but royal patronage (the princess of Wales was a convert) spread the practice, not least to other royal families. Among those inoculated were Maria Theresa of Austria, along with her children and grandchildren; Louis XVI and his children; Catherine II of Russia and her son, the future tsar Paul; and Frederick II of Prussia. A safer procedure was to use cowpox to vaccinate (from *vacca,* the Latin for cow) against smallpox, an experiment first run by a farmer named Benjamin Jesty in 1774, though history tends to give the credit to Edward Jenner, who performed his first vaccination twenty years later and published his findings in *An Inquiry into the Causes and Effects of the Variolae Vacciniae* (1798).[42]

If European royalty was prepared to take the chance of inoculation against smallpox, the plain people of New England were more skeptical. There were smallpox outbreaks in and around Boston in 1721–22, 1730, 1751–52, 1764, throughout the 1770s, in 1788, and in 1792, the first one being the most severe.[43] Proponents of inoculation—the Puritan minister Cotton Mather, the physician Zabdiel Boylston, and a Harvard tutor named Thomas Robie— encountered stiff opposition, despite being able to demonstrate a reduced fatality rate among the three hundred patients who had submitted to variolation.[44] During the 1730 epidemic, Samuel Danforth, a schoolmaster and Harvard alumnus, began inoculating in Cambridge. However, at town meetings, it was resolved that Danforth had "greatly endangered the town & disrupted sundrey families" and that he should "remove such inoculated persons into some convenient place whereby our town mayn't be exposed by them." Town officials also asked Harvard to discontinue inoculation, but a tutor, Nathan Prince, continued to treat those who wanted it. By the 1790s, when the practice was more widely accepted, Harvard encouraged students to be inoculated.[45] Massachusetts made smallpox vaccination compulsory in 1809. Sweden was the first European country to make it widely available, and then compulsory in 1816, followed by England in 1853, Scotland in 1864, the Netherlands in 1873, and Germany in 1874.[46] In the United States, however, vaccination became—and has since remained—a bone of contention. By 1930 opponents in Arizona, Utah, North Dakota, and Minnesota had succeeded in prohibiting compulsory vaccination, while thirty-five states left regulation to local authorities; only nine states and the District of Columbia had followed Massachusetts's lead. There, vaccination was enforced by imposing fines or by admitting to school only children who had been vaccinated, an approach validated by the Supreme Court in *Jacobson v. Massachusetts* (1905). As late as the 1840s, American doctors were treating cholera sufferers, variously, with bleeding, immense and highly toxic doses of mercury and mercury compounds such as calomel, tobacco smoke enemas, electric shocks, and the injection of saline solutions into the veins. The president of the New York State Medical Society recommended that the patient's rectum be plugged with beeswax or oilcloth to obstruct the diarrhea.[47] There were still plenty of clergymen ready to attribute the disease to divine chastisement, rather than the woefully unsanitary conditions in American cities.

The history of medical science as a tale of heroic Victorian researchers— of men and microscopes—is a familiar one. Charles Darwin had discerned as early as 1836 that disease could be transmitted by microscopic agents carried even by outwardly healthy people. Louis Pasteur proved that mold was airborne by placing filters over a dish of boiled broth. Ignaz Semmelweis showed in 1861 that doctors' dirty hands were a cause of puerperal fever in pregnant women. Joseph Lister developed methods of antisepsis in his operating theater, preventing the infection of wounds. Robert Koch identified the bacteria that caused anthrax, tuberculosis, and cholera; others using the methods from his seminal *Ätiologie der Tuberkulose* (1882)[48] soon isolated the microbes responsible for diphtheria, plague, tetanus, typhoid, leprosy, syphilis, pneumonia, and gonorrhea.[49] Carl Friedländer vied with Albert Fraenkel in the 1880s to identify the bacterium responsible for pneumonia.[50] Yet this story is intelligible only in an imperial context, for it was precisely the pressures generated by the exposure of Europeans to tropical illnesses that directed interest and resources toward such research. It was while working in British India in 1884 that Koch isolated *V. cholerae,* which only the previous year had killed Koch's French rival Louis Thuillier in Alexandria.[51] It was after an outbreak in Hong Kong in 1894 that the Swiss bacteriologist Alexandre Yersin identified and named the bacillus responsible for bubonic plague. It was a doctor in the Indian Medical Service, Ronald Ross, who first fully explained the etiology of malaria and the role of the mosquito in transmitting it; he himself suffered from the disease. It was three Dutch scientists based in Java—Christiaan Eijkman, Adolphe Vorderman, and Gerrit Grijns—who worked out that beriberi was caused by a dietary deficiency in polished rice (the lack of vitamin B1). And it was an Italian, Aldo Castellani, whose research in Uganda in 1902 identified the *Trypanosoma brucei* parasite in the tsetse fly that is responsible for sleeping sickness. There were errors as well as trials. Tuberculin, Koch's cure for TB, did not work. In 1906, his purported treatment for sleeping sickness irreversibly blinded one in five people who received it. On the whole, however, this was one of humanity's greatest winning streaks.

There were even breakthroughs on the peripheries of the Russian and American empires. In 1892, Dmitri Ivanovsky first identified pathogens smaller than bacteria—"filterable agents"—during his research into a disease (subsequently termed tobacco mosaic virus) that was causing widespread crop damage in Crimea, Ukraine, and Bessarabia.[52] A good illustration of the remarkable spirit of self-sacrifice often associated with this kind of work was the effort by American scientists working in Cuba—Walter Reed, James Carroll, Jesse Lazear, and Aristides Agramonte—to determine the exact cause of yellow fever. Following the lead of Carlos Finlay, a Cuban doctor who had written a dissertation on the subject, Carroll, Lazear, and Agramonte allowed themselves to be bitten by mosquitoes suspected of carrying the disease. Carroll became seriously ill but recovered (prompting Reed to "go out and get <u>boiling drunk</u>" in celebration). Lazear, however, was dead within three weeks. By the end of 1900, Reed and his colleagues were satisfied that mosquitoes were spreading a nonbacterial agent from person to person, but it was not until 1927 that Adrian Stokes isolated the virus in Asibi, a Ghanaian man who was sick with the disease.[53] Stokes himself died of yellow fever soon afterward, as did two of the other investigators on the ill-fated West African Yellow Fever Commission.[54] Nevertheless, identifying mosquitoes as the intermediaries was enough for William Gorgas, the chief sanitary officer in Havana, to design countermeasures—including the use of kerosene in pools of stagnant water—which were later deployed in Panama to protect workers digging the great canal.

These and other breakthroughs, clustered in the period from the 1880s to the 1920s, proved to be crucial in keeping Europeans, Americans, and hence the entire colonial project alive in the tropics. Africa and Asia had become giant laboratories for Western medicine. And the more successful the research—the more remedies like quinine, the antimalarial properties of which were discovered in Peru—the further the Western empires could spread and, with them, the supreme benefit of longer human life. The timing of the "health transition"—the start of sustained improvements in life expectancy—is quite clear. In Western Europe it came between the 1770s and the 1890s, first in Denmark, with Spain bringing up the rear. By the eve of the First World War, typhoid and cholera had effectively been eliminated in Europe, while diphtheria and tetanus were controlled by vaccine. In the twenty-three modern Asian countries for which data are available, with one exception, the health transition came between the 1890s and the 1950s. Between 1911 and 1950, Indian life expectancy rose from twenty-one to thirty-six years (though in the same period, British life expectancy increased from fifty-one to sixty-nine). In Africa the transition came between the 1920s and the 1950s, with just two exceptions out of forty-three countries. In nearly all Asian and African countries, then, life expectancy began to improve before the end of European colonial rule.[55] This effort also required a major advance in the institutionalization of scientific research. The Pasteur Institute, in Paris, founded in 1887,

was later matched by the Liverpool (1898) and London (1899) schools of tropical medicine and by the Hamburg-based Institute for Shipping and Tropical
Illnesses (1901).[56] Institutes in colonial centers, notably the Pasteur Institutes
in Dakar and Tunis, continued to be at the cutting edge of research. It was they
and their counterparts at the Rockefeller Institute for Medical Research, led by
Max Theiler, who finally devised a safe and effective vaccine for yellow fever.[57]

Yet there was more than self-sacrifice involved in what Boyce had called
"this practical conquest . . . of the tropic world." It was one thing to fathom
the causes of infectious disease. It was another to persuade ordinary people
to take the precautions recommended by the medical scientists. This had already become apparent in many European cities in 1830–31, when public ire
was directed at the very public officials trying to reduce the population's exposure to contaminated water. In Sevastopol, Crimea, tighter quarantine regulations in May and June of 1830 led to a bloody revolt in the Korabelnaya
suburb, in which several officials (including the military governor himself)
were killed and police posts and quarantine offices destroyed. In St. Petersburg a year later, by contrast, popular wrath was directed against foreigners
and doctors, as well as the police.[58] A similar eruption occurred in Iuzovka
(Donetsk), a mining and industrial town in the Donbass region of Ukraine, in
1892, when doctors were again threatened by the very migrant workers they
had been trying to help. As in the 1340s, there was an anti-Semitic element
to the unrest, with pitched battles against Cossack troops and the burning of
taverns giving way to a full-fledged pogrom.[59] Nor was it only in Russia that
infectious disease exacerbated ethnic divisions. An outbreak of smallpox in
Wisconsin in 1894, which was concentrated in the German and Polish neighborhoods of Milwaukee's South Side, led to violent clashes between untrust-
ing citizens and the local health authorities, culminating in the impeachment
of health commissioner Walter Kempster.[60] At the time of the bubonic plague
outbreak of 1900, Asian populations were targeted by discriminatory measures, which in Honolulu took the form of the incineration of Asian property,
culminating in the great fire of January 20, 1900. In San Francisco, Dr. J. J.
Kinyoun implemented quarantine measures that deliberately discriminated
against Chinatown.[61]

Perhaps not surprisingly, efforts at international cooperation had only limited success in the nineteenth century. The first International Sanitary Conference met in Paris in July 1851, but the representatives from twelve countries were unable to agree on standardized quarantine measures for dealing with cholera, yellow fever, and the plague.[62] Divisions among the medical experts on the causes of cholera did not help, but the main bone of contention was between Great Britain, whose spokesmen regarded traditional quarantine measures as medieval obstacles to free trade, and the Mediterranean states—France, Spain, Italy, and Greece—which blamed the British for bringing cholera to Europe from their outsized Oriental empire.[63] The "English system" favored inspections of ships, isolation of sick passengers, and tracking of infected persons over blanket quarantines. This probably was superior, but it fell far short of what was needed to contend with the resurgence of bubonic plague. The International Sanitary Conference of 1897—held in Venice—recommended that plague be controlled through isolation of the infected and incineration of their belongings. Unfortunately, the burning of property merely drove infected rats to seek new homes.[64]

In *Hind Swaraj* (*Indian Home Rule*), published in 1908, Mahatma Gandhi called Western civilization "a disease" and referred scornfully to the West's "army of doctors." "Civilization is not an incurable disease," Gandhi declared, "but it should never be forgotten that the English people are at present afflicted by it."[65] In an interview in London in 1931, he cited the "conquest of disease" as one of the purely "material" yardsticks by which Western civilization measured progress.[66] Such complaints seem faintly ridiculous, until one considers how brutally colonial governments implemented public health measures. In Cape Town, during the third bubonic plague pandemic, black residents were summarily rounded up and removed from the waterfront to Uitvlugt (Ndabeni), which became the city's first "natives location." When bubonic plague struck Senegal, the French authorities were ruthless in their response. The homes of the infected were torched, residents were forcibly removed and quarantined under armed guard, and the dead were unceremoniously buried in creosote or lime. Small wonder the indigenous population felt themselves to be more victims than beneficiaries of public health policy.

In Dakar there were mass protests and the first general strike in Senegal's history.[67]

In truth, the real advances of the nineteenth and early twentieth centuries were not scientific in the sense that many contemporaries imagined. For every advance by bacteriologists and virologists, there were erroneous steps in wrong directions, such as phrenology and eugenics. Progress took more humdrum forms. Public health benefited greatly from improved housing—the shift in Europe from wooden walls and thatch to brick walls and tiles—and regulations such as the UK Artisans' and Labourers' Dwellings Improvement Act of 1875.[68] Mistaken ideas such as miasmatism could have positive results: the draining of swamps, bogs, moats, and other sites of standing water, the introduction of hydraulic devices to circulate water in canals and cisterns, the clearing of trash from residential areas, the ventilation of living quarters and meeting places, and the use of disinfectants and insecticides in homes, hospitals, prisons, meeting halls, and ships. Such measures—the right things done for the wrong reasons—significantly reduced the exposure of European and American populations to pathogens and their carriers.[69]

John Snow is still a revered name in Soho because of his work in tracing the London cholera outbreak of 1854 back to a single water fountain on Broad Street that drew water from the sewage-filled Thames. But one did not need to accept Dr. Snow's argument that human feces were the problem to see the benefits of water filtration systems and separate sewage piping. Likewise, the creation of a Metropolitan Board of Health for New York City in 1866 allowed an unprecedented response to yet another cholera outbreak: 160,000 tons of manure were cleared from vacant lots, the apartments of infected people were promptly disinfected with chloride of lime or coal tar, and their clothing, bedding, and utensils were burned.[70] According to one estimate, clean-water technologies such as filtration and chlorination were responsible for nearly half the total mortality reduction in American cities in the first four decades of the twentieth century, three quarters of the infant mortality reduction, and nearly two thirds of the child mortality reduction.[71] Sanitation worked. As the playwright George Bernard Shaw put it in 1906, in a preface to *The Doctor's Dilemma* that was less than kind to the medical profession:

For a century past civilization has been cleaning away the conditions which favor bacterial fevers. Typhus, once rife, has vanished: plague and cholera have been stopped at our frontiers by a sanitary blockade. . . . The dangers of infection and the way to avoid it are better understood than they used to be. . . . Nowadays the troubles of consumptive patients are greatly increased by the growing disposition to treat them as lepers. . . . But the scare of infection, though it sets even doctors talking as if the only really scientific thing to do with a fever patient is to throw him into the nearest ditch and pump carbolic acid on him from a safe distance until he is ready to be cremated on the spot, has led to much greater care and cleanliness. And the net result has been a series of victories over disease.[72]

People in the industrialized world were eating better, too. By today's standards, no doubt, the working-class Englishman in around 1904 drank far too much alcohol—on average, seventy-three gallons of beer per year,* 2.4 gallons of spirits, and one gallon of wine. He also ate too little in the way of fruit and vegetables—which led to deficiencies in calcium, riboflavin, vitamin A, and vitamin C—and too much starchy carbohydrate. Nevertheless, "Britain was on the cusp of having a working population where very nearly all households had a diet that provided sufficient energy for sustained work."[73] And higher rates of female education and employment correlated with roughly simultaneous declines in fertility and infant mortality.[74]

Still, it is easy to see why the scientists were inclined to take so much credit for the general improvements in public health, which had produced an unprecedented increase in life expectancy at birth in the space of a century—in the case of the United Kingdom, from around forty at the time of the Battle of Waterloo to fifty-three in 1913. When the International Sanitary Conference was held in Venice in 1897, new breakthroughs seemed all but guaranteed. True, Waldemar Haffkine's attempt at a vaccine against bubonic plague had unpleasant side effects—including fever, swellings, and flushing

---

*The equivalent figure today is a paltry nineteen gallons. However, the alcohol content of modern beer tends to be higher than in the past.

of the skin—and did not provide complete protection against *Y. pestis,* but it was progress, as was the recognition that controlling rodents (and their fleas) through trapping and poisoning might be the most effective remedy of all. There were also the first steps to utilize the telegraph to track infectious passengers on board ships. In the words of the Austrian delegate at the 1892 conference (also held in Venice), "The telegram is a prophylactic measure in the largest sense of the word."[75] It was the same optimism that was later to inform Boyce's *Mosquito or Man.* But such faith in scientific progress was about to be dealt a very heavy blow indeed.

LADY INFLUENZA

So cometh now
My Lady Influenza, like a star
Inebriously wan, and in her train
Fever, the haggard soul's white nenuphur,
And lily-fingered Death, and grisly Pain
And Constipation who makes all things vain,
Pneumonyer, Cancer, and Nasal Catarrh.

Rupert Brooke's "To My Lady Influenza" (1906) was a facetious undergraduate work.[76] Yet "Lady Influenza" was never to be trifled with. The first well-described influenza outbreaks were in sixteenth-century Europe, but the earliest was probably in 1173. There had been significant influenza pandemics in 1729, 1781–82, 1830–33, and 1898–1900, with total mortality rising from 400,000 to 1.2 million (between 0.06 and 0.08 percent of the world's estimated population).[77] But the twentieth century was to be hit much harder.[78] A more populous world was also a more urban world and a more mobile world—a world in which low air quality in industrial towns may have made people more susceptible to respiratory illnesses. A year after Brooke wrote "To My Lady Influenza," his eldest brother, Dick, died of pneumonia, at the age of twenty-six. Brooke himself would live only a year longer, dying of an infected mosquito bite that led to sepsis, off the Greek island of Skyros, en route to the fatal beaches of Gallipoli. The twentieth century increased life expectancy, yet it was also extraordinarily wasteful of young men.

A predictable gray rhino, in the sense that danger of a general European war was well known, but also a surprising black swan, in the sense that contemporaries seemed bewildered by its outbreak, the First World War was a true dragon-king event in terms of its vast historical consequences.[79] It began with an act of terrorism on June 28, 1914, when shots fired by a tubercular nineteen-year-old Bosnian youth named Gavrilo Princip fatally severed the jugular vein of the archduke Francis Ferdinand, the Habsburg heir to the thrones of Austria and Hungary, as well as killing his wife. Those shots also precipitated a war that destroyed the Austro-Hungarian Empire and transformed Bosnia and Herzegovina from one of its colonies into a part of a new South Slav state. These were in fact the things Princip had hoped to achieve, making the assassination perhaps the single most effective act of terrorism in history, even if he cannot have anticipated such far-reaching success.[80] Yet they were only the intended consequences of his action. The war he triggered was not confined to the Balkans; it also drew broad and hideous scars across Northern Europe and the Near East. Like gargantuan abattoirs, its battlefields sucked in and slaughtered young men from all the extremities of the globe, claiming in all nearly ten million lives as a direct result of warfare. The war also furnished a pretext for the Ottoman regime's genocide against its Armenian subjects. Moreover, even when an armistice was proclaimed, the war refused to stop; it swept eastward after 1918, as if eluding the grasp of the peacemakers, into the Arctic, Siberia, Mongolia, and other regions previously untouched by the fighting. In Poland and Ukraine, for example, it was not easy to say exactly when World War I ended and when the Russian Civil War unleashed by the Bolshevik Revolution began.

World War I was enormously disruptive in economic terms, too. In the summer of 1914, the world economy was thriving in ways that look distinctly familiar. The mobility of commodities, capital, and labor reached levels comparable to those we know today; the sea lanes and telegraphs across the Atlantic were never busier, as capital and migrants went west and commodities and manufactures went east. The war sank globalization—literally: nearly thirteen million tons of shipping went to the bottom of the sea as a result of German naval action, most of it by U-boats. International trade, investment, and emigration all collapsed. In the war's aftermath, revolutionary regimes arose that were fundamentally hostile to international economic integration. Plans replaced the market; autarky and protection took the place of free trade. Flows of goods diminished; flows of people and capital all but dried up. In political terms, too, the war was transformative. The war swept away four dynasties that had ruled for centuries: the Romanovs, the Habsburgs, the Hohenzollerns, and the Ottomans. The European empires' grip on the world—which had been the political undergirding of globalization—was dealt a profound, if not yet quite fatal, blow. New nation-states were created. The process of democratization was accelerated: franchises were widened and, in many countries, women were granted the vote. Socialist parties came to power through revolutions or elections. The power of trade unions grew.[81]

At the same time, the experience of war convinced many veterans and civilians alike not just that dynasticism was dead but that liberalism, with its representative parliamentary institutions and law-based procedures, had also become obsolete. Not only socialists but also fascists proposed alternative political arrangements that radically diminished the roles of free elections and individual freedoms. Finally, efforts to "recast bourgeois Europe" and restore the prewar order were fatally undermined by the structural instability of the international order that emerged after the war.[82] The restored gold standard functioned poorly and finally degenerated into a global transmission mechanism for an American depression.[83] Significant elements of the peace treaties proved impossible to enforce. New institutions of collective security such as the League of Nations proved weak in the face of defiant nation-states. More broadly, the United States failed to match its greatly enhanced economic importance with a commensurate geopolitical role.[84] Power remained disproportionately in the hands of the victorious European empires, the British and the French, but both were so constrained fiscally and domestically that they could not preserve the fruits of their victory.

And yet, disastrous as the war was, its proximate impact in terms of lives lost was exceeded by that of the influenza pandemic that broke out in its final year. Where exactly the new strain of H1N1 first appeared is uncertain, but it is usually said to have been Fort Riley, Kansas, the site of Camp Funston, one of the network of Army camps where hundreds of thousands of young American men were being trained to fight in Europe as the American Expeditionary Forces. There is, however, evidence that the pandemic originated in the British Army in 1917, though the condition was initially identified as "purulent bronchitis with bronchopneumonia."[85] Here was the key to influenza's twentieth-century success. Never had armies been mobilized on such a scale before—more than seventy million men in uniform. Never had so many young men been taken from their homes and workplaces, crowded into primitive accommodations, and sent over long distances in ships and trains. The idea that the virus originated in pigs has been refuted (an avian origin seems more likely);[86] if anything, the direction of infection was from men to pigs.[87] And why not? Not for nothing were German conscripts known as *Frontschweine*.

The first American cases were recorded at Camp Funston on March 4.[88] A week later, a member of Fort Riley's catering staff entered the infirmary, followed in the coming days by a stream of infected soldiers. By the end of the month, more than a thousand cases had been recorded and forty-eight men had died of influenza. As if to mock the efforts of men to kill one another, the virus spread rapidly across the United States and then crossed to Europe on the jam-packed American troopships. It is possible that the pandemic explains the near doubling of the proportion of German soldiers reporting sick in the summer of 1918, which was a crucial factor in the imperial army's subsequent collapse.[89] Certainly, we have reports of German prisoners of war with the flu from July.[90] By that time it had reached India, Australia, and New Zealand. A few months later, a second and deadlier wave struck all but simultaneously in Brest, France; Freetown, Sierra Leone; and Boston.[91] The virus made a new landfall in the United States at Boston's Commonwealth Pier on August 27, 1918, when three cases of influenza appeared on the sick list. Eight cases emerged the next day, and fifty-eight the next, fifteen of whom were so ill they were transferred to the U.S. Naval Hospital in Chelsea. On September 8, influenza arrived at the Army's Camp Devens. Within ten days, thousands of feverish patients overwhelmed the camp's hospitals; within weeks, the morgue was full of blue-tinged, asphyxiated corpses. (Few patients who developed the distinctive heliotrope cyanosis survived.) The epidemic then traveled west and south across the country, reaching its high point in terms of mortality in the week of October 4.[92] A third wave affected some areas of the world in early 1919, principally England, Wales, and Australia. There was something like a fourth wave in Scandinavia in 1920. Combatant countries sought to suppress the news of the pandemic as potentially harmful to wartime morale; this hardly helped to keep the public informed. The disease came to be known as the Spanish flu because only the largely uncensored press of neutral Spain reported on it with any accuracy.

Between 40 and 50 million people died as a result of the pandemic, the majority of them suffocated by a lethal accumulation of blood and other fluid in the lungs. The absolute numbers were highest in India (18.5 million deaths) and China (between 4.0 and 9.5 million), but death rates varied widely from place to place. Close to half (44.5 percent) of the population of Cameroon was wiped out; in Western Samoa, nearly a quarter (23.6 percent). In Kenya and Fiji, more than 5 percent of the people died. The other sub-Saharan countries for which we have data suffered mortality of between 2.4 percent (Nigeria) and 4.4 percent (South Africa). In Central America, mortality was also high: 3.9 percent of the population of Guatemala, 2 percent of all Mexicans. Indonesia also had a high death rate (3 percent). The worst mortality rates in Europe were in Hungary and Spain (each around 1.2 percent), with Italy not far behind. By contrast, North America got off lightly: between 0.53 and 0.65 percent for the United States, 0.61 percent for Canada. Brazil had a similar death rate; Argentina and Uruguay were largely spared.[93] As these figures imply, the Spanish flu was indifferent as to a country's combatant status. While its initial spread may have been related to wartime accommodation and transportation, that soon ceased to be true.

In the United Kingdom, the official death toll was over 150,000, but a modern estimate is closer to 250,000, including associated deaths from encephalitis lethargica, plus another five thousand aborted births (pregnant women had a shockingly high mortality rate).[94] In the United States, the deaths of as many as 675,000 people were attributed to the Spanish flu, of which 550,000 were excess deaths (above what would have been expected in that period under normal circumstances). Equivalent mortality in 2020 would have been between 1.8 and 2.2 million Americans. The Spanish flu killed an order of magnitude more Americans than died in combat in the war (53,402). According to the War Department's figures, influenza sickened 26 percent of the Army—more than one million men—and killed almost thirty thousand trainees before they even got to France.[95] Ironically, unlike most flu epidemics, but like the war that preceded and spread it, the influenza of 1918 disproportionately killed young adults. Out of 272,500 male influenza deaths in the

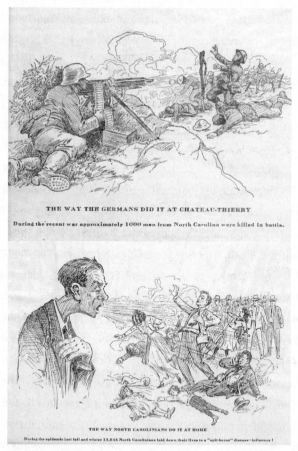

THE WAY THE GERMANS DID IT AT CHATEAU-THIERRY

During the recent war approximately 1000 men from North Carolina were killed in battle.

THE WAY NORTH CAROLINIANS DO IT AT HOME

During the epidemic last fall and winter 13,644 North Carolinians laid down their lives to a "spit-borne" disease—influenza !

"The way the Germans did it at Chateau-Thierry" and "The way North Carolinians do it at home."

United States, nearly 49 percent were aged twenty to thirty-nine, whereas only 18 percent were under five and 13 percent were over fifty.[96] The very young and very old were also (as usual) vulnerable, so that all countries for which age-specific death rates are available recorded a roughly W-shaped age distribution of mortality; this was also true in Australia, India, New Zealand, South Africa, and the United Kingdom, where 45 percent of all civilian deaths were people aged fifteen to thirty-five.[97] Death was not caused by the influenza virus itself so much as by the body's immunological reaction to the virus. Perversely, this meant that individuals with the strongest immune systems were more likely to die than those with weaker immune systems. A good illustration of the impact of the pandemic on young adults, as well as a vivid description of the hallucinogenic miseries of the illness itself, can be found in Katherine Anne Porter's short story "Pale Horse, Pale Rider" (1937), about a wartime romance cut cruelly short by the virus.[98]

Cholera had been class conscious. Influenza was thought not to be. In England, the registrar-general argued that the incidence of the Spanish flu varied "definitely, though not greatly with social class." His counterpart in Scotland asserted that "the most outstanding feature of the distribution of the mortality" was "its universality."[99] According to *The Times,* "the town-dweller fared no better than the peasant, the white man than the black or the yellow, the dweller among snows than the dweller in tropical jungles. The only immunity in all this slaying—and it was but relative—was enjoyed by the very young and the very old. For these, and for these alone, the monster seemed to have small appetite."[100] In truth, there were significant differences throughout the British Empire, but they had little to do with class. There was somewhat higher mortality in the poorest, least salubrious parts of London, but the correlation with wealth was not especially strong. The Tyneside towns of Hebburn and Jarrow were hit hard, but that reflected the high proportion of men employed in ships and boats, who were occupationally more likely to be exposed to the virus. In New Zealand, however, the Maori death rate was almost twice that of the white population.[101] The Inuit and other indigenous peoples in Canada also suffered much higher mortality than Canadians of European descent.

There was considerable regional variation in the United States.[102] Infection rates ranged widely, from 18.5 percent in New London, Connecticut, to 53.5 percent in San Antonio, with an overall infection rate of 29.3 percent, implying an infection fatality rate of 1.82 percent.[103] Mortality rates in Indiana and New York were three times higher than in a non-pandemic year, whereas in Montana the 1918 rate was more than six times higher. Colorado, Maryland, and Pennsylvania were also hit hard. The cities with the highest 1918 mortality rates (Pittsburgh, Scranton, and Philadelphia) were all located in Pennsylvania, and the cities with the lowest rates (Grand Rapids, Minneapolis, and Toledo) were all located in the Midwest. For no obvious reason, Darien and Milford, Connecticut, had no deaths at all. In all cities, the 1918 influenza mortality rate was at least twice the normal rate, but it was at least three times higher in Memphis, St. Louis, and Indianapolis and four times higher in Nashville and Kansas City. White influenza mortality rates were typically lower than those for blacks, but this difference decreased in the influenza pandemic of 1918. A Public Health Service survey of more than 100,000 individuals conducted in nine cities during the summer of 1919 indicated that the mortality rate of whites "was nearly twice as great among the 'very poor' as among the 'well-to-do' and those classified as in 'moderate' circumstances."[104]

How far did these differences reflect state or municipal policies? It has been suggested that, in the United States, non-pharmaceutical interventions at the local level not only reduced the public health impact of the pandemic but also expedited economic recovery, but on closer inspection the picture is somewhat less clear.[105] Except in New York and Chicago, state and local officials all across the country shuttered schools and churches. On the other hand, the campaign to sell the Fourth Liberty Loan—$6 billion of war bonds— meant that multiple public meetings and mass rallies took place in September and October. Restaurants were not closed.[106] New York kept not only schools but also theaters open. The city's principal innovation was the introduction of staggered business hours to keep crowding on subways to a minimum.[107] Matters were not helped by the insouciance of Dr. Royal Copeland, the New York

City health commissioner, who insisted in August that "there was not the slightest danger of an epidemic of Spanish Influenza in New York." An optometrist with little training in public health, Copeland felt obliged to understate the risk at every opportunity. When the first cases arrived from Norway in August, he did not quarantine them, asking breezily, "You haven't heard of our doughboys getting it, have you? You bet you haven't, and you won't. . . . No need for our people to worry over the matter." As the contagion spread in late September, Copeland insisted that the "situation was well in hand in all five boroughs, and . . . there was little fear that the disease would spread to any great extent." When the number of new cases doubled over a twenty-four-hour period in late September, he continued to take few precautions, aside from warning against coughing and sneezing in public. Even when 999 cases were reported on a single day in early October, Copeland refused to close schools, against the advice of his counterpart in Philadelphia.

The ineptitude of Copeland finally prompted a public intervention by a former health commissioner, Dr. S. S. Goldwater, who warned in *The New York Times* that conditions were "far worse than the public is aware and that unless help comes from the government, should the epidemic spread, there will be danger that many will suffer for lack of care." Two weeks later, the mayor of the city, John Hylan, publicly complained that "the Health Department [had] failed to check the spread of the disease" when it did not attempt to quarantine the city's first victims. By this time (October 27, 1918), the Public Health Committee of the New York Academy of Medicine estimated that "418,781 persons [had] been afflicted with influenza since it first appeared in the city." In a city of approximately 5.6 million people, this meant that at least one in every thirteen New Yorkers had the Spanish flu. When the pandemic was over, it had killed around 33,000 people in the city.[108] There seems little doubt that closing schools would have reduced this death toll. Cities that not only closed schools but also banned public gatherings early, notably St. Louis, fared appreciably better than those that delayed action, such as Pittsburgh.[109] In San Francisco, at the instigation of the health commissioner, Dr. William C. Hassler, mask wearing was made mandatory in October and November 1918 and again in January 1919, eliciting a familiar reaction from a motley coalition of civil libertarians, Christian Scientists, and economic interest groups that coalesced in the Anti-Mask League.[110]

The Spanish influenza was a public health disaster more than it was an economic disaster.[111] Clearly, there were adverse economic effects, especially in the countries that were hardest hit.[112] The Indian experience, though horrific, was in many ways Malthusian: the survivors in the most affected areas were left with additional land, which raised per capita wealth, which led not only to larger families but also to more investment in the education of children.[113] By contrast, the pandemic had enduring negative effects on Brazil's interwar economic development.[114] In the United States, newspapers reported steep declines in the retail sector (aside from the drugstores) in Little Rock and "crippling" industrial labor shortages due to illness in Memphis.[115] But the net impact was a recession of "exceptional brevity and moderate amplitude," according to a 1946 review of U.S. business cycles, not least because such interventions in economic life as took place were of very short duration (around four weeks).[116] There was a postwar recession in 1920–21, but it had nothing to do with the pandemic two years earlier and everything to do with fiscal and monetary tightening.[117] The Second Federal Reserve District's monthly reports, which covered New York, Chicago, and New England, show that economic activity was relatively strong in 1919. The percentage of firms failing declined in 1918 and 1919. There was a surge of building activity in New York and northern New Jersey in 1919. All indicators show that it was in 1920–21 that the economy contracted. The only clear connection between the pandemic and the recession was the fact that above-average influenza deaths among prime-age adults were associated with above-average business failures in 1919 and 1920. Paradoxically, the epidemic was positively correlated with subsequent economic growth in the 1920s.[118] However, such correlations fail to capture a much longer-lasting adverse effect of the pandemic: the fact that Americans who were in utero during the pandemic had, over the course of their lives, reduced educational attainment, higher rates of physical disability, and lower income relative to those who went through fetal development immediately before or after.[119] Those born at the crests of the three waves also had higher lifetime risk from respiratory and cardiovascular diseases.[120] Similar impacts on fetal development have also been found for other countries, including Brazil, Italy, Norway, Sweden,[121] Switzerland, and Taiwan.[122] There is also some evidence that the Spanish flu eroded social trust in the countries most adversely affected.[123]

TWIN CONTAGIONS

The influenza pandemic of 1918–19 shattered the illusion of inexorable medical progress as completely as the war that preceded it (and perhaps caused it) had shattered the illusion of inexorable economic and political progress. Numerous vaccines against the Spanish flu were devised and distributed in the United States in 1918–19; in truth, they were at best placebos.[124] Science had won some significant victories in the preceding century. The men with the microscopes had found vaccines or therapies, however imperfect, for smallpox, typhoid, malaria, yellow fever, cholera, and diphtheria. But they had no answer for the new strain of influenza, as Dr. William Henry Welch, of Johns Hopkins University, realized when he performed his first autopsy on a Spanish flu victim at Camp Devens, Massachusetts, in late September 1918. Contemplating the blue, swollen lungs filled with a thin, bloody, frothy fluid, Welch could say only, "This must be some new kind of infection or plague."[125] The German bacteriologist Richard Pfeiffer claimed to have identified the bacillus responsible; he was wrong. The only real remedies—quarantines, masks, prohibitions on meetings—were the old ones that long predated microscopes. Not until 1933 did a team of British scientists succeed in isolating the virus that had caused the Spanish flu.[126]

It has been suggested that "the pandemic of 1918, horrifying as it was, did little to affect political and social alterations already made by the war."[127] This is difficult to accept. The impact of the First World War on India, to take just one example, was modest, though 1.5 million Indian servicemen played an important part in the defense of the British Empire, serving in almost every theater of the conflict.[128] The impact of the pandemic, by contrast, was catastrophic, killing 240 times more Indians (18 million, as compared with around

74,000). In Britain itself, the ineffectual response of the medical authorities—under the Local Government Board since 1871—shattered the myth that Britain led the world in public health. It is no coincidence that a Ministry of Health was created in June 1919. Moreover, to an extent that should not be forgotten, the Spanish flu also afflicted the world's political and intellectual elite. Among the millions of victims of the pandemic were Louis Botha, the first prime minister of the Union of South Africa; Yakov Sverdlov, the Bolshevik chairman of the All-Russian Central Executive Committee (very likely the man who ordered the execution of Tsar Nicholas II and his family); the German sociologist Max Weber, one of the architects of the Weimar Republic's constitution; the Austrian artists Gustav Klimt and Egon Schiele; and the Brazilian president-elect, Francisco de Paula Rodrigues Alves, who early in his career had faced riots against public health measures in Rio. (Frederick Trump, the German-born paternal grandfather of the forty-fifth president of the United States, was another victim, though hardly a member of the elite.)

The years 1918 and 1919 were years of sickness as well as death. John Maynard Keynes, the most influential economist of his generation, was among those who fell ill. Keynes was in Paris, attending the peace conference that would ultimately produce the Treaty of Versailles. On May 30, 1919, he wrote to his mother, "Partly out of misery and rage for all that's happening and partly from prolonged overwork, I gave way last Friday and took to my bed from sheer nervous exhaustion, where I have remained ever since." He remained prostrate for close to a week, getting up only for meetings with the prime minister, David Lloyd George, and "a daily stroll in the Bois" de Boulogne. Did Keynes have the dreaded Spanish flu, as Lloyd George did? We cannot be sure. If so, he was lucky to survive it.[129] A later bout of influenza would undoubtedly contribute to the heart condition that cut Keynes's life short.

The most eminent person who contracted Spanish flu was President Woodrow Wilson, who fell ill on April 3, 1919, at a crucial stage in the four-power negotiations over the Versailles Treaty. For three days he lay in bed, unable to move. Wilson recovered, but he was a changed man. ("He manifested peculiarities," as his secretary put it, a view shared by Herbert Hoover, among others.) On a number of points of disagreement with the European leaders, Wilson now abruptly yielded.[130] The president returned from Europe exhausted and suffered a severe stroke in October 1919. He was largely incapacitated in 1920 and deemed by his own party unfit to run for reelection that year. Some historians blame the failure of the United States to ratify the Versailles Treaty and join the League of Nations on Wilson's illness, but the main obstacle was the febrile popular mood, agitated by the influenza pandemic, a postwar "Red Scare," the passage of women's suffrage, widespread race riots and lynchings, and the enactment of Prohibition, over Wilson's veto. Wilson had already lost control of both houses of Congress in 1918, when the Republicans gained a narrow majority of two in the Senate. Among the senators elected was Albert B. Fall, a New Mexico Republican whom Wilson had made the mistake of criticizing—at a time when Fall was grieving over the deaths from influenza of his only son and one of his daughters.[131] Two years later, with 60 percent of the popular vote and 404 electoral votes, the Republican candidate, Ohio senator Warren G. Harding, resoundingly won the 1920 election with the slogan "Return to Normalcy." The Democratic candidate, James M. Cox, was swept away in the largest electoral landslide since James Monroe's uncontested 1820 bid for the presidency. The Republicans also bolstered their majorities in both the Senate and the House.

There was an inescapable dualism about the way the First World War ended. Even as a viral contagion swept the world, so, too, did an ideological pandemic. The ideas of Vladimir Ilyich Lenin and his fellow Bolsheviks spread across the Russian Empire and seemed capable of producing outbreaks all over the world, even as Wilson's own principle of national self-determination threatened to undermine colonial rule from Egypt to Korea. In the eyes of many contemporaries, these two phenomena were intertwined. At the height of the Russian Civil War, during which typhus claimed up to three million lives, Lenin declared that "either socialism will defeat the louse or the louse will defeat socialism."[132] It was not long before anti-Bolsheviks in Europe— among them an abrasive orator named Adolf Hitler—were using biological metaphors to characterize the ideology of the Soviet regime as well as the Jews within their own countries, whom they regarded as Lenin's confederates. "Don't think that you can combat racial tuberculosis," Hitler declared in

August 1920, "without seeing to it that the people is freed from the causative organ of racial tuberculosis. The impact of Jewry will never pass away, and the poisoning of the people will not end, as long as the causal agent, the Jew, is not removed from our midst."[133] In *Mein Kampf,* the rambling tract Hitler wrote in prison after the failed Beer Hall Putsch of 1923, he elaborated on the theme, denouncing "the Jew" as "the typical parasite, a sponger who like a noxious bacillus keeps spreading as soon as a favorable medium invites him. And the effect of his existence is also like that of spongers: wherever he appears, the host people dies out after a shorter or longer period."[134] The book is shot through with lurid imagery drawn from the realm of medicine. Germany, Hitler argued, was diseased, and only he and his followers knew how to cure it. In this sadistic synthesis of racial prejudice and pseudoscience lies the origins of the most terrible of all man-made disasters—most terrible because it was carried out by a highly educated people, employing the most advanced technologies, and often claiming to act on the basis of science. There was a bitter irony when, in 1941 and again in 1942, in the midst of the Holocaust, Hitler likened himself to Robert Koch. "He discovered the bacillus and thereby ushered medical science onto new paths," declared Hitler. "I discovered the Jew as the bacillus and fermenting agent of all social decomposition."[135] It is easy to forget that, once upon a time, eugenics and racial hygiene also seemed to be embraced, near universally, as "settled science."[136]

6

===

THE PSYCHOLOGY OF
POLITICAL INCOMPETENCE

Mit der Dummheit kämpfen Götter selbst vergebens. (Against stupidity even the gods struggle in vain.)

—Friedrich Schiller

TOLSTOY VS. NAPOLEON

There is a well-understood psychology of military incompetence.[1] Is it possible to define a similar psychology of political incompetence? Norman Dixon argued that military life, with all its tedium, repels the talented, leaving mediocrities, lacking in intelligence and initiative, to rise through the ranks. By the time they reach senior decision-making positions, these people tend to have suffered some intellectual decay. A bad commander, Dixon observed, is unwilling or unable to change course when he has made the wrong decision. To reassure himself of the rightness of his decision, and to try to resolve his cognitive dissonance, he will be inclined to pontificate.[2] Symptoms of military incompetence include the tendencies to waste human and other resources; to cling to outworn traditions without profiting from past experience; to misuse or neglect to use available technology; to reject or ignore information that conflicts with one's preconceptions; to underestimate the enemy and overestimate one's own side; to abdicate from the role of decision maker; to persist in a given strategy despite strong evidence that it is defective; to "pull punches" rather than push home an attack; to neglect reconnaissance; to order frontal assaults, often against the enemy's strongest point; to prefer brute force over surprise or deception; to seek scapegoats for setbacks; to suppress or distort news from the front; to believe in mystical forces such as fate and luck.[3] Dixon identifies two distinct types of incompetents in British military history: the "mild, courteous and peaceful men who, though no doubt caring deeply about the fearful losses which their armies suffered, seemed quite incapable of ame-liorating the situation," and those "whose besetting sin was an overweening ambition coupled with a terrifying insensitivity to the suffering of others."[4] It may already have struck the reader that at least some of these characteristics are to be found in the realm of civilian administration, too.

At the same time, we must not make a fetish of leadership, whether mil-itary or civilian. As Carl von Clausewitz long ago argued persuasively, the mo-rale of an army is as important a variable in battle as the quality of its generals. In the language of a more recent writer, the defeat of an army is above all a result of its "organizational breakdown," which may come about because of heavy casualties, or surprising setbacks, or difficulties with the terrain or the weather.[5] As we shall see, the phenomenon of organizational breakdown can afflict "frock coats" as well as "brass hats." How far can or should any catas-trophe be attributed to one individual? In a striking passage in *War and Peace,* Tolstoy tries to show how little of the events of 1812 could be explained with reference to the emperor Napoleon's will. The French invasion of Russia, Tol-stoy writes, was "an event . . . opposed to human reason and to human nature":

> Millions of men perpetrated against one another such innumerable crimes, frauds, treacheries, thefts, forgeries, issues of false money, bur-glaries, incendiarisms, and murders as in whole centuries are not re-corded in the annals of all the law courts of the world, but which those who committed them did not at the time regard as being crimes.
>
> What produced this extraordinary occurrence? What were its causes? The historians tell us with naive assurance that its causes were the

wrongs inflicted on the Duke of Oldenburg, the nonobservance of the Continental System, the ambition of Napoleon, the firmness of [Tsar] Alexander, the mistakes of the diplomatists, and so on. . . .

To us, to posterity who view the thing that happened in all its magnitude and perceive its plain and terrible meaning, these causes seem insufficient. . . . We cannot grasp what connection such circumstances have with the actual fact of slaughter and violence: why because the Duke was wronged, thousands of men from the other side of Europe killed and ruined the people of Smolensk and Moscow and were killed by them.

In reality, Tolstoy proposes, "the actions of Napoleon and Alexander, on whose words the event seemed to hang, were as little voluntary as the actions of any soldier who was drawn into the campaign by lot or by conscription."

This could not be otherwise, for in order that the will of Napoleon and Alexander (on whom the event seemed to depend) should be carried out, the concurrence of innumerable circumstances was needed without any one of which the event could not have taken place. It was necessary that millions of men in whose hands lay the real power—the soldiers who fired, or transported provisions and guns—should consent to carry out the will of these weak individuals, and should have been induced to do so by an infinite number of diverse and complex causes.

Ultimately, argues Tolstoy, "A king is history's slave.

History, that is, the unconscious, general, hive life of mankind, uses every moment of the life of kings as a tool for its own purposes.

Though Napoleon at that time, in 1812, was more convinced than ever that it depended on him . . . he had never been so much in the grip of inevitable laws, which compelled him, while thinking that he was acting on his own volition, to perform for the hive life—that is to say, for history—whatever had to be performed. . . . In historic events the so-called great men are labels giving names to events, and like labels they have but the smallest connection with the event itself.[6]

This is not a fashionable view of the historical process nowadays, and it is easy to see why. "Inevitable laws" of history are generally scoffed at; the public remains wedded to the "great man" school of history, even if academic historians eschew it. There is a mystical aspect to Tolstoy's reasoning, as if the "power that moves nations" is a supernatural force. Yet his argument can easily be updated. Formally, a leader sits atop a hierarchical organizational chart, issuing edicts that are transmitted down to the lowliest functionary. In reality, leaders are hubs in large and complex networks. The extent of their power is in fact a function of their centrality. If they are well connected to the political class, the bureaucracy, the media, and the wider public—if information flows in both directions, so that they can be informed as well as command—then they can be effective leaders. To be isolated within the structure of power is to be doomed to impotence, no matter how grand one's title. To be sure, political uses can be made of expert knowledge. Career bureaucrats and academic advisers can be manipulated into legitimizing a partisan objective.[7] But it is also true that bureaucrats can manipulate their supposed masters, presenting them—in a way memorably described by Henry Kissinger—with three alternatives, only one of which is plausible, namely the one the civil servants have already decided on.[8] And it is true, too, that in a democracy the electorate may decline to be manipulated. A civilian leader nominally stands at the head of a motley, unruly, untrained army. But the line of least resistance may be to admit, echoing the radical republican Alexandre-Auguste Ledru-Rollin in 1848, "I am their leader; I must follow them!" ("Je suis leur chef; il faut que je les suive!")[9]

We think, without reflecting too deeply, that we understand the difference between a natural and a man-made disaster. We classify volcanic eruptions, earthquakes, floods, and famines as natural disasters, and wars, violent revolutions, and economic crises as man-made, allowing that some man-made disasters are more deliberate than others. Thus, most historians would now

agree that Hitler's extermination of the Jews was intended and for years premeditated. Yet if we consistently apply the Tolstoyan principle, even the Holocaust becomes hard to represent as solely the result of one man's psychopathic
anti-Semitism. An entire school of historiography—unattractively referred to
as "structural functionalists"—sought to explain that the attempted extermination of the Jews of Europe took place because, in the abnormal circumstances created by the Second World War, a great many Germans, whether
out of ideological conviction, a hunger for loot, or simple moral cowardice, actively "worked towards the Führer" without needing direct written orders to
perpetrate genocide. And why had the war begun? The official reason was
that Hitler had demanded the handover of the "free city" of Danzig and a pleb-
iscite in the "corridor" of Polish territory taken from Germany in 1920, Poland
had refused, and Britain and France were then obliged to honor their treaty
commitments to Warsaw. This seems as satisfactory as the theory, mocked by
Tolstoy, that France had invaded Russia in 1812 over "the wrongs inflicted on
the Duke of Oldenburg."

DEMOCRACY VS. FAMINE

How truly natural are natural disasters? In two seminal works—*Poverty and
Famines* (1983) and *Development as Freedom* (1999)—the Indian economist
Amartya Sen challenged the widespread view of famines as natural rather
than man-made disasters. Far from being caused by insufficient food supply,
Sen argued, famines occur when the price of food rises beyond the means of
lower-income groups—they are, in short, entitlement failures. Most famines
could therefore be prevented by boosting wages through schemes of public
works, or by banning hoarding and speculation.[10] "No famine has ever taken
place in the history of the world in a functioning democracy," Sen argued,
because democratic governments "have to win elections and face public
criticism, and have [a] strong incentive to undertake measures to avert famines and other catastrophes."[11] Reflecting on the disastrous famine Mao Zedong's government inflicted on China, Sen argued that even a fraction of the

Chinese death toll "would have immediately caused a storm in the newspapers and a turmoil in the Indian parliament, and the ruling government would almost certainly have had to resign."[12]

Sen's arguments are largely borne out by the examples of the worst famines of the past three centuries. In *The Wealth of Nations,* Adam Smith made the bold claim that in the two centuries prior to his writing, no famine had arisen in "any part of Europe . . . from any other cause but the violence of Government attempting, by improper means, to remedy the inconveniences of a dearth."[13] However, the French famines of 1693–94 and 1709–10—during the reign of the absolutist "Sun King," Louis XIV—seem to have been classic Sen-type examples of markets failing in the wake of disastrously bad harvests, and of unaccountable authorities doing too little in the way of relief for the starving. In the earlier of the two crises, an estimated 1.3 million people died—around 6 percent of the French population.[14] The rapacity of the East India Company—which was accountable only to its stockholders and, in the end, the British Parliament—bore almost the entirety of the blame for the catastrophic Bengal Famine of 1770, which killed between one and two million people, or up to 7 percent of the population.[15]

The proximate cause of the disastrous Irish Famine of the late 1840s was a fungal spore named *Phytophthora infestans,* which destroyed potato crops with devastating speed, at a time when potatoes accounted for 60 percent of Ireland's food supply and 40 percent of households depended almost entirely on potatoes for subsistence. The "blight" arrived in Ireland from North America via Belgium in 1845 and recurred in all but one year until 1850. Around three quarters of the potato crop was lost in 1846. By 1848, acreage under potatoes was barely more than 15 percent of its 1845 level. Because of this disruption of the rural population's principal source of calories, production of other crops such as wheat and oats also declined. Between 1846 and 1849, the number of pigs in Ireland fell by 86 percent. The rural population had little or no access to credit to offset the shock, apart from what was provided by around three hundred Irish Loan Funds, an early form of microfinance.[16] The death toll is estimated to have been around one million, or about 11 percent of the pre-famine population of approximately 8.75 million.[17] Another million people emigrated from Ireland, most to North America.

Ireland was not Bengal. Irishmen sat in both houses at Westminster. True, the Irish aristocracy was Anglo-Irish, separate in religious, cultural, and often linguistic terms from the mass of people. True, the franchise was more restricted than in England in both urban and rural constituencies: there were only around ninety thousand voters after the electoral reforms of 1829 and 1832.[18] Still, there were elected Irish representatives in the House of Commons, including the impressive Daniel O'Connell—"the Liberator"—who in January 1847 presided over a meeting in Dublin of Irish landowners and politicians to demand a government response to the disaster.[19] Yet key decision makers, such as Charles Trevelyan, the assistant secretary of the Treasury, subscribed to doctrines of evangelical Christianity and political economy that argued against government intervention. "It is hard upon the poor people that they should be deprived of knowing that they are suffering from an affliction of God's providence," Trevelyan wrote on January 6, 1847. As God had ordained the famine "to teach the Irish a lesson, that calamity must not be too much mitigated. . . . The real evil with which we have to contend is not the physical evil of the Famine, but the moral evil of the selfish, perverse and turbulent character of the people."[20] On the basis of such arguments, exports of grain (mostly oats) from Ireland were not suspended.

To be sure, some steps were taken to alleviate starvation and the diseases that followed hard on its heels. In 1846 Sir Robert Peel's Conservative government had repealed the Corn Laws, protectionist tariffs that had hitherto impeded cheap grain imports to the United Kingdom. There were imports to Ireland of maize and cornmeal from America, some public works schemes, and substantial charitable donations: with the support of the royal family and the Rothschilds, the British Association for the Relief of the Extreme Distress in the Remote Parishes of Ireland and Scotland raised some £470,000 in the course of its existence. The government itself raised an £8 million Irish Famine Loan in 1847.[21] But these measures were not nearly enough to offset the collapse of rural incomes at a time of severe dearth. The prevailing mood in

London after Peel's downfall over the Corn Laws was one of indifference, if not contempt, toward the Irish. "Rotten potatoes have done it all," complained the Duke of Wellington at the time of the Tory schism over the Corn Laws. "They put Peel in his damned fright."[22] "For our parts," commented *The Times*, "we regard the potato blight as a blessing. When the Celts once cease to be potatophagi, they must be carnivorous. With the taste for meats will grow the appetite for them; with the appetite the readiness to earn them. With this will come steadiness, regularity, and perseverance; unless, indeed, the growth of these qualities be impeded by the blindness of Irish patriotism, the short-sighted indifference of petty landlords, or the random recklessness of Government benevolence."[23] As the chancellor of the Exchequer, Sir Charles Wood, explained to the House of Commons, "No exertions of a Government, or, I will add, of private charity, can supply a complete remedy for the existing calamity. It is a national visitation, sent by Providence."*[24]

It might be thought that no two ideologies had less in common than the classical liberalism of the Victorians and the bloody Marxism of the Bolsheviks; yet each in its different way could rationalize mass starvation. Nevertheless, there were important differences. There were two serious famines in the history of the Soviet Union: one in 1921–23, the other in 1932–33. As a Ukrainian historian has written, "Grain requisition and export—not drought and poor harvest—were the real causes of the first great famine in Soviet Ukraine which occurred in 1921–1923."[25] A hot, rainless spring in 1920 set the stage, but the principal drivers of famine were a shortage of labor due to the ongoing civil war and a reluctance on the part of the peasantry, fearful of grain requisitions, to plant the fields. The twenty most productive agricultural prov-

---

*In fairness to the much-maligned Wood, he acknowledged "the awful calamity which has visited Ireland" and was at pains to explain the government's efforts, through public works, to "put into the hands of the people of Ireland the means of purchasing that food which heretofore they had raised for themselves, but which, through the failure of the potato crop, they had no longer the means of providing for themselves, and were, therefore, under the necessity of buying." The fact that public works schemes had proved insufficient because many people were too famished to work had persuaded Wood of the necessity to distribute imported food. His peroration therefore deserves to be quoted more fully than is usual: "We cannot conceal from ourselves that hundreds are dying every week from want. I can assure the House, that it is with pain I can ill attempt to describe, that I peruse the accounts which day after day reach us of the deaths by starvation in the west of Ireland. No exertions of a Government, or, I will add, of private charity, can supply a complete remedy for the existing calamity. It is a national visitation, sent by Providence; and we must, if not to the extent which some hon. Gentlemen have contemplated, still, to a large extent . . . come forward and assist our suffering brethren in Ireland. Sir, I do not believe this country will refuse to render assistance, or will be disposed to withhold its aid under such an extremity."

inces in imperial Russia had annually produced 22 million tons of grain before the revolution. By 1921 output was down to 2.9 million. The crisis was
especially acute in Ukraine. In 1921 the amount of grain harvested in the
province of Odessa dropped to 12.9 percent of its pre-revolutionary level.[26]
Herbert Hoover's American Relief Administration estimated that around two
million people died—perhaps 1.3 percent of the pre-famine population. The
ARA withdrew from Russia in protest against the Bolsheviks' sales of grain in
exchange for hard currency, at a time when famine was ravaging large parts
of the territory they controlled. Unlike Victorian ministers, Bolshevik commis-
sars were accountable to no opposition. There was no free press in Russia to
condemn their conduct. But worse was to come.

The spring of 1931 was cool and dry throughout the Soviet Union: the
Volga region, Kazakhstan, Siberia, and central Ukraine all suffered episodes
of drought. However, the bad harvests of 1931 and 1932 would not have sufficed to cause a disastrous famine without the confusion caused by Stalin's policy of collectivization, which he had convinced himself was the only way to
expedite the industrialization (and proletarianization) of Russia and to stamp
out the supposedly counterrevolutionary kulak class. Far from increasing agricultural output, the abolition of private property and the herding of the peasantry into state collective farms obliterated incentives. Rather than lose it to
the state, farmers slaughtered and devoured their livestock. At the same time,
Stalin ramped up exports from 187,000 tons in 1929 to 5.7 million tons in
1931.[27] As famine ravaged Ukraine, the Politburo issued two decrees that explicitly blamed falling agricultural output on the 1920s policy of "Ukrainiza-
tion," which had granted a measure of autonomy to the Ukrainian Soviet
Republic. This led to a mass purge of Communist Party of Ukraine officials, as
well as verbal and then physical attacks on suspect academics and intellectuals. Under the leadership of Lazar Kaganovich,* the first secretary of the Ukrainian party, teams of "activists" marauded through the Ukrainian countryside
searching farmhouses from top to bottom for anything and everything edible.

---

*"Iron Lazar" had been born into a Jewish family in 1893. A ruthlessly murderous disciple of Stalin, he was
the longest-lived of the original "Old Bolshevik" revolutionaries. He died, aged ninety-seven, on July 25,
1991, just one month before the dissolution of the Communist Party of the Soviet Union, for which he had
sacrificed so many other people's lives.

Desperate neighbors informed on one another in the hope of being rewarded with a few crusts.[28] The mortality rate was three times higher in Ukraine than in Russia,[29] but things were even more desperate in Kazakhstan.

Some historians insist that it was not Stalin's intention to conduct a genocidal policy against the Ukrainians and Kazakh herders. Perhaps not, but Stalin's conception of class war implied not just terror but mass murder. As he put it to Mikhail Sholokhov, the author of *And Quiet Flows the Don,* in May 1933, "The esteemed grain growers of your region (and not only your region) carried out a sit-down strike (sabotage!) and would not have minded leaving the workers and the Red Army without bread. The fact that the sabotage was quiet and apparently harmless (bloodless) does not alter the fact that the esteemed grain growers were basically waging a 'quiet' war against Soviet power. A war by attrition (*voina na izmor*), dear Comrade Sholokhov . . ."[30] In all, an estimated five million Soviet citizens died, around 3 percent of the pre-famine population, but the proportion of Ukrainians who died was closer to 18 percent, making it the worst famine of modern times. The birthrate also collapsed. Had these policies not been adopted by Stalin, the Soviet population at the beginning of 1935 would have been around eighteen million higher. The difference between Victorian liberals and Soviet Communists should now be clear. Nature, in the form of a new pathogen, played a much larger role in the Irish Famine. The Ukrainian Holodomor, by contrast, was largely manmade and with malice aforethought.

The 1930s were a time of trouble for agriculture all over the world, to be sure. Beginning in 1932, persistent drought conditions on the North American Great Plains caused widespread crop failures and exposed the region's recently cultivated soil to strong winds. A large dust storm on May 11, 1934, swept soil particles as far as Washington, D.C., and three hundred miles out into the Atlantic Ocean. More intense and frequent storms swept the Plains in 1935. On March 6 and again on March 21, dust clouds passed over Washington. This was a disaster for farmers in Kansas, Oklahoma, Texas, New Mexico, and Colorado. Such droughts had affected the Great Plains in previous centuries;[31] indeed, the 1856–65 drought may have been even more severe. What made the 1930s so catastrophic was the unintended effects of the overhasty conversion of large tracts of the Great Plains to wheat and cotton fields.[32] Here was a different kind of politically caused disaster. The antithesis of the Soviet system, U.S. agriculture policy encouraged the private ownership and settlement of land. Legislation—the Homestead Act of 1862, the Kinkaid Act of 1904, the Enlarged Homestead Act of 1909—gave land away to the pioneering types who were willing to cultivate it. "The soil is the one indestructible, immutable asset that the nation possesses," the Federal Bureau of Soils declared. "It is the one resource that cannot be exhausted, that cannot be used up." Private developers made their own contribution. "Riches in the soil, prosperity in the air, progress everywhere. An Empire in the making!" proclaimed W. P. Soash, a real estate salesman from Iowa. "Get a farm in Texas while land is cheap—where every man is a landlord!" The Santa Fe Railway published a map that purported to show the "rain line"—rainfall of twenty inches or more annually—moving westward at the rate of eighteen miles a year. If they sowed the land, the rain would come. Towns such as Boise City, Oklahoma, a boomtown in the 1920s, were built on such promises.[33] Between the Civil War and the start of the 1930s, approximately a third of the U.S. Great Plains was converted to cropland. The high commodity prices caused by World War I and the availability of farm machinery on credit further encouraged the "great plow-up."[34] As prices fell in the 1920s and collapsed after 1929, the scrabbling grew suddenly harder.

The result was an environmental disaster. Deep plowing and other methods used to prepare the land for cultivation eliminated those native prairie grasses that held the soil in place and retained moisture during periods of drought. When arid conditions caused crops to wither and die, topsoil lay exposed to the elements.[35] The first "black duster" or "black blizzard" occurred on September 14, 1930. The worst came on April 14, 1935, when multiple storms in a single afternoon moved twice as much dirt as had been dug in seven years to create the Panama Canal.[36] All this reduced the Great Plains farmers to a wretched poverty and forced many to migrate westward in a thankless quest for work (as depicted in John Steinbeck's *Grapes of Wrath*). Yet there was no mass starvation. And those who expressed their opposition to government policy—notably Hugh Hammond Bennett, the author of *Soil*

Erosion: A National Menace—were not persecuted but promoted. The National Industrial Recovery Act, passed in June 1933, established the Soil Erosion Service in the Department of the Interior. Bennett was put in charge of it in September 1933.[37] He also sat on the Great Plains Drought Area Committee, the interim report of which, on August 27, 1936, stated unequivocally, "Mistaken public policies have been largely responsible for the situation." Here was a level of accountability undreamt of by Ukrainians.

Which was worst: American capitalism, Soviet Communism, or British imperialism? One historian has gone so far as to describe famines in India in the 1870s and 1890s as "Late Victorian Holocausts."[38] This seems a bad analogy. Hitler set out to annihilate the Jews and could rely on German scientists, engineers, soldiers, and his own security services to devise the most ruthlessly efficient way to commit genocide. By contrast, as one of India's leading economic historians has shown, before 1900 "the prospect of devastating famines once every few years was inherent in India's ecology. . . . Famines were primarily environmental in origin," and after 1900 the problem had been somewhat mitigated by the greater integration of the Indian market for foodstuffs. The Indian mortality rate declined steeply between the 1920s and the 1940s, as did the death toll attributable to famines.[39] What went disastrously wrong in Bengal in 1943 cannot therefore be compared to what happened in Ukraine or Kazakhstan ten years before. Stalin was waging class war against Soviet citizens, threatening those who resisted with a bullet in the back of the head or the gulag. The British government of India was waging a defensive war against Imperial Japan, which enjoyed support from at least some Indian nationalist leaders, notably Subhas Chandra Bose and his Indian National Army. Nor was Gandhi's anti-British "Quit India" campaign exactly helpful in the fight against Japan. The fall of Burma to the Japanese in early 1942 was the first blow, as Bengal had come to rely quite heavily on Burmese rice imports. The poor wheat harvest in the Punjab and North India was the second blow. Then, on October 16, 1942, the coast of Bengal and Orissa was hit by a cyclone, flooding the rice paddies up to forty miles inland. The sea brought with it the fungal disease known as rice blast.[40] (The impact on Bengal's total food supply was in fact modest.) The government of India asked London for assistance, or at least to halt the export of food from India. However, the British War Cabinet declined. It also refused to make shipping available for relief supplies to India.

There were certainly other priorities to be considered, at a time when the British Empire was fighting for its life on multiple fronts. Still, Prime Minister Winston Churchill's lack of compassion for the Bengalis is undeniable. When Leo Amery, the secretary of state for India and Burma, pleaded for ships for India, Churchill replied with a reference to "Indians breeding like rabbits and being paid a million a day by us for doing nothing about the war."[41] Amery "lost patience and couldn't help telling him that I didn't see much difference between his outlook and Hitler's, which annoyed him no little."[42] (Amery later remarked that Churchill knew as much about India as George III had known about the American colonies.)[43] Only when the incoming viceroy, Field Marshal Archibald Wavell, threatened to resign did Churchill agree to send more food. The prime minister "seemed to regard sending food to India as an 'appeasement' of Congress," Wavell noted with unease.[44] Yet despite his cavils, Churchill delivered. By January 1944 a total of 130,000 tons of barley had been shipped from Iraq, 80,000 from Australia, 10,000 from Canada, and a further 100,000 more from Australia. By the end of the year a million tons of grain had been dispatched from Australia and the South East Asia Command.[45]

In seeking to lay the blame for the famine on Churchill, some historians have failed to heed the Tolstoy principle. The problem in Bengal was not simply the distant and hostile British prime minister but also the weakness of key British officials on the spot and the corruption of some local Bengali politicians, to whom much power had been delegated by the 1935 Government of India Act. The governor of Bengal, Sir John Herbert, was dying of cancer in Government House; the outgoing viceroy, the Marquess of Linlithgow, acquiesced as the other provincial governments kept their food to themselves, while price-fixing measures simply encouraged wholesalers to hoard. One of the villains of the piece was the minister for civil supplies, an Oxford graduate named Huseyn Shaheed Suhrawardy, who was suspected by Linlithgow's successor of having "siphoned money from every project that was undertaken to ease the famine, and awarded to his associates contracts for warehousing, the sale of grain to governments, and transportation."[46] (Hoary old arguments that the indigenous elites would treat the Indian masses worse than the British began to ring true.) As *The Statesman* put it on September 23, "This sickening catastrophe is man made"—the result of a "shameful lack of planning capacity and foresight by India's own civil Governments, Central and Provincial."[47] What changed the situation was in fact Churchill's decision to appoint Wavell as viceroy. Though Erwin Rommel had defeated him in the North African desert in 1941, Wavell was an intelligent and effective soldier and administrator. Having seen for himself the dire state of affairs in Calcutta, he ordered consignments of food from the rest of India, the creation of properly managed relief camps in the countryside around Calcutta, and military deliveries of "food for the people" to outlying villages. The death toll was still shockingly high: between 2.1 and 3 million people—up to 5 percent of the population of Bengal, though around 0.8 percent of the population of British India (see table below).

By contrast, when Stalinist strategy and tactics were imported into China by Mao Zedong, the results of a premeditated domestic policy to replace the market altogether were an order of magnitude worse. According to one recent account, forty-five million Chinese citizens died in the famine caused by Mao's "Great Leap Forward" between 1959 and 1961—just under 7 percent of the entire Chinese population—although estimates range from thirty to sixty million.[48] Convinced that collectivization and industrialization must be achieved in China, as they had been achieved by Stalin in the Soviet Union in the 1930s, the Communist Party elite encouraged officials in the provinces to set impossibly high procurement quotas. Grain was extracted from the provinces and sold by the central government for foreign currency that was then used to purchase manufacturing equipment. At the same time, peasants were diverted into crude forms of industrial production.[49] As in other famines, bad weather played a part, but a small one. "The illusion of superabundance" created by previous exaggerated reports of bumper harvests led some provinces (notably Sichuan) to face especially high procurement quotas.[50] The result was chaos and catastrophe: deforestation, demolition of buildings, the reckless overuse of pesticides, and the introduction of counterproductive farming methods such as "deep plowing" and excessively heavy concentrations of seed.[51] While driving down official rations to just twenty-nine to thirty-three pounds of grain per head each month, the party continued not only exporting food but also providing unrequited aid in the form of food to Albania and Guinea, and in the form of cash to Burma, Cambodia, and Vietnam.[52] Because China's storage-and-transport infrastructure was unequal to the task, there was colossal waste: crops were ruined by rats, by insects, by rot, by fire. In Hunan, the pig population shrank from 12.7 million to 3.4 million in 1961. Locusts infested fifty square miles in the Xiaogan region of Hubei alone. In Zhejiang Province, 10 percent of the harvest was lost in 1960 to snout moths, leafhoppers, pink bollworms, and red spiders. Deforestation and clumsy irrigation projects led to flooding.[53] A host of diseases flourished in a society profoundly weakened by hunger: polio, hepatitis, measles, malaria, diphtheria, meningitis, and even leprosy. The party encouraged brutal, humiliating violence against rule breakers. As in other (though not all) famines discussed here, there were numerous reports of cannibalism.[54]

MODERN FAMINES, 1770–1985[55]

		DEATHS (MILLIONS)			POPULATION			
	Year(s)	Minimum	Maximum	Best	Regional	Percent*	National	Percent†
Bengal (India)	1770	1.0	2.0	2.0	28.6	7.0%	180	1.1%
Ireland (UK)	1845–50	1.0	1.5	1.0	8.8	11.4%	27	3.7%
Soviet Union	1921–23	1.0	2.0	2.0	n/a	n/a	152.8	1.3%
Ukraine (USSR)	1932–33	3.9	5.0	5.0	28.0	17.9%	162	3.1%
Bengal (India)	1943–46	2.1	3.0	3.0	60.3	5.0%	389	0.8%
People's Republic of China	1958–62	30.0	60.0	45.0	n/a	n/a	653.2	6.9%
Ethiopia	1984–85	0.4	1.2	1.2	n/a	n/a	44.5	2.7%

*Affected region where applicable (e.g., Bengal, Ireland, Ukraine).

†Wider unit (e.g., India, UK, USSR).

These examples would seem to bear out Sen's core point that famines are at root political disasters, i.e., the authorities fail to mitigate market failures in conditions of dearth and acute poverty. Yet "market failure" hardly describes the Soviet and Chinese cases; in both, the market had been entirely abolished. The same applies to North Korea, which experienced famine as recently as the 1990s. In the case of Ethiopia, where up to 1.2 million people died between 1984 and 1985 (around 2.7 percent of the population), the culprit was again Marxism, not market failure. The Derg military dictatorship, led by Mengistu Haile Mariam, had come to power in the wake of the 1973–74 famine in the province of Wollo. After a campaign of "Red Terror" against its political rivals, the Derg had adopted the disastrous Stalin-Mao strategy of agricultural collectivization.[56] It instrumentalized the mid-1980s drought[57] as part of a counterinsurgency strategy directed mainly against the Tigray People's Liberation Front, the Oromo Liberation Front, and the Eritrean Liberation Front. As in the Soviet and Chinese cases, the goal was "social transformation" via deliberate starvation of politically suspect regions. Not coincidentally, the Marxist-Leninist Workers' Party of Ethiopia (WPE) was founded in early 1984, with Mengistu* as general secretary.[58] As a million Ethiopians starved, the streets of Addis Ababa were festooned with posters that read "The oppressed masses will be victorious," "Marxist Leninism is our guideline!" and "Temporary natural setbacks will not deter us from our final objective of building Communism!"[59] This reality was often missed in the emotive European response to the Ethiopian Famine, which culminated in the 1985 Live Aid concert, organized by the Irish singer Bob Geldof.[60] Nevertheless, Sen's broader point stands that the accountability of governments makes a difference. The other major famines in the world since 1945—Biafra in 1967–70, Bangladesh in 1974, Sudan in 1985, and Somalia in 1992 and 2011–12—were all closely associated with dictatorship, civil war, or state failure.

An interesting question, however, is why Sen's theory does not apply to all forms of disaster. If famines can be successfully avoided, or at least miti-

---

*Mengistu visited the United States three times between 1964 and 1970, attending officer training courses at the Savanna Army Depot, in Illinois, the Aberdeen Proving Ground, in Maryland, and the U.S. Army Combined Arms Center, in Fort Leavenworth, Kansas. According to one account, his experiences of racial prejudice did nothing to endear capitalism and democracy to him.

gated, when governments are more accountable, why is the same not true of earthquakes, floods, wildfires, or pandemics? Why should voters be effective in holding democratic governments responsible for ensuring a supply of affordable food, but not for keeping the air or water supply free from lethal viruses, or preventing people from building their homes on fault lines or floodplains? Or, to put it differently, why do democratic governments avoid one kind of disaster—famines—more successfully than others? Great Britain had representative government earlier than most countries. Yet the population of its capital city suffered recurrent, toxic "pea-souper" fogs during the nineteenth and twentieth centuries, which were attributable to the large-scale burning of coal for manufacture and domestic heating and cooking in the mist-prone setting of the banks of the river Thames. The Smoke Nuisance Abatement (Metropolis) Act of 1853, passed shortly after Dickens published the memorably foggy opening to Bleak House, failed to avert a major calamity in the severe winter of 1879–80, when a temperature inversion caused a thick layer of coal smog made up of sulfur dioxide, nitrogen dioxide, and other combustion particles to sit over the capital for three days, leading to nearly twelve thousand deaths.[61] Even an indignant pamphlet on the subject by Francis Albert Rollo Russell, the son of the former prime minister Lord John Russell, had little effect.[62] A similar disaster struck in December 1952, with a comparable death toll and 150,000 people hospitalized.[63] Recent research has shown that the naturally moist air and sunlight led to the formation of "very concentrated sulfuric acid droplets" in the fog.[64] Democratic pressures finally led to the passage of the Clean Air Act of 1956. But it is worth noting that socialism had played its part in the "Great Smog" four years before. The National Coal Board—a government-run monopoly established when the coal industry was nationalized, in 1947—had been marketing an exceptionally dirty and smoky coal derivative ("nutty slack") for use in household heating.[65] As recently as December 1991, London had another dire smog episode, though by this time traffic fumes had taken the place of coal as the primary pollutant. The monitoring site at Bridge Place, Victoria, recorded an hourly average nitrogen dioxide reading of 423 parts per billion, more than twice the WHO guideline level.[66]

Approaching disasters within this broader framework makes it clear that democratic institutions by themselves are far from a sufficient safeguard against disasters of all kinds—especially those that are not normally distributed but follow power-law distributions—regardless of whether we insist on classifying them as either natural or man-made.

DEMOCRACY AND WAR

Like many other statesmen of the time, Churchill was tempted to explain the First World War as a kind of natural disaster. "One must think of the intercourse of the nations in those days not as if they were chessmen on the board," he wrote in *The World Crisis* (1923), but as

> prodigious organisations of forces active or latent which, like planetary bodies, could not approach each other in space without giving rise to profound magnetic reactions. If they got too near, the lightnings would begin to flash, and beyond a certain point they might be attracted altogether from the orbits in which they were restrained and draw each other into dire collision. . . . In such grave and delicate conjunctions one violent move by any party would rupture and derange the restraints upon all, and plunge Cosmos into Chaos.[67]

The wartime prime minister, David Lloyd George, wrote in his memoirs of a "typhoon" and a "cataclysm." "The nations slithered over the brink into the boiling cauldron of war. . . . [They] backed their machines over the precipice."[68] In reality, the First World War was neither a natural disaster nor an accident. It came about because politicians and generals on both sides miscalculated. The Germans believed (not unreasonably) that the Russians were overtaking them militarily and so risked a preemptive strike before the strategic gap grew any wider. The Austrians failed to see that stamping on Serbia, useful though that might be in their war against Balkan terrorism, would embroil them in a Europe-wide conflagration. The Russians overestimated their own military capability almost as much as the Germans did; they also stubbornly ignored the evidence that their political system would crack under the strain of another war, so soon after the fiasco of defeat by Japan in 1905. Only the French and the Belgians had no real choice. The Germans invaded them; they had to fight.

The British, too, had the freedom to err. At the time, the government claimed that intervention was a matter of legal obligation, because the Germans had flouted the terms of the 1839 treaty governing Belgian neutrality, which all the great powers including Prussia had signed. In fact, Belgium was a useful pretext. The Liberals went to war for two reasons. First, they feared the consequences of a German victory over France, imagining the kaiser as a new Napoleon, bestriding the continent and menacing the Channel coast. That may or may not have been a legitimate fear, but if it was, then the Liberals had not done enough to deter the Germans, and the Conservatives had been right to argue for conscription. The second reason for going to war was a matter of domestic politics, not grand strategy. Since their electoral triumph in 1906, the Liberals had seen their electoral support wither away. They stayed in power after 1910 only with the support of the Irish Home Rulers. By 1914 Herbert Asquith's government was on the verge of collapse over Ulster Protestants' militant opposition to a devolved government in Dublin. Given the abject failure of their foreign policy to avert a European war, Asquith and his Cabinet colleagues ought to have resigned. But they dreaded the return to opposition. More, they dreaded the return of the Conservatives to power. They therefore went to war partly to keep the Tories out; had they not done so, two or three members of the Cabinet, including Churchill, would have resigned and the government would have fallen. The central strategic problem, in short, was that the Liberal foreign secretary had privately committed Britain to intervention in the event of a German attack on France, but his party had consistently opposed conscription, which would have established the kind of large standing army that might have deterred the Germans. The British intervention in 1914 was therefore a direct consequence of democratic politics. The war was genuinely popular; those who condemned intervention, like the Scottish socialist James Maxton, were a reviled minority. But the combination of a continental commitment without a credible military capability produced the worst possible outcome: a force capable of defeating the huge and well-trained German army had to be assembled and trained while the war was being fought.

War killed many more Britons in the twentieth century than fog did, much less famine. It is notable that democracy entirely failed to prevent this. True, in 1914 Britain was not a full democracy in the modern sense, in that women did not yet have the vote and there were still property qualifications for men, but nearly 7.8 million men—roughly three fifths of adult males—were eligible to vote in 1910, the last election before the war. Germany had a broader franchise—all adult males had the vote in elections to the imperial parliament (Reichstag)—but the power of the legislature was more circumscribed than in the United Kingdom, and the chancellor and secretaries of state were answerable to and removable by the kaiser. Nevertheless, the democratic elements in each constitution did nothing to prevent Britain and Germany from fighting a protracted and immensely bloody four-year war, ostensibly over the arcane question of Belgian neutrality.

An entire book could quite easily be devoted to the ensuing military disasters of the years 1914 to 1918 (Kut al-Amara and Gallipoli spring readily to mind), but it will suffice for our purposes to focus on the battle most notorious to British readers: the Somme. This was the moment of truth, when the new army that had been assembled after the declaration of war was sent into battle against the well-entrenched Germans. The Somme is remembered, with good reason, as one of the worst disasters in British history. On the first day of the offensive, July 1, 1916, the British Expeditionary Force suffered 57,000 casualties, of whom 19,000 were killed. The full significance of this figure becomes clear when it is realized that the German defenders lost only 8,000 men. This was just the beginning of a four-month attritional struggle, which may have resulted in as many as 1.2 million British, French, and German casualties. The Allies advanced, at most, seven miles.

One indication of the ghastliness of the Somme is the amount of black humor it has generated. As early as 1916, Siegfried Sassoon's fellow officers joked about commuting by train from England to the front, as if to a civilian office job. A year later an officer calculated that it would take until the year

2096 to reach the Rhine if the pace of advance achieved at the Somme, Vimy Ridge, and Messines was maintained.[69] By 1969 the Somme had become the butt of antiwar mockery in the film *Oh! What a Lovely War.* Twenty years later, the television series *Blackadder Goes Forth* took the ridicule further still ("Haig is about to make yet another gargantuan effort to move his drinks cabinet six inches closer to Berlin"). The image of British soldiers as "lions led by donkeys"—or by "butchers and bunglers"—has proved indelible.[70] Ever since Churchill's disastrous bid to win the war by defeating the Ottoman army at Gallipoli, the argument has been made that battles like the Somme were avoidable. Basil Liddell Hart—who fought at the Somme, where he was hit three times and badly gassed—contended that Germany could have been defeated without embroiling Britain in a prolonged and bloody continental stalemate. The indirect approach, relying on naval power and only a "limited liability" army, would have been far less costly.

Yet British military historians have mounted a tenacious defense of Douglas Haig, the British commander in chief, and his conduct of the Somme offensive. According to John Terraine, there was no alternative to sending the British Expeditionary Force in 1914; no substitute for the offensives at the Somme and Passchendaele; no reason to impugn Haig's "educated" generalship.[71] Gary Sheffield has argued that the Somme was an essential phase in the BEF's "learning process," "an attritional success for the Entente powers, [and] an essential step on the road to eventual victory."[72] For William Philpott, the Somme itself was a "bloody victory."[73] The debate illustrates the need for precision in assessing disaster. For the point of failure at the Somme was not at the top—or at least not entirely.

To begin with, the date, time, and place of the Somme offensive were decided not by Haig but by the French. Then the German attack at Verdun drew French forces away from the Somme offensive, increasing the onus on Britain's raw recruits. Haig had two plans in mind for the Somme: one was to break through the German positions and restore mobile warfare; the other was a more limited "attritional" offensive, a second-best option if no breakthrough was achieved. "When a break in [the German] line is made," Haig wrote, "cavalry and mobile troops must be at hand to advance at once to make a bridgehead (until relieved by infantry) beyond the gap. . . . At the same time our mounted troops must cooperate with our main attacking force in widening the gap."[74] Haig intended General Hubert Gough's Reserve Army to play a key role in this scenario.

The problem was that General Sir Henry Rawlinson, commander of the Fourth Army, had a different conception. "What we want to do now," he had written in 1915, "is what I call, 'bite and hold.' Bite off a piece of the enemy's line, like [at] Neuve Chapelle, and hold it against all counter-attack. . . . There ought to be no difficulty in holding it against the enemy's counter-attacks & inflicting on him at least twice the loss that we have suffered in making the bite."[75] This was a theory of attrition, not breakthrough. Rawlinson's draft plan for the Somme was "to kill as many Germans as possible with the least loss to ourselves" by seizing points of tactical importance and waiting for the Germans to counterattack.[76] When Haig questioned this, Rawlinson felt unable to stand his ground and appeared to acquiesce: "It is a gamble to go for an unlimited offensive," he wrote, "but D. H. apparently wants it and I am prepared to undertake anything within reason."[77] After the initial advance on the first day, however, he failed to order local reserves forward, paid no attention to Gough, and at midday issued an order for the Reserve Army to stand down, noting in his diary, "There is of course no hope of getting cavalry through today."[78]

One justification for Rawlinson's skepticism about a breakthrough was the failure of Haig's preliminary artillery bombardment to cut the German barbed-wire defenses. "Poor Haig—as he was always inclined to—spread his guns," recalled Major General J. F. N. "Curly" Birch, artillery adviser at general headquarters. The frontage of the German positions attacked was already too wide for the number of guns available, but Haig also ordered that the artillery should target a depth (i.e., width) of up to 2,500 yards, further diluting the impact of the bombardment. More seriously, ammunition was found to be defective (up to 30 percent of shells did not explode) and a quarter of the British guns were simply worn out through overuse. There were too few high-explosive shells, as well as numerous technical shortcomings: calibration was a matter of guesswork, map surveying was inaccurate, poor communications prevented corrections, and counter-battery work was ineffective. In addition, the British fire plan was too rigid. Worst of all, the bombardments of 1916 not only failed in their primary task but also hindered the subsequent infantry advance. The need for briefer bombardments to ensure surprise was still not yet realized, while adhesion to a rigid plan prevented the exploitation of early success.[79]

To be sure, the Germans did not have an easy time of it at the Somme, as is clear from Ernst Jünger's diary description of the German front line at Guillemont in August 1916: "Among the living lay the dead. As we dug ourselves in, we found them in layers stacked up on top of one another. One company after another had been shoved into the drum-fire and steadily annihilated." It was this experience, he wrote, which "first made me aware of the overwhelming effects of the war of material (*Materialschlacht*)."[80] Had the

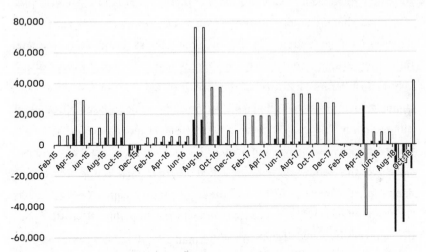

■ Surplus/deficit of British killed, missing or POWs

□ Surplus/deficit of British casualties including wounded

The British-German "net body count," February 1915–October 1918: British casualties minus German casualties in the British sector of the Western Front.

Source: War Office, *Statistics of the Military Effort of the British Empire During the Great War, 1914–1920* (London: HMSO, 1922), pp. 358–62.

Note: The figures are not always for individual months, so in a number of cases average monthly figures are given. This may understate the impact of certain military events in particular months.

shell that fell at his feet not been a dud, Jünger would not have written another word; as it was, he missed the annihilation of his company only because
of a leg wound. But the truth was that, from the British standpoint, the Somme
achieved neither breakthrough nor attrition. The reality was that at best—if
one accepts the British official figure for German casualties of 680,000—the
Somme was a draw. (The British suffered 419,654 casualties, the French
204,253.) If, as is much more likely, the German figure for casualties was correct (450,000), then the strategy of attrition was self-defeating. Even Haig
began to divine that, by remaining on the defensive, it was the Germans who
were "wear[ing] out our troops."[81] J. E. B. Seely, the former secretary of state
for war who commanded the Canadian Cavalry Brigade between 1915 and
1918, summed up the absurdity of attrition when he remarked in 1930, "Some
foolish people on the allied side thought that the war would be ended on the
Western Front by killing off the Germans. Of course this method could only
succeed if we killed a great many more of them than we lost ourselves."[82]

To say that the Somme set Britain on a path to victory makes sense only
if any certainty existed in 1916 that the United States would ultimately enter
the war on Britain's side, thereby tipping the balance of manpower irretriev-
ably against Berlin. That was not the case. It took major German errors—the
campaign of unrestricted submarine warfare against neutral shipping and the
Zimmermann Telegram seeking a German-Mexican military alliance—to
bring America into the war (on April 6, 1917). Even after that, Haig still presided over the bloody failure of the Allied offensive at the Battle of Passchendaele (July to November 1917) and the frantic retreat caused by the German
"Michael" offensive (March to July 1918), which achieved precisely the breakthrough that had eluded him. If there was a "learning curve" between the
Somme and the spring of 1918, it was invisible to investors, who felt anything
but confident of an Allied victory. And the Germans were learning throughout that time, too, perfecting their storm-troop tactics and defense in depth.[83]

A common theme of the literature about the war is that those on the
"home front" had no inkling of the realities of the Western (or any other)
Front. This is the central theme of the Viennese satirist Karl Kraus's dramatic
masterpiece *The Last Days of Mankind* (1918). R. H. Tawney, the English eco-

nomic historian, fulminated at British civilians as he convalesced after being
badly wounded at the Somme:

> I read your papers and listen to your conversation, and I see clearly
> that you have chosen to make to yourselves an image of war, not as it is,
> but of a kind which, being picturesque, flatters your appetite for novelty,
> for excitement. . . . You have chosen, I say, to make an image, because
> you do not like, or cannot bear, the truth.[84]

Yet the British public flocked to see the official documentary film *The Battle of
the Somme* (August 1916), which offered a startlingly unvarnished depiction
of the British side's experience of the *Materialschlacht*. No less than 13 percent of the film's seventy-seven-minute running time was given over to shots
of the dead and wounded; in the case of the last quarter of the film, more than
40 percent. The titles, too, were unflinching: "British Tommies rescuing a
comrade under shell fire. (This man died twenty minutes after reaching a
trench.)" Despite its candor—which was too much for American audiences—
the film was a huge success in Britain. *Kine Weekly* called it "the most wonderful battle picture that has ever been written." By October 1916 it had been
booked by more than two thousand cinemas across the country, nearly half
the total of forty-five hundred.[85] It was only with hindsight that the Somme
came to be seen as a disaster, and Haig as a callous butcher. At the time there
was mass support for offensive operations on the Western Front.

SAME AGAIN

The extraordinary feature of British history in the twentieth century was that
precisely the same mistake was made in the 1920s and '30s as had been made
in the 1900s and '10s. No serious effort was made to maintain a military capability sufficient to deter potential aggressors, principally Germany but also
Japan and Italy. Yet diplomatic commitments ended up being made—to Poland and others—that led (despite Liddell Hart's best efforts) to another
continental commitment. This time, however, the British Expeditionary Force

was routed by the Germans and forced to cast down its weapons and flee from the beaches at Dunkirk. Similar catastrophes befell British forces in multiple locations, perhaps most humiliatingly in Singapore. Democracy may insure a country against a famine; it clearly does not insure it against military disaster.

"*Si vis pacem, para bellum*"—If you want peace, prepare for war—is ancient lore.* Britain's classically educated political elite knew its meaning. The arguments that prevailed against it in the 1930s were mostly economic. Under pressure from voters to honor wartime pledges to build "homes fit for heroes," while at the same time struggling to service a bloated national debt and to restore the pound to its prewar value in terms of gold, British politicians first neglected and then largely forgot about imperial defense. In the ten years ending in 1932, the defense budget was cut by more than a third, at a time when Italian and French military spending rose by, respectively, 60 and 55 percent. At a meeting of the War Cabinet in August 1919, a convenient rule had been adopted:

> It should be assumed, for framing revised Estimates, that the British Empire will not be engaged in any great war during the next ten years, and that no Expeditionary Force is required for this purpose. . . . The principal function of the Military and Air Forces is to provide garrisons for India, Egypt, the new mandated territory and all territory (other than self-governing) under British control, as well as to provide the necessary support to the civil power at home.[86]

Every year until 1932, this "Ten Year Rule" was renewed, and every year new spending was put off. The rationale was straightforward: as Neville Chamberlain admitted in 1934, "it was impossible for us to contemplate a simultaneous war against Japan and Germany; we simply cannot afford the expenditure involved."[87] As chief of the Imperial General Staff between 1928 and 1940, General Archibald Montgomery-Massingberd had "one thought . . . to post-

---

*The original can be found in Publius Flavius Vegetius Renatus's tract *De re militari:* "Igitur qui desiderat pacem, praeparet bellum."

pone a war—not look ahead."[88] The corollary of this was the policy of appeasement, which meant putting off war ("cunction," in the words of Sir Robert Vansittart, the permanent undersecretary at the Foreign Office) by making concessions to Germany and other belligerent states. The most notorious of these concessions was the partial dismemberment of Czechoslovakia agreed to by Chamberlain and his French counterpart, Édouard Daladier, at Munich in September 1938.[89]

On October 5, Churchill gave a speech in the House of Commons that eviscerated the policy of appeasement:

> I will begin by saying what everybody would like to ignore or forget but which must nevertheless be stated, namely, that we have sustained a total and unmitigated defeat, and that France has suffered even more than we have. . . .
>
> It is the most grievous consequence of what we have done and of what we have left undone in the last five years—five years of futile good intentions, five years of eager search for the line of least resistance, five years of uninterrupted retreat of British power, five years of neglect of our air defences. . . .
>
> There can never be friendship between the British democracy and the Nazi power, that power which spurns Christian ethics, which cheers its onward course by a barbarous paganism, which vaunts the spirit of aggression and conquest, which derives strength and perverted pleasure from persecution, and uses, as we have seen, with pitiless brutality the threat of murderous force. That power cannot ever be the trusted friend of the British democracy.[90]

Although twenty-nine other Conservative MPs joined him in abstaining from the vote at the end of the Munich debate, Churchill's speech was deeply unpopular. Nancy Astor interrupted Churchill with a cry of "Nonsense!" The *Daily Express* dismissed the speech as "an alarmist oration by a man whose mind is soaked in the conquests of Marlborough."[91] An influential constituent and former supporter, Sir Harry Goschen, complained to the chairman of the

Conservative Association in Epping, Churchill's constituency, that "he broke up the harmony of the House by the speech he made. . . . I think it would have been a great deal better if he had kept quiet and not made a speech at all." So great was the disapproval of Churchill's speech among Epping Tories ("a mockery and a shame," "a menace in Parliament") that he might well have faced deselection before the next election had not subsequent events entirely vindicated him.[92]

The naval base at Singapore had been built in the 1920s as the linchpin of Britain's position in the Far East. Throughout the interwar period, the declared strategy for defending Singapore in the event of an attack was to send the fleet. On the eve of the Japanese invasion, however, the fleet was otherwise engaged. There were just 158 first-line aircraft in Malaya, where a thousand were needed, and three and a half divisions of infantry, where eight divisions plus two armored regiments would barely have sufficed. Above all, there had been a woeful failure to build proper fixed defenses (minefields, pillboxes, and anti-tank obstacles) on the land approaches to Singapore. When they attacked it, the Japanese thus found that the supposedly impregnable citadel was a sitting duck. At 4:00 p.m. on February 15, 1942, despite Churchill's desperate exhortation to fight "to the death," Lieutenant-General Arthur E. Percival and his garrison of 16,000 Britons, 14,000 Australians, and 32,000 Indians surrendered, unaware of the exhausted condition of their 30,000 adversaries, who had pedaled down the Malay Peninsula on bicycles and had all but run out of food and ammunition. Two weeks before the surrender, a Singaporean student named Maurice Baker was walking along the corridors of Raffles College with his friend Lee Kuan Yew. Suddenly they heard a huge explosion—the sound of the destruction of the causeway linking Singapore to the Malayan mainland. Lee Kuan Yew, the future prime minister of Singapore, turned to Baker and said simply, "That is the end of the British Empire."

Who was to blame for the fall of Singapore? Churchill? "It had never entered my head," Churchill wrote in his war memoirs, "that no circle of detached forts of a permanent character protected the rear of the famous fortress. I cannot understand how it was I did not know this. . . . My advisers ought to have known and I ought to have been told, and I ought to have asked."[93] This illustrates an important point. Churchill's historically framed analysis of the British Empire's predicament in the 1930s had been broadly correct and was borne out by events. He had been quite right to argue that Britain would have done better to fight in 1938 than in 1939, for Hitler made much better use of the intervening year than Chamberlain did. But he had been ignored and widely reviled at that time. It seems reasonable to ask if he could really be blamed for not knowing the precise nature of the fortifications around Singapore.

The British Empire did not, in truth, end in 1942 with the fall of Singapore. In February 1945, Churchill still bestrode the world stage as one of the "Big Three," dividing up the world with Roosevelt and Stalin at Yalta. No sooner had the war ended, however, than he was swept from office. Within a decade, Britain had conceded independence to India, Pakistan, Burma, and Ceylon and had given up its mandate in Palestine. Ministers and officials in the 1950s still sought to perpetuate British influence in what remained—often with the support of traditional elites, who had no desire to see colonial "protectorates" replaced by self-styled nationalists who had acquired a taste for Marxism at the London School of Economics.[94] But the Suez debacle in 1956 set the seal on the end of empire, a mere fourteen years after the fall of Singapore, even if it was not until the 1960s—and in some cases the 1970s—that the "winds of change" reached sub-Saharan Africa, the Persian Gulf, and the remnants of colonial rule "East of Suez," and not until 1997 that Hong Kong was handed over to the Chinese.

Nevertheless, the ignominious surrender of Singapore was a microcosm of the empire's malaise, a trailer for the longer feature that lay ahead. Alan Brooke, who as chief of the Imperial General Staff was among Churchill's harshest critics, was dismayed. "It is hard to see why a better defence is not being put up," he confided in his diary as the Japanese closed on Singapore. "I have during the last 10 years had an unpleasant feeling that the British Empire was decaying and that we were on a slippery slope. I wonder if I was right? I certainly never expected that we should fall to pieces as fast as we are." With the Japanese threatening to overrun Burma too, he became distraught: "Cannot work out why troops are not fighting better. If the army cannot fight better than it is doing at present we shall deserve to lose our Empire!"[95] The disintegration of a complex system can happen all at once, with breathtaking speed, or it can take the form of successive, convulsive phase transitions. To lay the responsibility for the British imperial crisis of the 1940s on one individual therefore makes little sense. It was no more all Churchill's fault than the Bengal Famine would be the following year.

HOW EMPIRES FALL

Harry Truman—in alliance with whom Churchill and Stalin brought the Second World War to a victorious conclusion—had a sign on his White House desk that read THE BUCK STOPS HERE.* In an address at the National War College on December 19, 1952, Truman explained its significance to him: "You know, it's easy for the Monday morning quarterback to say what the coach should have done, after the game is over. But when the decision is up before you—and on my desk I have a motto which says, 'The Buck Stops Here'—the decision has to be made." In his farewell address, in January 1953, Truman reverted to this point: "The president—whoever he is—has to decide. He can't pass the buck to anybody. No one else can do the deciding for him. That's his job."[96] These admirable sentiments have often been echoed by Truman's successors. Yet they return us to the simplified world in which politics is a matter of presidential decision making, and all disasters must be attributable to bad presidential decisions.

Nominally, most great empires have a central authority figure, whether it is a hereditary emperor or an elected president. In practice, the power of such individuals is a function of the complex network of economic, social, and political relations over which they preside. Empires are the most complex of all political units that humans have constructed, precisely because they seek to exert power over very large areas and diverse cultures. It is not surprising,

---

*The sign was made by prisoners in the federal reformatory at El Reno, Oklahoma, and was a gift to Truman from his friend Fred A. Canfil, then marshal for the western district of Missouri. On the other side were the words "I'm from Missouri."

then, to find that they exhibit many of the characteristics of other complex adaptive systems—including the tendency for apparent stability to give way quite suddenly to disorder.

Take the most famous imperial decline and fall, that of ancient Rome. In his *History of the Decline and Fall of the Roman Empire,* published in six volumes between 1776 and 1788, Edward Gibbon covered no fewer than 1,400 years, from AD 180 to 1590. This truly is history over the long run, in which the causes of decline range from the personality disorders of individual emperors to the power of the Praetorian Guards to the rise of the great monotheistic religions. Yet few modern historians of Rome's decline feel the need or have the skill to paint on such a broad canvas. True, civil war was a recurrent problem after the death of Marcus Aurelius, in 180, as would-be emperors competed for the spoils of supreme power.[97] Humiliatingly, the emperor Valerian was captured in battle by the Sassanid Persians in 260, though Aurelian won for himself the title "restorer of the world" (*restitutor orbis*) by recapturing the territory lost to the Sassanians. The empire was divided by Diocletian, Christianized by Constantine. Barbarian invasions or migrations began in the fourth century and intensified as the Huns moved westward, displacing Gothic tribes like the Tervingi. All this may still be presented as a Gibbonian narrative of long-term decline. Alternatively, however, Roman history can be understood as the normal working of a complex adaptive system, with political strife, barbarian migration (and integration), and imperial rivalry as integral features of late antiquity, and Christianity as a cement, not a solvent. Rome's *fall,* by contrast, was quite sudden and dramatic—just as one would expect when such a complex system goes critical. Cooperation with the Visigoths against the Huns broke down, leading to the Battle of Adrianople in 378, at which the main imperial army was routed and the emperor Valens killed. The final breakdown in the Western Roman Empire came in 406, as Germanic invaders poured across the Rhine into Gaul and then Italy. Four years later, Rome itself was sacked by the Visigoths, led by their king, Alaric—the first time the city had fallen since 390 BC. Between 429 and 439, Genseric led the Vandals to victory after victory in North Africa, culminating in the fall of Carthage. Fatally, Rome's southern Mediterranean breadbasket was lost, and with it a vital source of tax revenue. Only with the support of the Visigoths were the Romans able to defeat Attila's Huns as they swept westward, having ransacked the Balkans. By 452 the Western Empire had lost all of Britain, most of Spain, the richest provinces of North Africa, and southwestern and southeastern Gaul. Not much was left except Italy.[98] The Eastern Roman Empire (Byzantium) lived on—indeed, the emperor Basiliscus attempted to recapture Carthage in 468—but the Western Empire was dead. Beginning in 476, Rome was ruled over by Odoacer, a German who deposed the child emperor Romulus Augustulus and proclaimed himself king. In all this, the striking thing is the speed of the Western Empire's collapse. The population of the Eternal City itself fell by three quarters in the space of just five decades. Archaeological evidence from the rest of Western Europe—inferior housing, more primitive pottery, fewer coins, smaller cattle—suggests that "the end of civilization" came within the span of a single generation.[99] And all this was long before the Plague of Justinian, in the mid-sixth century.

It is not difficult to show that other great empires have suffered similarly swift collapses. The Ming dynasty in China had been born in 1368, when the warlord Zhu Yuanzhang renamed himself Hongwu, meaning "vast military power." For most of the next three centuries, Ming China was the world's most sophisticated civilization by almost any measure. But then, in the middle of the seventeenth century, the wheels came off. This is not to exaggerate its early stability. Yongle had succeeded his father, Hongwu, only after a period of civil war and the deposition of the rightful successor, his eldest brother's son. But the mid-seventeenth-century crisis was unquestionably a bigger disruption. Political factionalism was exacerbated by a fiscal crisis as the falling purchasing power of silver eroded the real value of tax revenues.[100] Harsh weather, famine, and epidemic disease opened the door to rebellion within and incursions from without.[101] In 1644, Beijing itself fell to the rebel leader Li Zicheng. The last Ming emperor, the Chongzhen Emperor, hanged himself. This dramatic transition from Confucian equipoise to anarchy took little more than a decade.

The consequences of the Ming collapse were devastating. Between 1580 and 1650, conflict and epidemics reduced the Chinese population by 35 to 40 percent. What had gone wrong? The answer is that the Ming system had created the appearance of a high equilibrium—impressive outwardly, but fragile inwardly. The countryside could sustain a remarkably large number of people, but only on the basis of an essentially static social order that ceased to innovate. It was a kind of trap, and when the least little thing went wrong, the trap snapped shut. There were no external resources to draw on. True, a considerable body of scholarship has sought to represent Ming China as a prosperous society, with considerable internal trade and a vibrant market for luxury goods.[102] More recent Chinese research, however, shows that Chinese per capita income stagnated in the Ming era and the capital stock shrank.[103] Many of these pathologies simply continued under new management after the Manchus successfully established the Qing dynasty, but with even larger disasters—notably the White Lotus and Taiping rebellions—and a final, irrevocable collapse of the imperial system in 1911.[104]

In much the same way, Bourbon France passed from triumph to terror with astonishing rapidity. What seemed like a good idea at the time—intervention on the side of the colonial rebels against British rule in North America—tipped the finances of absolutism into a critical state. The summoning of the Estates General in May 1789 unleashed a political chain reaction and a collapse of royal legitimacy so swift that within four years the king had been decapitated by guillotine, a device invented only in 1791. Just over a century and a quarter later, the disintegration of the dynastic land empires of Eastern Europe came with comparable swiftness, despite the narrative fallacies that the Habsburgs, Ottomans, and Romanovs were doomed for decades before the First World War broke out. The truly remarkable thing was in fact how well these ancient empires withstood the test of total war, with the unraveling commencing only after the Bolshevik Revolution of October 1917. A mere seven years after his armies had triumphed at Gallipoli, Mehmed VI departed Constantinople aboard a British warship. By then, all three dynasties were defunct.

The half-life of empire grew shorter in the twentieth century. The attempt to restore the German Empire—the "Third Reich"—ended in the utter destruction and partition of Germany just over a dozen years after Hitler's appointment as Reich chancellor on January 30, 1933. The moment when Hitler came to power—surely the biggest disaster democracy has ever produced—had been postponed by the members of the old political elite around the eighty-five-year-old president Paul von Hindenburg; the Nazi leader should really have become chancellor after his party's electoral triumph in July 1932. Few in 1933 saw as clearly as the East Prussian conservative Friedrich Reck-Malleczewen that Hitler would be Germany's nemesis, a terrifying reincarnation of the sixteenth-century Anabaptist John of Leiden:

> As in our case, a misbegotten failure conceived, so to speak, in the gutter, became the great prophet, and the opposition simply disintegrated, while the rest of the world looked on in astonishment and incomprehension. As with us . . . hysterical females, schoolmasters, renegade priests, the dregs and outsiders from everywhere formed the main supports of the regime. . . . A thin sauce of ideology covered lewdness, greed, sadism, and fathomless lust for power . . . and whoever would not completely accept the new teaching was turned over to the executioner.[105]

Reck-Malleczewen died of typhus at Dachau as his prophecy of disaster was being fulfilled.

The most recent and familiar example of imperial collapse is, of course, the dissolution of the Soviet Union shortly before its sixty-ninth birthday. With the benefit of hindsight, historians can see all kinds of dry rot within the Soviet system, dating back to the Brezhnev era and beyond. Perhaps, as the historian Stephen Kotkin has argued, it was only the high oil prices of the 1970s that "averted Armageddon."[106] But that was not how it seemed at the time. When Mikhail Gorbachev became general secretary of the Communist Party of the Soviet Union, in March 1985, the Soviet economy was still estimated by the CIA to be around 60 percent the size of the U.S. economy; the Soviet nuclear arsenal was larger than the American. The Third World had been going the Soviets' way for much of the previous twenty years, with clients and proxies scattered across the globe. In the words of the historian Adam Ulam,

"In 1985, no government of a major state appeared to be as firmly in power, its policies as clearly set in their course, as that of the USSR."[107] Yet within four and a half years of Gorbachev's appointment, the Russian imperium in Central and Eastern Europe had fallen apart, followed by the Soviet Union itself by the end of 1991. Only a very few dissidents had the temerity to foresee anything like this—notably Andrei Amalrik, whose 1970 essay asked, "Will the Soviet Union Survive Until 1984?" (Amalrik correctly anticipated that a bureaucratic elite cut off from the reality of economic stagnation and "moral weariness," and concerned only with perpetuating their comfortable lives, would eventually lose control of the centrifugal tendencies of the imperial periphery, "first in the Baltic area, the Caucasus and the Ukraine, then in Central Asia and along the Volga.")[108] If ever an empire fell off a cliff, rather than gently declining, it was the one founded by Lenin.

Note, finally, the differing durations of each of the empires referred to here. The Roman Empire proper (excluding Byzantium) lasted just over five hundred years. The Ottoman Empire was not far behind, at 469 years. The British Empire has no obvious start date, but 350 years seems a fair approximation of its life span. The Ming dynasty managed 276 years. The Soviet Union was formally established at the end of 1922 but was dissolved before the end of 1991; Hitler's Third Reich lasted a mere dozen years. Quite apart from the erratic incidence of geological disasters, those seeking cyclical patterns in history have a serious difficulty if the periodicity of empire is so variable. The challenge becomes even greater when one realizes that some of these empires—notably the Russian and the Chinese—have proved capable of reconstituting themselves even after seeming to collapse. The political geography of the world today can appear to be a patchwork quilt of nation-states, all based on the template of the standard nineteenth-century Western European polity imagined by Giuseppe Mazzini. On closer inspection, the emperors live on in both Beijing and Moscow.[109] General Secretary Xi Jinping incessantly seeks to legitimize the Communist Party's rule with allusions to China's imperial past, the fifteenth-century voyages of Admiral Zheng He being an especial favorite with propagandists of Xi's "One Belt One Road" strategy.[110] Vladimir Putin quite explicitly sees the Russian Federation as the heir of the Soviet Union, to the extent of delivering long, thoroughly researched, and tendentious defenses of Soviet conduct in 1939–40.[111] What are we to make of empires that rise, fall, and then rise again? In a similar way, the second-most-populous country in the world, India, is in many respects the heir of the British Raj. As Indian prime minister Manmohan Singh acknowledged in a remarkable address at Oxford University in 2005,

> Our notions of the rule of law, of a Constitutional government, of a free press, of a professional civil service, of modern universities and research laboratories have all been fashioned in the crucible where an age-old civilization met the dominant Empire of the day. . . . Our judiciary, our legal system, our bureaucracy and our police are all great institutions, derived from British-Indian administration, and they have served our country exceedingly well. Of all the legacies of the Raj, none is more important than the English language and the modern school system. That is, of course, if you leave out cricket! . . . The founding fathers of our Republic were also greatly influenced by the ideas associated with the age of enlightenment in Europe. Our Constitution remains a testimony to the enduring interplay between what is essentially Indian and what is very British in our intellectual heritage.[112]

In Ankara, meanwhile, Recep Tayyip Erdoğan fondly dreams of an Ottoman revival, casting aspersions on the Treaty of Lausanne (1923) and reviving the territorial claims of the "National Oath" adopted in the last session of the Ottoman parliament in 1920.[113] In decrepit Tehran, too, they harbor delusions of grandeur. "Since its inception, Iran has had a global [dimension]," declared Ali Younesi, a former intelligence minister and adviser to President Hassan Rouhani on minority issues, in 2015. "It was born an empire. Iran's leaders, officials and administrators have always thought in the global [dimension]." Younesi defined the territory of "Greater Iran" as extending from the borders of China to Babylon (Iraq)—the historic capital of the Achaemenid Empire—and including the Indian subcontinent, the North and South

Caucasus, and the Persian Gulf.[114] Even if not many Iranians share that vaulting ambition, the widespread aspiration to lead a regional "Shia Crescent" has similar imperial implications.

The collapse of an empire is a tragedy only to the imperialists, it is usually assumed. And yet it is often in the moments of imperial disintegration that violence reaches new heights, usually to the detriment of the people supposedly being liberated—think only of the violence that attended the Romanov, Habsburg, and Ottoman dissolutions, or the horrors of partition as the British Raj was wound up. Of all the forms catastrophe can take, the death agony of an empire may be the most difficult to fathom, precisely because it is the most complex.

7

═══

FROM THE BOOGIE WOOGIE FLU
TO EBOLA IN TOWN

I had just gotten over a serious illness that I won't bother to talk about.

—Jack Kerouac, *On the Road*

ROCKIN' PNEUMONIA

To be young was very heaven in the United States of 1957. That summer, Elvis Presley topped the charts with "(Let Me Be Your) Teddy Bear," followed in September by Buddy Holly & the Crickets' "That'll Be the Day" and in October by the Everly Brothers' "Wake Up Little Susie." Jack Kerouac's *On the Road* was published in the fall. *Cat on a Hot Tin Roof*, starring Paul Newman and Elizabeth Taylor, won the Oscar for Best Picture. The folk memory of those idyllic "happy days" omits the racial cleavages of that time: 1957 was just three years after *Brown v. Board of Education* had sounded the death knell of racial segregation in public schools, two years after Emmett Till's murder and Rosa Parks's refusal to give up her bus seat, and the same year federal troops had to be sent to Little Rock to escort nine black students into the Arkansas capital's Central High School. That history is now taught in schools, but we still tend to forget that 1957 also saw the outbreak of one of the biggest pandemics of the modern era—the eighteenth largest in history, according to one recent survey.[1] It is not without significance that another hit of that year was

Huey "Piano" Smith & the Clowns' "Rockin' Pneumonia and the Boogie Woo-gie Flu."*

> *I wanna squeeze her but I'm way too low.*
> *I would be runnin' but my feet's too slow.*

Having been defeated in the presidential election of November 3, 2020, President Donald J. Trump might possibly, if incongruously, be compared to Woodrow Wilson, whose chances of reelection—not to mention his health—were undermined by the Spanish flu pandemic of 1918–19. However, a more illuminating comparison (and contrast) might be to Dwight D. Eisenhower. Eisenhower had two encounters with pandemics in his exemplary career of public service. The first saw him promoted to lieutenant colonel for his actions in command of a ten-thousand-man Army tank force at Camp Colt, in Gettysburg, Pennsylvania, during the Spanish flu. The second came when he was president during the 1957–58 Asian flu pandemic. The first episode has been the subject of several books and numerous papers. When seeking historical analogies in 2020, commentators referred more often to 1918–19 than to any other case. The more recent episode, by contrast, is now largely forgotten other than by historians and historically minded epidemiologists. And yet it deserves to be much better known. For, as a public health crisis, it looks much more like the COVID-19 pandemic of our own time than does the 1918–19 pandemic, which was one of the ten deadliest in all history.[2]

The policy response in 2020 could hardly be more different from the response of the Eisenhower administration to the pandemic that struck sixty-three years before. Indeed, it was almost the exact opposite. Eisenhower did not declare a state of emergency in the fall of 1957. There were no state lockdowns and no school closures. Sick students simply stayed at home, as they usually did. Work continued more or less uninterrupted. Nor did the Eisen-

---

*The single sold more than one million copies, achieving gold disc status, and got to number 52 on the *Billboard* chart.

hower administration borrow to the hilt to fund transfers and loans to citizens and businesses. The president asked Congress for a mere $2.5 million ($23 million in today's inflation-adjusted terms, and around 0.0005 percent of 1957 GDP, which was $474 billion) to provide additional support to the Public Health Service.[3] True, there was a recession that year, but it had little if anything to do with the pandemic. Eisenhower's job approval rating did deteriorate, sliding from about 80 to 50 percent between January 1957 and March 1958,[4] and his party sustained heavy losses in the 1958 midterms. But no serious historian of the period would attribute these setbacks to the pandemic. Huey "Piano" Smith & the Clowns would appear to have correctly judged the national mood of insouciance, which was summed up in a phrase coined the year before: "What, me worry?"*

TEENAGE CONTAGION

The "Asian flu"—as it was then uncontroversial to call a contagious disease that originated in Asia—was an antigenically novel strain (H2N2) of influenza A, possibly similar to the strain that had caused a pandemic in 1889 (the "Asiatic" or "Russian" flu).[5] This virus was different from the coronavirus that causes COVID-19 (both are riboviruses, but from different phyla), but its impact was comparable. It was first reported in Hong Kong in April 1957, having originated in mainland China two months before, and—like COVID-19—it swiftly went global. It spread throughout East Asia and into the Middle East in April, May, and June, leading to outbreaks at U.S. military bases in Korea and Japan. By June, more than twenty countries, including the United States mainland, had experienced their first cases. The virus reached South America and Africa in July and August. In September, epidemics began in North America and Europe.[6] Unlike carriers of SARS-CoV-2 today, H2N2 carriers traveled mainly by ship, the dominant mode of long-

---

*"Alfred E. Neuman" had been christened in 1956 by *Mad* magazine's second editor, Al Feldstein, and painted by Norman Mingo. Thereafter, the tousle-headed, gap-toothed youth invariably appeared on the magazine's cover with his familiar signature phrase, "What, me worry?"

haul transport in those days. The spread of the virus was still remarkably rapid.

Like COVID-19, the Asian flu led to significant excess mortality. The most recent research concludes that around 1.1 million (700,000–1.5 million) people worldwide died in the pandemic.[7] A recent but pre-COVID study of the 1957–58 pandemic concluded that if "a virus of similar severity" were to strike in our time, around 2.7 million deaths might be anticipated worldwide.[8] Like COVID-19, it hit some countries much harder than others. Latin American nations—notably Chile—suffered especially high excess mortality rates, as did Finland. In the United States there were between 14,000 and 115,700 excess deaths.[9] Adjusting for today's higher population, that would be between 26,000 and 215,000 excess deaths.

These comparisons are important because it is now clear that, in terms of its likely fatality rate, the 2020–21 pandemic more closely resembles the 1957–58 pandemic than the much more catastrophic Spanish flu, which may have killed 2.2 to 2.8 percent of the world's population and 0.65 percent of the U.S. population (see chapter 5).[10] The pandemic of 1918–19 was one of history's worst, comparable in its impact to the *cocoliztli* epidemic (of multiple Eurasian diseases) that devastated the peoples of Central and South America in the sixteenth century. In 1918, life expectancy for both men and women in the United States declined by 11.8 years.[11] One influential but questionable British epidemiological model predicted in March 2020 that, in the absence of both social distancing and economic lockdowns, COVID-19 had the potential to kill up to forty million people worldwide and 2.2 million Americans.[12] That now seems implausible. In the United States, the infection fatality rate (IFR) of the Spanish flu was around 2 percent. It seems likely, on the basis of the serological studies published to date, that the IFR of COVID-19 is less than half that.[13] A scenario of universal infection is hard to imagine.

Excess mortality in the United States may end up being higher in 2020–21 than in 1957–58: the IFR of the Asian flu was probably no more than 0.26 percent. Unlike COVID-19, however, the Asian flu killed appreciable numbers of young people. As in most influenza pandemics—in 1892 and 1936, for example—significant numbers not only of the very old (over sixty-five) but also of the very young (under five) died. In terms of excess mortality relative to baseline expected mortality rates, however, the age groups that suffered the heaviest losses globally were fifteen- to twenty-four-year-olds (34 percent above average mortality rates), followed by five- to fourteen-year-olds (27 percent above average). In the United States, too, although the highest excess death rates were in the age groups under five, sixty-five to seventy-four, and seventy-five and over, and although around two thirds of excess deaths were of people older than sixty-five,[14] the relative excess death rate in the fifteen-to-nineteen age group was more than four times the expected rate.[15] In other words, contemporaries would have anticipated higher mortality among the elderly at the time of year the Asian flu struck; they would not have anticipated it among teenagers. The fact that so many young people succumbed to the 1957–58 pandemic means that, even if the death toll of 2020–21 ends up being a larger share of the U.S. population, the number of quality-adjusted life years (QALYs) lost may still have been higher in the earlier case. According to one recent estimate, the cost of the Asian flu in terms of QALYs was 5.3 times higher than that of an average flu season between 1979 and 2001 and 4.5 times higher than that of the 2009 "swine flu," but just one twentieth of the cost of the Spanish flu.[16]

The first cases of Asian flu in the United States occurred early in June 1957, among the crews of ships berthed at Newport, Rhode Island. Naval bases on the West Coast were soon reporting thousands of cases. At the end of June, there was an outbreak among high school girls on the campus of the School of Veterinary Medicine at the University of California, Davis. A student exposed to the Davis outbreak traveled to Grinnell, Iowa, to attend a Westminster Fellowship Conference that commenced on June 28. The student developed the flu en route, exposing 1,680 delegates from more than forty states and ten foreign countries to the virus. A few cases also appeared among the 53,000 boys attending the Boy Scout Jamboree at Valley Forge, Pennsylvania.[17] As Boy Scout groups traveled around the country in July and August, they, too, disseminated the flu widely.[18] In July there was a "massive outbreak" in Tangipahoa Parish, Louisiana. The illness was said to be "sudden in onset and marked by high fever, malaise, headache, generalized myalgia [muscle pain], sore throat, and cough. . . . Nausea and vomiting were not unusual among the younger children." Two people died. There soon followed a series of outbreaks throughout Louisiana and adjacent areas of Mississippi.[19] By the end of the summer, cases had also appeared in California, Ohio, Kentucky, and Utah.

It was the start of the school year at the end of the summer that made the Asian flu an epidemic in the United States. As soon as pupils returned from vacation, the virus spread rapidly throughout the country. The Communicable Disease Center, as the CDC was then called, had established a new Influenza Surveillance Unit in July, which received county reports covering 85 percent of the population, a weekly National Health Survey of a representative sample of two thousand people, and reports on absenteeism from AT&T, covering sixty thousand telephone workers in thirty-six cities. These data give us a more detailed picture of the 1957 epidemic than is possible for any previous episode. The CDC estimated that approximately forty-five million people—equivalent to about 25 percent of the population—had become infected with the new virus in October and November 1957. County-level data showed attack rates ranging from 20 to 40 percent. The peak of morbidity was in week 42; the peak in influenza and pneumonia deaths came three to four weeks later. The highest attack (i.e., infection) rates were in the age groups from school-age children to young adults up to thirty-five or forty years of age. Adults over sixty-five accounted for 60 percent of influenza deaths, an abnormally low share. (In 1960, they represented fully 80 percent of all excess pneumonia and influenza deaths.)[20]

Why were young Americans disproportionately vulnerable to the Asian flu? Part of the explanation is that they had not been as exposed as older Americans to earlier strains of influenza. There had been a total of nine type A H1N1 influenza epidemics since 1934 (1934–35, 1937, 1939, 1940–41, 1943–44, 1947, 1950, 1951, and 1953). All of these were cases of above-average "seasonal flu" resulting from an antigenic "drift" of the virus. The 1957–58 flu was a new H2N2 strain, but older Americans may have had some residual immunity.[21] As one authority noted,

> With the exception of persons >70 years of age, the public was confronted by a virus with which it had had no experience, and it was shown that the virus alone, without bacterial coinvaders, was lethal. . . .
>
> The virus was quickly recognized as an influenza A virus by complement fixation tests. However, tests defining the HA antigen of the virus showed it to be unlike any previously found in humans. This was also true for the neuraminidase (NA) antigen. The definitive subtype of the Asian virus was later established as H2N2.[22]

However, there is a second explanation for the unexpectedly high susceptibility of young Americans to the 1957 pandemic. As we saw in chapter 4, the scale and incidence of any contagion are functions of the properties of the pathogen itself and the structure of the social network that it attacks.[23] The year 1957 was in many ways the dawn of the American teenager. The first baby boomers born after the end of World War II turned thirteen the following year. Prosperous as their parents had most certainly not been in their teens, this generation enjoyed not only an economic life but also a social life that was quite novel and—as Hollywood projected it in a spate of films devoted to teenage antics—the envy of the world. The heady whirl of proms, parties, and games of chicken had its shadow side, however. As the historian of the CDC has noted, teenagers at that time "experienced the highest contact rate of any segment of the population, far surpassing the number of contacts of the housewife, the preschool children, or her husband at work."[24]

Summer camps, school buses, and unprecedented social mingling after school ensured that between September 1957 and March 1958 the proportion of teenagers infected with the virus rose from 5 percent to 75 percent. The triggering event in Tangipahoa had been the opening of twenty of the parish schools in mid-July (after the annual strawberry harvest). The nationwide epidemic in the fall was driven primarily by schools reopening at the end of the

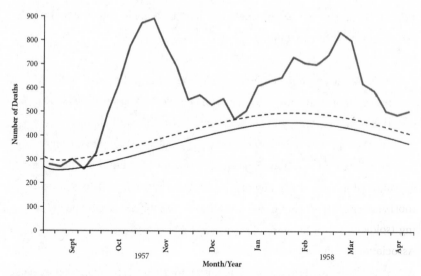

The 1957–58 pandemic in the United States; weekly pneumonia and influenza deaths in 108 U.S. cities.

Note: The upper solid line represents the number of pneumonia and influenza deaths reported from 108 cities weekly from September 1957 to April 1958. The lower solid line is the number of such deaths that would be expected based on previous years' experience with pneumonia and influenza. The dashed line is the "epidemic threshold," which is almost never exceeded except during influenza epidemics.

summer. The CDC estimated that more than 60 percent of students had clinical illnesses that autumn. Data from twenty-eight U.S. school systems showed absenteeism running at 20 to 30 percent above the usual 5 percent average. In New York, school absenteeism reached its maximum on October 7, with 280,000 absences. This amounted to 29 percent of all school attendees, and 43 percent in Manhattan.[25] As we shall see, in 1957 the U.S. authorities had tacitly opted for what we would now call a herd immunity strategy. Yet this did not avert a second wave in February 1958—something that took the CDC by surprise. This second wave saw almost as big a spike in excess mortality, but this time it was concentrated in older age groups (forty-five to seventy-four). There were subsequent epidemics of influenza in January–March 1960 (influenza A2) and again in early 1962 and 1963 (influenza B). There were also mild epidemics in 1965 and 1966.[26] Then came the bigger "Hong Kong flu" of 1968–70 (influenza A/H3N2), though it was only half the size of the 1957–58 pandemic in terms of excess mortality.[27]

HILLEMAN'S WAY

President Eisenhower's decision to keep the country open in 1957–58 bore the imprint of his time as a young officer at Camp Colt during the Spanish flu, when he had overseen mitigation efforts so successfully that the Army had not only promoted him but also sent thirty doctors from Camp Colt around the country to teach others. Eisenhower's strategy in 1918 had been simple: trust doctors (he deputized the camp's chief surgeon to lead the response and authorized him to perform experimental treatments) and employ social distancing (soldiers were split into tents of three across an open field).[28] When the Association of State and Territorial Health Officials (ASTHO) concluded on August 27, 1957, that "there is no practical advantage in the closing of schools or the curtailment of public gatherings as it relates to the spread of this disease," Eisenhower listened.[29] As a CDC official later recalled:

> Measures were generally not taken to close schools, restrict travel, close borders, or recommend wearing masks. Quarantine was not considered to be an effective mitigation strategy and was "obviously useless because of the large number of travelers and the frequency of mild or inapparent cases." . . .
>
> In early October, the Nassau County Health Commissioner in New York stated that "public schools should stay open even in an epidemic" and that "children would get sick just as easily out of school." . . .
>
> ASTHO encouraged home care for uncomplicated influenza cases to reduce the hospital burden and recommended limitations on hospital admissions to the sickest patients. . . . Most were advised simply to stay home, rest, and drink plenty of water and fruit juices.[30]

This decision meant that the onus shifted entirely from non-pharmaceutical to pharmaceutical interventions. As in 2020, there was a race to find a vaccine. Unlike in 2020, however, the United States had no real competition, thanks to the acumen of one exceptionally talented and prescient scientist.

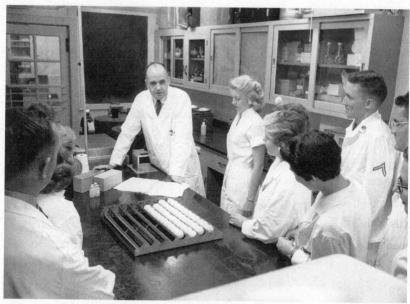

Maurice Hilleman (1919–2005) talks with his research team as they study the Asian flu virus in a lab at Walter Reed Army Medical Center, Silver Spring, Maryland, 1957.

From 1948 to 1957, Maurice Hilleman—born in Miles City, Montana, in 1919—was chief of the Department of Respiratory Diseases at the Walter Reed Army Medical Center. The Commission on Influenza of the Armed Forces Epidemiological Board had been studying the flu and its prevention by vaccines since the 1940s.[31] Early in his career, Hilleman had discovered the genetic changes that occur when the influenza virus mutates, known as shift and drift. It was this work that enabled him to recognize, when reading reports in the press of "glassy-eyed children" in Hong Kong, that the outbreak had the potential to become a disastrous pandemic. He and a colleague worked nine fourteen-hour days to confirm that this was a new strain of flu that could potentially kill millions, as had happened in 1918—although, as we shall see, antibiotics were now available to combat the secondary infections that had killed so many people then. The Army Medical Center received its first influenza specimens from Hong Kong on May 13, and Hilleman had definitively identified the new strain by May 22.[32]

Speed was of the essence. Hilleman was able to work directly with vaccine manufacturers—bypassing "the bureaucratic red tape," as he put it. The Public Health Service released the first cultures of the Asian influenza virus to manufacturers even before Hilleman had finished his analysis. A key role was played by the CDC's Montgomery, Alabama, laboratory, which was the World Health Organization's International Influenza Center for the Americas. In the 2020 pandemic, as we shall see, the WHO did not cover itself in glory. In 1957, however, it facilitated cooperation between the CDC and its British counterpart, the World Influenza Center in London. In Montgomery, as well as at CDC headquarters in Atlanta, staff members volunteered for the first trials of the vaccine. H. Bruce Dull, of the Epidemic Intelligence Service—which had been set up in 1951 in response to the threat of biological weapons during the Korean War—led a trial at the Atlanta United States Penitentiary, which was 80 to 90 percent effective in the first round. By the late summer, six companies were producing a vaccine, including Merck Sharp & Dohme.

The rapidity with which the United States went from detection of pandemic risk to mass vaccination was astonishing. The first *New York Times* report of the outbreak in Hong Kong—three paragraphs on page 3—was on April 17.[33] As early as July 26, little more than three months later, doctors at Fort Ord, California, began to inoculate recruits to the military. Three days later, Lowry Air Force Base, in Colorado, did so, too. Next in line were doctors, nurses, and other healthcare workers. President Eisenhower was duly inoculated, as were Queen Elizabeth and Prince Philip, ahead of their planned visit to the United States and Canada. In the eyes of public health officials, this vaccination drive was the core of the U.S. response to the pandemic. Surgeon General Leroy Burney announced on August 15 that the vaccine was to be allocated to states according to population size but distributed by the manufacturers through their customary commercial networks. At its late August meeting in Washington, ASTHO declared that prevention "in the absence of effective means to stop the spread of infection resolves itself into an immunization program." Approximately four million one-milliliter doses were released in August, nine million in September, and seventeen million in October.[34]

"It didn't let me down, the pandemic of 1957, it began on time," Hilleman reminisced in a 2005 interview. As a result, the much-feared repeat of 1918–19 was largely avoided. "That's the only time we ever averted a pandemic with a vaccine," Hilleman recalled.[35]

Yet this amounted to enough vaccine for just 17 percent of the population. Moreover, vaccine efficacy was found to range from 53 to 60 percent. Inevitably, there were mistakes. Football players—not only the San Francisco 49ers but also the college teams at the University of California and Stanford—got their shots before policemen and firemen. The sales manager at Merck explained, "You got twenty-five people wanting apples and you got one apple. So who gets the apple? The guy who's got his hand out first."[36] All this led one former CDC official to conclude that the vaccine "had no appreciable effect on the trend of the pandemic."[37] This underestimates Hilleman's achievement, however. The net result of his rapid response to the Asian flu was surely to limit the excess mortality suffered in the United States. For, on closer inspection, the public health policy that had emerged was one of herd immunity for young Americans combined with selective vaccination of military and health-care personnel. There was continued experimentation and research in the subsequent years. It was found that "more vaccine was required to initiate a primary antibody response than with the earlier H1 vaccines. . . . In 1958, 1959, and 1960 (as recurrent infections occurred), mean initial antibody levels in the population increased (i.e., subjects were primed) and response to vaccination was more readily demonstrated. Divided doses given at intervals of <4 weeks were more beneficial than a single injection. Less benefit was derived from this strategy as years passed." Studies of Navajo schoolchildren and New York City medical students found that "subclinical infections occurred each year" but "clinically manifested infections" decreased in conjunction with an increasing level of H2N2-specific antibodies.[38] In light of these and later findings, policy shifted to one of regular vaccination of the elderly population, who, during most flu seasons, were and are the most vulnerable to most strains of influenza.

In the course of 1957, Hilleman joined Merck as head of its new Virus and Cell Biology Research department, in West Point, Pennsylvania. What followed was prodigious. It was at Merck that Hilleman developed most of the forty experimental and licensed animal and human vaccines with which he is credited. Of the fourteen vaccines routinely recommended in current vaccine schedules, he developed eight: those for measles, mumps, hepatitis A, hepatitis B, chickenpox, meningitis, pneumonia, and *Haemophilus influenzae* bacteria. In 1963, his daughter Jeryl Lynn came down with the mumps. Hilleman cultivated viral material from her and used it as the basis of a mumps vaccine. The Jeryl Lynn strain of the mumps vaccine is still used today. Hilleman and his team invented a vaccine for hepatitis B by treating blood serum with pepsin, urea, and formaldehyde. This was licensed in 1981 (though superseded in the United States in 1986 by a vaccine that was produced in yeast) and was still the preferred option in 150 countries as recently as 2003.

Reading accounts of Hilleman's life, one is reminded that the culture of scientific research in the Cold War era was a good deal more combative than is tolerated today. "He ran his laboratory like a military unit," wrote his biographer, "and he was the one in command. For a time, he kept a row of 'shrunken heads' (actually fakes made by one of his children) in his office as trophies that represented each of his fired employees. He used profanity and tirades freely to drive his arguments home, and once, famously, refused to attend a mandatory 'charm school' course intended to make Merck middle managers more civil."[39]

THE BIOCHEMISTRY OF COLD WAR

The 1957–58 Asian flu pandemic had some economic effects, of course. By early November 1957, 82 million Americans had been ill, losing 282 million days to sickness. Yet the most that can be said is that the pandemic coincided with a recession. The economic contraction had in fact begun before the virus started spreading in the United States, in the summer of 1957. The proximate causes of the recession were rising market interest rates, which the Federal Reserve had half-heartedly followed,[40] and cuts in defense spending. In any case, the recession was short—it lasted just nine months—and shallow. Unemployment rose moderately, from 4.1 percent in August 1957 to a peak of

7.5 percent the following July, below the peak of 7.9 percent in the 1948–49 recession. Personal income and personal consumption expenditures did not contract. An August 1958 Federal Reserve review of the recession did not even mention the pandemic as a potential cause of the downturn, noting that restaurants, bars, and malls had been among the least impacted sectors.[41] AT&T's data on its employees in thirty-six cities showed that the epidemic peaked during the week ending October 19 with an excess absenteeism rate of just 2.7 percent. In the larger number of cities that the CDC tracked itself, excess absenteeism during each city's peak week varied from 3 percent to 8 percent. Data from Canada tell a similar story.[42] The Congressional Budget Office has described the Asian flu as an event that "might not be distinguishable from the normal variation in economic activity."[43]

The economic consequences of the pandemic of 1957–58 were thus minimal compared with those of 2020. But the same might not be said of the political aftermaths. In 1958, Republicans suffered one of the greatest rebukes in midterm history, losing 13 Senate and 48 House seats, by a popular vote margin of 13 percent. Yet the pandemic was probably a minor variable in the election. *The New York Times* did not even mention the Asian flu in its 1958 midterm postmortem.[44] National security concerns almost certainly loomed larger. The previous year, the Soviets had successfully launched their Sputnik satellite, causing consternation among Americans, who had assumed their country had an innate technological advantage in both the Cold War and the space race. Civil war was raging in Cuba; Fidel Castro was just a few months from victory; and in July a coup d'état had overthrown King Faisal II of Iraq, the prelude to the Baathist takeover of power in that country in 1963. American troops had been dispatched to Lebanon in response.

The Asian flu pandemic thus cannot be seen apart from its geopolitical context. It helped Maurice Hilleman a great deal, for example, that by 1957 the American CDC was a leading node in an international network of public health agencies. This network had its origins in the early 1900s, which had seen the creation of the PanAmerican Sanitary Bureau (1902) and the Paris-based Office International d'Hygiène Publique (1907), but it was only after the First World War that it became truly global. In December 1920, the Assembly of the League of Nations approved a resolution to create a Health Committee under Ludwik Rajchman, a Polish bacteriologist who had resisted the eastward spread of typhus as successfully as his military counterpart, Józef Piłsudski, had resisted the spread of Bolshevism. Created in 1921, the Epidemiological Intelligence Service was a central part of Rajchman's organization. The next year, it started to issue a variety of periodical reports. Until 1923, the Health Committee was designated as "provisional," then, from 1923 to 1928, it became the Permanent Health Committee, before being renamed the League of Nations Health Organization (LNHO), though in practice it relied heavily on funding from the Rockefeller Foundation. A Far Eastern Bureau (also known as the Eastern Bureau) was opened in Singapore in 1925. It produced two standard weekly bulletins, one that was sent through the mail and one that was broadcast on the radio. By the early 1930s, the LNHO's network spanned forty-five countries and two thirds of the world's population.

Not everyone joined. Latin American governments preferred to work within the Pan American Health Organization, arguably for fear of "epidemiological imperialism," but in reality the spirit of LNHO was more liberal than imperial. Frank Boudreau, the Canadian physician who became the organization's director, captured this spirit in January 1940: "The truth shall make men free, said the prophet, and to know the truth about disease means freedom for passenger and freight traffic, freedom from disease and from unnecessary restrictions." For Boudreau, the Singapore bureau was "a central fire-station in a municipal system of fire prevention," overseeing "the world's alarm system."[45] To an amazing extent, the LNHO kept working even as the world slid back into war. Germany continued to send out epidemiological bulletins even after Hitler rescinded the country's League membership in October 1933.[46] The weekly bulletin continued to be issued from Singapore despite the Japanese invasion of China in 1937 and the outbreak of World War II in Europe in 1939. As Boudreau observed in 1939, "It is one of to-day's paradoxes that the world which is destroying international co-operation by every means in its power is being saved from possibly devastating epidemics by international co-operation in health matters." By 1940, it is true, the system broke down as American and then British officials began withholding information, for fear that it would assist the Germans and their allies. Yet the LNHO survived World War II and "laid the groundwork for the system that the World Health Organization still uses today," providing several of the WHO's founding officials.[47] The spirit of Frank Boudreau lived on in that agency's first director, Brock Chisholm, another Canadian with a utopian vision of "a new kind of citizen [who] is necessary if the human race is going to survive."[48]

Beginning in the late 1930s, there was a transformation in American attitudes toward national security that ensured international public health would remain a priority after 1945. In a speech in October 1937, President Franklin D. Roosevelt referred to an "epidemic of world lawlessness" and warned that "war is a contagion, whether it be declared or undeclared, [that] can engulf states and peoples remote from the original scene of hostilities."[49] Roosevelt and the New Dealers became convinced that international security— and thus U.S. security—depended upon economic and political development.[50] As Vice President Henry A. Wallace put it in 1942, "War is seen as part of a continuous process whose roots lie deep in poverty, insecurity, starvation and unemployment. A world from which these evils have not been banished is a world in which Hitlers and wars will perpetually recur."[51] This logic was seamlessly carried forward into the Cold War, not least because the Soviet Union represented a much more plausible rival as a sponsor of Third World economic development than Germany, Japan, or Italy ever had before 1945.[52] As the director of a U.S. technical cooperation mission to Iran explained to the president of the Iranian parliament in 1952, "I did not wake up each morning thinking, 'How can I fight communism?' but I woke up each morning thinking, 'How can I assist in fighting the diseases, hunger, and poverty that plague the people of Iran?' . . . If this was an attack on the roots of communism, then communism was a diseased plant and ought to be rooted out."[53]

The United States brought to this competition the formidable advantage of the world's most advanced pharmaceutical industry. It was not so much that American scientists were ahead of their competitors; in terms of Nobel Prizes they were not. Between 1901 and 1940, U.S. scientists won just 8 percent of science Nobels, Germans 22 percent.[54] But when it came to developing and distributing a new drug, the United States was unrivaled. Sulfonamide drugs were pioneered as antibacterials by the German company Bayer AG, then part of the chemical trust IG Farben, but it turned out that the active ingredient in Bayer's trademarked Prontosil was a widely available compound called sulfanilamide. "Sulfa" drugs were soon being mass-produced in the United States and to remarkable effect, both good and ill. In the fall of 1937, one hundred people were poisoned with diethylene glycol after taking "the elixir sulfanilamide," a disaster that led to the passage of the Federal Food, Drug, and Cosmetic Act in 1938 and the beginning of serious pharmaceutical regulation in the United States. On the other hand, in 1941 alone, between ten and fifteen million Americans were being treated with sulfa drugs. The results were a 25 percent decline in maternal mortality, a 13 percent decline in pneumonia/influenza mortality, and a 52 percent decline in scarlet fever mortality.[55]

In the same way, it was a Scotsman, an Australian, and a German—Alexander Fleming, Howard Florey, and Ernst Chain—who, between 1929 and 1940, discovered and developed penicillin, but it was American companies that were mass-producing antibiotics by the end of World War II. In the United States between 1937 and 1952, the infectious disease mortality rate fell by 8.2 percent a year, as compared with an average of 2.8 percent a year between 1900 and 1936. Antibiotics alone were responsible for a decrease in the mortality rate of around 5.4 percent a year for fifteen years, for an overall reduction of more than 56 percent. Not all the improvement in mid-twentieth-century mortality should be attributed to sulfa and antibiotics, of course: as we have seen, improved hygiene, nutrition, and sanitation also played a major part, in both the United States and the United Kingdom, as did social policies designed to reduce poverty.[56] Novel non-pharmaceutical interventions such as contact tracing, pioneered in British schools and adopted by the U.S. Army in 1937, also contributed.[57] But—like most of the vaccines widely discovered and distributed in the mid-twentieth century—these other factors had a much bigger impact in reducing mortality among the young; for older people, sulfa and antibiotics were what made the difference.[58] Propelling medical research forward was the simultaneous British and American adoption of the randomized controlled trial in 1948 and the double-blind method in 1950.[59] In short, Maurice Hilleman's success in 1957–58 was not only the result of heroic, high-speed American innovation; it was also based on the fact that cooperation among Hong Kong, London, and Washington, D.C., had been institutionalized for years prior to the Asian flu outbreak, as well as the fact that the U.S. population had never been healthier than in the summer they were hit by the "boogie woogie flu."

At the same time, in 1957 the Soviet Union was approaching the peak of its self-confidence under Nikita Khrushchev. It is worth reiterating that the Soviet launch of Sputnik came on October 4, 1957, in the midst of the Asian flu pandemic. That may help explain why the memory of the Asian flu has faded. After all, the Cold War posed such an unprecedented threat of disaster— the threat of thermonuclear war—that the traditional threats posed to humanity by microbes somewhat receded in popular consciousness. Asked during the fifties and sixties whether they thought there would be a world war in the next five years, between 40 and 65 percent of Americans who had an opinion answered yes. By the 1980s that percentage had risen to 76. Asked if, in the event of a world war, the hydrogen bomb would be used against the United States, between 60 and 75 percent of Americans again said yes. How far this truth was internalized is debatable. The argument made by the economist Joel Slemrod in the 1980s was that fear of Armageddon had depressed the American private savings rate—because why save for a future that might never come? Slemrod's prediction was that in a post–Cold War world, with the risk of nuclear war suddenly reduced, savings would recover,* especially in the United States.[60] In any case, from the 1950s to the 1980s, people thought more about World War III than about any other threat to humanity. In the words of the WHO's Brock Chisholm, "The destructive potentialities of man have become so great that his inferiorities, anxieties, fears, hates, aggressive pressures, fanaticisms, and even his unreasoning devotions and loyalties, which are among the common symptoms of physical, mental or social ill health, may now constitute a serious threat to the continued existence of large numbers of people."[61]

---

*Unfortunately for Slemrod's hypothesis, they did nothing of the kind. Even as the atomic scientists' Doomsday Clock was wound back to seventeen minutes to midnight in the wake of the Soviet collapse, the personal savings rate continued to slump, from 9.4 percent of disposable income in 1983—when the world teetered on the brink of disaster—to 2.5 percent in 2005.

Even without nuclear Armageddon, the Cold War was distinctly hot in places. Conventional warfare continued to rage in multiple zones of conflict from Indochina to Central America. The "brinkmanship" of the Eisenhower era was succeeded by even more alarming showdowns under Presidents Kennedy and Johnson: Berlin in 1961, Cuba in 1962, and then the disastrous escalation of the U.S. commitment to South Vietnam thereafter. Détente made only a slight improvement. By almost any measure, the Nixon-Ford-Carter years were far more violent than the Bush-Obama-Trump years. There were more than 2 million battle deaths due to state-based armed conflict in the 1970s, as compared with approximately 270,000 in the 2000s.[62] Vietnam was a vastly more lethal war than Iraq (47,424 U.S. combat deaths versus 3,527). According to the Peace Research Institute of Oslo (PRIO), which estimates total battle deaths arising from state-based armed conflict, the peak years of conflict between 1956 and 2007 were 1971 (around 380,000 fatalities) and 1982 to 1988, when the annual average was close to 250,000. Between 2002 and 2007, by contrast, the average was just under 17,000.[63] The "war magnitude" index calculated by the Center for Systemic Peace, in Vienna, Virginia, rose steadily from the 1950s to the mid-1980s, then fell steeply—by more than half—after the end of the Cold War in 1991, as did the CSP's estimate for the percentage of states experiencing warfare and the number of armed-conflict events. A broader measure of "annual deaths from political violence," which includes the victims of genocide, ethnic cleansing, and the like, tells a similar story, with the global death rate peaking in the early 1970s and then declining more or less steadily, aside from the spike resulting from the 1994 genocide in Rwanda.[64] The frequency of revolutions, military coups, and political assassinations is also lower now than it was in the late twentieth century.

In the context of their nuclear rivalry, the superpowers behaved in contradictory ways toward other potential threats. On the one hand, American and Soviet scientists cooperated during the Cold War in the development of two hugely successful vaccines.[65] The University of Cincinnati's Albert Sabin (who had been born in Białystok when it was still part of the Russian Empire) teamed up with the Soviet virologist Mikhail Chumakov to run a large-scale test of Sabin's live attenuated oral vaccine against polio, which they administered to ten million children.[66] Superpower cooperation was also the essential basis for the successful campaign to eradicate smallpox via mass vaccination that culminated in 1978.[67] This was one of a number of global initiatives that transcended the Cold War divide, along with the 1973 International Convention for the Prevention of Pollution from Ships, which aimed to reduce pollution of the world's oceans by making oil tankers less prone to spillage, and the Montreal Protocol of 1987, which aimed to protect the stratosphere's ozone layer by restricting the production and use of chlorofluorocarbons.[68]

At one and the same time, however, the Soviet Union was engaged in a massive program of research into biological weapons, in violation of the Biological Weapons Convention that it signed in 1972. According to Kenneth Alibek, a former Soviet scientist who worked at Biopreparat in the late 1980s, the Soviets developed antibiotic-resistant strains of plague, glanders, tularemia, and anthrax, including the highly virulent 836 strain. Its operational biological weapons were capable of delivering tularemia, glanders, Venezuelan equine encephalitis, and brucellosis about a hundred miles behind enemy lines, while its strategic biological weapons were designed to carry plague and smallpox to targets in the United States. Other pathogens being developed for use in biological weapons, according to Alibek's testimony, included Q fever, the Marburg, Ebola, and Machupo viruses, hemorrhagic fever, Lassa fever, and Russian encephalitis.[69]

SAYING PRAYERS, TAKING CHANCES

A striking contrast between 1957 and the present is that Americans today would appear to have a much lower tolerance for risk than their grandparents and great-grandparents six decades ago. As one contemporary recalled,

> For those who grew up in the 1930s and 1940s, there was nothing unusual about finding yourself threatened by contagious disease. Mumps, measles, chicken pox, and German measles swept through entire schools and towns; I had all four. Polio took a heavy annual toll, leaving thousands of people (mostly children) paralyzed or dead. . . . Growing up

meant running an unavoidable gauntlet of infectious disease. For college students in 1957, the Asian flu was a familiar hurdle on the road to adulthood. . . . We took the Asian flu in stride. We said our prayers and took our chances.[70]

D. A. Henderson, who as a young doctor was responsible for establishing the CDC Influenza Surveillance Unit, recalled a similar sangfroid in the medical profession:

> In early October, the *New York Times* reported that "extra beds were being prepared" at one hospital, and at Bellevue Hospital extra physicians were assigned to cope with the "upper respiratory epidemic" and elective surgeries were suspended. . . . However, a physician at Bellevue referred to the pandemic as a "newspaper epidemic," and "the Hospitals Department . . . [saw] it as only a large number of cases." . . .
>
> There were no [newspaper] reports that major events were canceled or postponed except for high school and college football games, which were often delayed because of the number of players afflicted. . . .
>
> From one watching the pandemic from very close range . . . it was a transiently disturbing event for the population, albeit stressful for schools and health clinics and disruptive to school football schedules.[71]

Compare these stoical attitudes with the hesitancy of many voters in 2020 to end the lockdowns and return to work and social normalcy. According to Gallup data from late April 2020, only 21 percent of American adults were ready to return to normal activities "right now." More than a third—36 percent—said they would return to their activities once the number of new cases of coronavirus in their state had declined significantly, while 31 percent said they would return to normal life only once there are *no* new cases in their state. More than one in ten (12 percent) said they would wait for a vaccine to be developed.[72] Polling in late September showed that nearly half of U.S. adults were either very worried (10 percent) or somewhat worried (39 percent) about contracting the coronavirus, down from 59 percent a month before, and that these worries continued to discourage people from going to offices, restaurants, and airports.[73]

Other changes in public attitudes are striking. In 1957, a man as mercurial as Maurice Hilleman could work with a fearless single-mindedness for both the government and a corporation. No doubt such people still exist: vaccines for COVID-19 were discovered almost as swiftly as a vaccine for Asian flu in 1957. But it is certainly not easy to imagine Hilleman, with his strong language and shrunken heads, thriving in the academy of the 2020s. Finally, it seems plausible that a society with a stronger fabric of family life, community life, and church life was better equipped—"tighter," in the terminology of Michele Gelfand[74]—to withstand the anguish of excess mortality than a society that has in so many ways "come apart."[75]

A further contrast between 2020 and 1957 is that the competence of government would appear to have diminished even as its size has expanded in the past six decades. In 1957, to be sure, the total number of federal civilian employees was just under 1.87 million, as compared with 2.1 million in early 2020; in that sense, the government has shrunk in relative terms.[76] However, all government employees, including those in state and local governments, numbered 7.8 million in November 1957, and reached around 22 million in 2020.[77] Federal net outlays were 16.2 percent of GDP in 1957, versus 20.8 percent in 2019.[78] The gross federal debt rose from 57.4 percent of GDP in 1957 to 58.1 percent of GDP in 1958; it declined as a share of GDP every year thereafter until 1974.[79] The gross federal debt in 2019 was 105.8 percent of GDP; it is projected to increase by as much as 19 percent of GDP in 2020.[80] In 1957 there was no Department of Health and Human Services, but a Department of Health, Education, and Welfare. HEW had been created in 1953 to take over the responsibilities of the Federal Security Agency, established in 1939. The Communicable Disease Center, the forerunner of today's CDC, had been established just eleven years before the 1957 pandemic, with the eradication of malaria as its principal objective. These relatively young institutions appear to have done what little was required of them in 1957, namely to reassure the public that the disastrous pandemic of 1918–19 was not about to be repeated while helping the private sector to test, manufacture, and distribute the vaccine. The contrast with the events of 2020 is once again striking.

However, we should not understate the risk aversion of 1950s Americans, nor overstate the competence of the government of that era. While they were singularly sanguine about the Asian flu, Americans were anything but sanguine about poliomyelitis (polio, for short), an enteric (intestinal) infection caused by the poliovirus, which is spread through contact with fecal waste. In a small number of cases—perhaps one in a hundred—the virus gets beyond the gut and invades the brain stem and the central nervous system, destroying the motor neurons that stimulate the muscles to contract and causing irreversible paralysis, most often in the legs. Even more rarely, polio can kill when it paralyzes the breathing muscles.[81] Partly because polio had deprived Franklin Roosevelt of the use of his legs, and partly because the man who ran the National Foundation for Infantile Paralysis (NFIP), Basil O'Connor, was such an effective organizer, polio became a national obsession, beginning in the late 1930s.[82] Employing the latest techniques in advertising and fundraising, O'Connor succeeded in turning a horrific but relatively rare disease into the most feared affliction of the age, a fear that culminated in 1952, when reported cases of polio reached a peak of 37 per 100,000.[83]

The polio pandemic panic exposed serious weaknesses in the American system of public health. First, rejecting government support or oversight on principle as a "Communistic, un-American . . . scheme," the NFIP gave all its financial support to Jonas Salk's killed-virus vaccine, which was designed to stimulate the immune system to produce the desired antibodies without creating a natural infection. The results of the trials—which involved two million elementary-school children throughout the country—showed Salk's vaccine to be 60 to 70 percent effective against the type 1 polio virus and 90 percent or more effective against the type 2 and type 3 viruses.[84] In April 1955, within hours of the results' publication, the Public Health Service approved the Salk vaccine for commercial production. But the popular demand for the vaccine took the secretary of health, education, and welfare, Oveta Culp Hobby, by surprise.[85] The Eisenhower administration had simply assumed that the entire process would remain in private hands, with the vaccine going "from the manufacturer to the wholesaler to the druggist to the local doctor."[86] The scramble to produce enough doses of the vaccine led to the distribution of a faulty batch from Cutter Laboratories, in Berkeley, California. Some children who were given the defective vaccine contracted polio; a number developed paralysis. In the end, it turned out that Albert Sabin's orally administered live vaccine was superior, though Salk's was also effective.[87] It is in this context that Maurice Hilleman's race for a flu vaccine must be understood. The events of 1957 occurred in a quite distinctive context: just two years before, the dangers of a purely market-driven approach and the need for effective federal oversight had been conclusively demonstrated, leading to a significant increase in funding and power for the National Institutes of Health as well as the CDC.

Did the U.S. government learn the right lessons from the pandemic of 1957–58—and indeed from that of 1968? It is tempting to say that it did. Preparedness for the next influenza pandemic remained at a high level throughout the subsequent decades. Indeed, it appeared to tip over into overpreparedness in 1976, when an outbreak of influenza A, subtype H1N1, at Fort Dix, New Jersey, caused one death and hospitalized thirteen. Fearing a return of the 1918–19 influenza strain, CDC director David Sencer recommended mass immunization against what was now referred to as "swine flu." Persuaded, but mindful of the Cutter debacle, President Gerald Ford urged Congress to pass legislation giving the manufacturers indemnity in case any problems arose with their vaccine. However, the program had to be halted amid reports that some vaccine recipients had developed Guillain-Barré syndrome, which can cause paralysis and respiratory arrest.[88]

When reports reached Washington of an outbreak of H5N1 "bird flu" in Asia in 2005, the administration of George W. Bush was ready to implement another emergency response, with vaccines once again at its core.[89] Bush himself had been alerted to the perils of an influenza pandemic by reading John M. Barry's *The Great Influenza*. Health and human services secretary Michael O. Leavitt told the *Los Angeles Times* that of all the threats he had to prepare for, "the one that keeps me awake at night is influenza."[90] But the 2005 epidemic did not reach the United States. By contrast, the 2009 swine flu outbreak, which originated in Mexico in February of that year, did. The administration of Barack Obama is sometimes lauded for its pandemic preparedness,[91] but it was unable to provide a vaccine against the 2009 strain of H1N1 until the following year, after two distinct waves of infection, of which the second (in the fall) was the larger.[92] The only reason mortality was no higher than in an average flu season was simply that the virus was not especially lethal. Early estimates of the fatality rate for the virus were much higher than the roughly 0.01 to 0.03 percent that transpired, which was still enough to kill 12,469 Americans and hospitalize 274,304 in the space of twelve months. The global death toll was around 300,000.[93] But the 2009 swine flu infected between 43 and 89 million Americans. If its IFR had been ten times higher, mortality could have been proportionately higher. Moreover, swine flu killed young as well as old: mean age at death was half that in the average 1970–2001 flu season, so more QALYs were almost certainly lost. Early in the COVID-19 pandemic, the epidemiologist Larry Brilliant suggested to me that, to get a sense of the new disease's potential impact, we might imagine an attack rate similar to that of the influenza of 2009, but with an IFR of 0.1–0.4 percent. Such an epidemic would have killed up to 183,000 Americans in 2009 and up to 385,000 in 2020. The mere fact that the Obama administration had a pandemic preparedness plan[94] tells us nothing about how well it would have been implemented if COVID-19 had struck during his presidential tenure. As we shall see, his successor's administration had no shortage of such plans.

FAREWELL, FREDDIE

Thirty years after Huey "Piano" Smith's "Rockin' Pneumonia and the Boogie Woogie Flu," another rock star—one more in Elvis Presley's league than Huey Smith's—encountered a very different kind of virus. Freddie Mercury, the flamboyant, bisexual lead singer of the British band Queen, was diagnosed with the human immunodeficiency virus (HIV) in 1987. He was forty-one. Four years later he was dead.

In the period between 1957 and 2020, the United States—and the world—faced only one historically significant pandemic, and that was the one caused by HIV and the lethal disease it can lead to, acquired immunodeficiency syndrome (AIDS). The policy response was dismal: the initial reaction of most world leaders was to avoid talking about the virus, which was mostly (though not entirely) sexually transmitted. Not much more impressive was the response of medical science, which failed altogether to devise an effective vaccine and took fifteen years to find a therapy that could prevent HIV-infected people from developing AIDS. Nor, for that matter, was the public response especially edifying. Long after they understood the risks associated with the spread of HIV, people continued to act in ways that increased their chances of infection. As a result, AIDS has now killed thirty-two million people around the world. At the height of the pandemic, in 2005–6, fifteen years after the death of Freddie Mercury, nearly two million people a year were dying of AIDS.

The virus responsible for the vast majority of AIDS cases, HIV-1, appears to have crossed from chimpanzees in central Africa in the 1920s or earlier, probably because of the trade in and consumption of "bushmeat." It spread slowly for decades, before transmission accelerated—perhaps as a result of African urbanization—and went global in the 1970s.[95] But "slowly" is the operative word. (In Cameroon they call the disease *le poison lent,* the slow poison.) Compared with an influenza pandemic, HIV/AIDS moved at a snail's pace. Why, then, was the national and international response so ineffectual? According to the San Francisco–based journalist Randy Shilts, who himself died of AIDS in 1994, it was because of a systemic failure: in the United States, the medical and public health bodies, federal and private scientific research establishments, the mass media, and the gay community's leadership all failed to respond in the ways they should have.[96]

In 1981, the *New York Native* published the first article about gay men being treated in intensive care units for a strange new illness. The headline was "Disease Rumors Largely Unfounded." The earliest American patients, most of whom lived in San Francisco, New York, or Los Angeles, were diagnosed with one of a number of unusual illnesses: Kaposi's sarcoma, a rare cancer that in these patients proved unusually aggressive and fatal; *Pneumocystis* pneumonia, a rare form of pneumonia; cryptosporidiosis, a disease usually found in sheep; cytomegalovirus, a herpes virus that spread rapidly through patients with severe immunodeficiency; toxoplasmosis, a disease resulting from infection by the *Toxoplasma gondii* parasite, usually found in cat feces or infected meat; and cryptococcal meningitis. On June 5, 1981, the CDC's *Morbidity and Mortality Weekly Report* published (on page 2) the first report on the epidemic, under the headline "*Pneumocystis* Pneumonia—Los Angeles."[97] Eleven days later, at the CDC hepatitis laboratory in Phoenix, Dr. Don Francis suggested that a form of "feline leukemia," likely caused by a retrovirus that spread via sex, was causing immune deficiencies in gay men.[98] Just over a year later, Bruce Evatt identified that there was a risk to hemophiliacs from blood transfusions that might be contaminated by the new virus.[99] In January 1983, Françoise Barré-Sinoussi, a young researcher at the Pasteur Institute in Paris, found in a biopsied lymph node taken from an AIDS patient a new retrovirus so deadly that it killed its host cells. Her boss, Luc Montagnier, identified it as a lentivirus, a type of virus more commonly found in animals.[100]

Yet such valuable findings by researchers failed to translate into an effective public health policy response. It was not until 1983 that the Public Health Service advised "high-risk groups . . . that multiple sexual partners increase the probability of developing AIDS" and modified its policy on blood donation.[101] Why? Part of the answer is that the administration of Ronald Reagan turned a blind eye. If polio-stricken children in leg braces had gripped the American imagination in the 1950s, gay men with a sexually transmitted wasting disease had the opposite effect in the 1980s. "The poor homosexuals— they have declared war upon nature, and now nature is exacting an awful retribution," remarked the conservative Pat Buchanan, a Reagan adviser.[102] Reagan did not even mention AIDS until 1985. Indeed, in 1987 Congress explicitly banned the use of federal funds for AIDS prevention and education campaigns that "[promoted] or [encouraged], directly or indirectly, homosexual activities," legislation sponsored by Senator Jesse Helms.[103] But this was not the sole reason for the overall policy failure. In addition, there was bureaucratic infighting among the CDC, the NIH, and the National Cancer Institute (NCI),[104] to say nothing of the questionable attempt by Robert Gallo at the NCI to claim the credit for identifying the virus that caused AIDS.[105] The name finally agreed upon—human immunodeficiency virus (HIV)—was a compromise between the rival French and American teams.[106] There was friction at the World Health Organization, too, where the director general, Hiroshi Nakajima, forced the resignation of Jonathan Mann as head of the Global Programme on AIDS.[107] Infighting continued until 1990 between the GPA and the much smaller WHO program on sexually transmitted diseases, to say nothing of the uncoordinated competition for donor dollars among the World Bank, UNICEF, UNESCO, the United Nations Population Fund (UNFPA), and the UN Development Program (UNDP).[108] The media gave much more coverage to stories about toxic shock syndrome, Legionnaires' disease, and contaminated Tylenol. In 1981 and 1982, *The New York Times* ran a total of six stories about AIDS. None made the front page.[109]

There was also division within the gay community. "[Larry] Kramer is telling us that something we gay men are doing (drugs? kinky sex?) is causing Kaposi's sarcoma," complained playwright Robert Chesley, in one of several letters attacking Kramer in the *New York Native*. "The concealed meaning of Kramer's emotionalism is the triumph of guilt: that gay men deserve to die for their promiscuity. . . . Something else is happening here, which is also serious: gay homophobia and anti-eroticism."[110] There was a reluctance to acknowledge that the hyperactive sex lives of a relatively small proportion of gay men were responsible for a very large share of infections. Only a few epidemiologists and network scientists grasped the essential point about HIV/AIDS: that the role of superspreaders in scale-free sexual networks made it quite different from previous pandemics.[111] Gaëtan Dugas, an Air Canada flight attendant who "estimated that he had had approximately 250 different male sexual partners each year from 1979 through 1981," was one of the first identified superspreaders.[112] Dugas was the heir to "Typhoid Mary" Mallon, the Irish cook who had infected an unknown number of New Yorkers with *Sal-*

monella typhi between 1900 and 1907 and again between 1910 and 1915, until she was forcibly quarantined.[113]

The result of all this was that the number of deaths from HIV/AIDS went up steadily—in the United States from around twelve thousand a year in 1987 to more than forty thousand in 1994, by which time heterosexuals and intravenous drug users made up a rising share of the victims.[114] However, if in America AIDS was a tragedy, in Africa—where the virus is overwhelmingly spread via heterosexual sex—it was a catastrophe.[115] More than a fifth of adult residents of capitals such as Kampala and Lusaka were HIV-positive by 1990. By 1996 AIDS was the most common cause of death in sub-Saharan Africa. In Botswana, South Africa, and Zimbabwe, life expectancy at birth had been above sixty in 1987. By 2003 it had fallen to fifty-three, fifty, and forty-four, respectively. Why was this? High levels of prostitution and promiscuity were part of the explanation: that was why truck drivers and miners were especially at risk. Another was misinformation. In Francophone Africa, SIDA (the acronym for AIDS in French) was said to stand for "syndrome imaginaire pour décourager les amoureux" (imaginary syndrome to discourage lovers).[116] In South Africa, successive presidents—Thabo Mbeki, who succeeded Nelson Mandela as president of South Africa in 1999, and Jacob Zuma, who took over from Mbeki ten years later—publicly denied the nature of the threat posed by the virus, the latter boasting that a postcoital shower offered protection enough. Matters were made worse by a Soviet disinformation campaign, which planted in a KGB-controlled Indian newspaper the story that AIDS had been deliberately engineered by the United States, and then amplified the lie with bogus research by a retired East German biophysicist, Jakob Segal, which was widely cited in newspapers around the world, including the *Sunday Express*.[117] Aside from the human suffering of millions of premature deaths, the economic consequences have been incalculable. AIDS kills slowly, weakening workers and lowering their productivity. The orphans it leaves behind have worse life chances. Sub-Saharan Africa is much poorer today than it would have been without AIDS.

The lesson of HIV/AIDS is not quite that it "changed everything"—the title of a celebratory book by UNAIDS published five years ago.[118] The most striking feature of the history of the AIDS pandemic is that behavior only partly changed after the recognition of a new and deadly disease spread by sex and needle sharing. An early American report noted "rapid, profound, but . . . incomplete alterations in the behavior of both homosexual/bisexual males and intravenous drug users," as well as "considerable instability or recidivism."[119] By 1998 just 19 percent of all U.S. adults reported some change in their sexual conduct in response to the threat of AIDS.[120] The advent, in 1996, of combination antiretroviral therapy (ART or cART), the use of a cocktail of HIV-suppressing drugs to prevent HIV carriers from succumbing to AIDS, somewhat diminished the fear factor. Even so, one might have expected a bit more fear to persist, especially given that ART at first cost $10,000 a year. A 2017 paper showed that fewer than half of at-risk men had used a condom the last time they had sex.[121] According to a recent British study, sustained campaigns of public and individual education are necessary to discourage gay men from having sex without condoms.[122] Meanwhile, in Africa, the "ABC" (abstain, be faithful, and condomize) approach has had only limited success. Between 2000 and 2015, according to the UN, "in eastern and southern Africa . . . condom use increased from 21.1% to 22.2% among boys and 21.6% to 32.5% among girls."[123] That scarcely constitutes victory, though there is some more encouraging evidence that young Africans are delaying having sex and turning away from traditional practices such as the ritual "cleansing" of a widow through sex with a relative of the deceased husband.[124]

In the absence of an effective vaccine, and with therapies at first unavailable and then expensive, containment of a pandemic is wholly dependent on behavioral change. In the case of a sexually transmitted disease, this is almost impossible for public health authorities to enforce: the best they can do is inform people and hope they listen. Without a doubt, there have been changes in sexual behavior over the past thirty years. According to the psychologists Brooke Wells and Jean Twenge, millennials have fewer sex partners on average than earlier generations.[125] Another U.S. study concluded that "promiscuity hit its modern peak for men born in the 1950s."[126] Condom use would also appear to have risen.[127] A 2020 analysis of responses to the General Social Survey between 2000 and 2018 revealed higher rates of sexual inactivity among the most recent cohort of twenty- to twenty-four-year-olds than among their predecessors born in the 1970s and '80s. Between 2000–2002 and 2016–18, the proportion of eighteen- to twenty-four-year-old men who reported having had no sexual activity in the past year increased from 19 to 31 percent. Sexual inactivity was also up for twenty-five- to thirty-four-year-olds, and there were declines in the proportion reporting sexual frequency as weekly or more.

However, these declines were most pronounced among students and men with lower incomes and with part-time or no employment, suggesting that declining sexual activity is an economically determined phenomenon. Other possible explanations for the decline include the "stress and busyness of modern life," the supply of "online entertainment that may compete with sexual activity," elevated rates of depression and anxiety among young adults, the detrimental effect of smartphones on real-world human interactions, and the lack of appeal to women of "hooking up."[128] The most recent version of the UK National Survey of Sexual Attitudes and Lifestyles revealed a similar marked decline in the frequency of sex in Britain, but once again this had little if anything to do with HIV/AIDS.[129] The return of the "No sex please, we're British" ethos mainly affects married or cohabiting couples and—according to a careful analysis in *The BMJ*—is most likely due to "the introduction of the iPhone in 2007 and the global recession of 2008."[130] Remarkably, there is no sign in the most recent U.S. General Social Survey of a decline in sex among men and women identifying as gay, lesbian, or bisexual, who were more likely than heterosexuals to report three or more sexual partners. More than two fifths of gay or bisexual American men said they had had sex weekly or more frequently in the preceding year. More than a third said they had had three or more sexual partners.[131]

Meanwhile—perhaps not surprisingly in light of these data—HIV lives on. In 2018, 37,968 Americans received an HIV diagnosis, 69 percent of them gay or bisexual men, keeping the total number of HIV-positive people above a million, just over half of whom are "virally suppressed" through ART.[132] But HIV accounted for just a fraction of the nearly 2.5 million total new cases of sexually transmitted disease, up for the fifth consecutive year. Chlamydia led (nearly 1.8 million cases), followed by gonorrhea (more than 580,000) and syphilis (115,000). Gay and bisexual men accounted for more than half of all syphilis cases.[133] Nothing could better illustrate the extreme difficulty of altering human behavior, even in the face of dangerous, if no longer deadly, pathogens. Those who hoped that in the time of COVID-19 face masks would be "the new condoms" failed to understand what a discouraging analogy that was.[134] If SARS-CoV-2 is to social life what HIV was to sex life, many more people are going to fall sick in the months after this book is completed.

REES VS. PINKER

Another pandemic at some point in the first twenty years of the twenty-first century was not difficult to predict. In 2002, the Cambridge astrophysicist Martin Rees publicly bet that "by 2020, bioterror or bioerror will lead to one million casualties* in a single event."[135] The Harvard psychologist Steven Pinker took the other side of the bet in 2017,[136] arguing that material "advances have made humanity more resilient to natural and human-made threats: disease outbreaks don't become pandemics." As Pinker argued,

> advances in biology . . . make it easier for the good guys (and there are many more of them) to identify pathogens, invent antibiotics that overcome antibiotic resistance, and rapidly develop vaccines. An example is the Ebola vaccine, developed in the waning days of the 2014–15 emergency, after public health efforts had capped the toll at twelve thousand deaths rather than the millions that the media had foreseen. Ebola thus joined a list of other falsely predicted pandemics such as Lassa fever, hantavirus, SARS, mad cow disease, bird flu, and swine flu. Some of them never had the potential to go pandemic in the first place. . . . Others were nipped by medical and public health interventions. . . . Jour-

---

*Given that the bet defined "casualties" as including "victims requiring hospitalization," Rees had won the bet even before the global death toll passed one million in September 2020. Unfortunately for him, the stake was a meager $400.

nalistic habits and the Availability and Negativity biases inflate the odds [of a pandemic], which is why I have taken Sir Martin up on his bet.[137]

Pinker was implicitly subscribing to the theory of the epidemiological transition—the belief that advances in living standards and public health had largely conquered infectious disease, leaving chronic conditions such as cancer and heart disease as the principal obstacles to longer life spans. However, by the time of their bet, Rees found himself in exceedingly good company. Among those who also correctly foresaw a pandemic were Laurie Garrett (2005),[138] George W. Bush (2005),[139] Bill Frist (in a Bohemian Grove Lakeside Talk), Michael Osterholm (2005),[140] Larry Brilliant (2006),[141] Ian Goldin (2014),[142] Bill Gates (2015),[143] Robert G. Webster (2018),[144] Ed Yong (2018),[145] Thoughty2 (2019),[146] Lawrence Wright (2019),[147] and Peter Frankopan (2019).[148] If ever there was a gray rhino, COVID-19 was it.

Why was this? First, as we have seen, the optimism of Maurice Hilleman's generation of vaccine pioneers had foundered on the rocks not only of HIV/AIDS but of tuberculosis and malaria, for which no effective vaccines had yet been found.[149] Second, infectious diseases once thought to have been vanquished had made comebacks, notably diphtheria, plague, and cholera, which had a devastating impact on war-torn Yemen in 2016–17. *Streptococcus pyogenes,* which caused fatal pandemics of scarlet fever and puerperal fever in the nineteenth century, had reemerged to cause new conditions such as streptococcal toxic shock syndrome, rheumatic fever, and necrotizing fasciitis. Zoonotic infectious diseases such as monkeypox, Lyme disease, tick-borne encephalitis, dengue fever, and West Nile virus were also becoming more widespread.[150] More than three fifths of emerging infectious diseases were known to be caused by zoonotic pathogens, of which 70 percent originated in wild rather than domestic animals, indicating that human contact with wildlife was increasing as a result of settlement of marginal land and the persistence in East Asia of "wet" markets for live wild animals.[151] Third, the continued rapid growth of international air travel represented an increase in contagion risk equal to, and quite possibly greater than, any concurrent advances in medical science.[152] In the words of the virologist Stephen Morse, humanity had changed the rules of "viral traffic." This, as the molecular biologist Joshua Lederberg said, was making our species "intrinsically more vulnerable than before."[153] Fourth, climate change was creating new hunting grounds for diseases—notably malaria and diarrheal infections—previously confined to tropical regions.[154]

It was easy to predict a pandemic when pandemics kept nearly happening. Before 2003, coronaviruses were known, but known not to be especially harmful. HKU1, NL63, OC43, and 229E were all associated with mild symptoms. Then, beginning in a food market in Shenzhen in late 2002, came SARS (SARS-CoV).[155] True, there was no SARS pandemic. In all, there were just 8,098 reported cases and 774 deaths. But the appearance of SARS revealed six troubling things. First, the new coronavirus was deadly, with a case fatality rate (CFR) of just under 10 percent. Second, this was a virus especially lethal to older people: the CFR for patients over sixty-four was 52 percent.[156] (As there appear to have been no asymptomatic cases, the CFR for SARS was essentially the same as the infection fatality rate.) Third, many infections were nosocomial, that is, they occurred in hospitals, suggesting that treatment of the sick, unless managed with great care, could end up spreading their illness. Fourth, even more than AIDS, SARS had a low dispersion factor, meaning that a high proportion of infections could be traced to a few superspreaders. A physician from Guangdong Province, in southern China, who checked into the Metropole Hotel in Hong Kong on February 21, 2003, directly or indirectly infected half of all the documented cases. No fewer than 144 of the 206 SARS patients diagnosed in Singapore (70 percent) were traced to a chain of five individuals that included four superspreaders.[157] Jamie Lloyd-Smith and coauthors spelled out the significance of this in a seminal article in *Nature*. A virus like SARS-CoV, with a low dispersion factor (k)—meaning that a lot of transmission comes from a small number of people—was likely to produce fewer but more explosive outbreaks than one with a higher k. The k of SARS was 0.16, as compared with 1.0 for the 1918 Spanish flu. That made a SARS epidemic less likely to start than a flu epidemic, but capable of growing explosively with enough superspreader events.[158] This meant that epidemiological models assuming a homogeneous population and a single reproduction number (R_0) were likely to get the trajectory of a coronavirus pandemic wrong.

The fifth troubling feature of the SARS outbreak was the international response.[159] The WHO itself performed well in the crisis, under the steely leadership of Gro Harlem Brundtland, the former Norwegian prime minister. Michael Ryan's Global Outbreak Alert and Response Network (GOARN) was impressively quick off the mark, and Brundtland approved an early global alert. The German virologist Klaus Stöhr did an effective job of coordinating international research, avoiding the petty competition that had hampered HIV research. (Perhaps the WHO's only misstep was naming the new virus "severe acute respiratory syndrome," overlooking that the acronym SARS is only one letter different from SAR, which denotes Hong Kong's official status as a "special administrative region" of the People's Republic of China.)[160] However, the real problem was the extreme difficulty the WHO had in getting speedy and frank information from Beijing. On April 9, 2003, Brundtland told the press that "it would have been better if the Chinese government had been more open in the early stages, from November to March." This had the desired effect, leading to the replacement of Chinese health minister Zhang Wenkang and notably more cooperative behavior by the Chinese leadership, allowing Western and Chinese researchers to collaborate in tracing the virus back to a species of horseshoe bat.[161] Sixth, and finally, the SARS outbreak revealed the high economic costs of such an outbreak to the countries affected.[162] The cost to the East Asian region was between $20 and $60 billion, as fear of SARS caused drastic declines in foreign visitors and retail sales. If such a small outbreak could be so costly, a 2005 study concluded, a pandemic affecting 25 percent of the world's population could lead to losses of up to 30 percent of world GDP.[163]

The threat posed by a novel coronavirus was underlined in 2012 with the appearance of Middle East respiratory syndrome (MERS) in Saudi Arabia, Jordan, and South Korea. Again it was a new zoonotic virus, this time originating in dromedary camels. Again it was a contained outbreak, with 2,494 reported cases and 858 deaths in twenty-seven countries. Again the case fatality rate was high: around 34 percent. Again most infections were nosocomial. Again the dispersion factor was low, around 0.25. In South Korea, 166 out of 186 cases did not lead to any secondary cases, but five superspreaders were responsible for a total of 154 secondary cases. The index case (patient zero) transmitted the MERS virus to twenty-eight people, three of whom themselves became superspreaders, infecting eighty-four, twenty-three, and seven people, respectively.[164]

Both SARS and MERS were deadly and readily detectable diseases. In the case of SARS, the incubation period was two to seven days, and the interval between symptom onset and maximum infectivity was five to seven days.[165] This was why the outbreaks were containable. The same was true of a very different disease that seized the world's attention in 2014. Ebola is one of a group of viral hemorrhagic fevers (the others are Marburg virus disease, Lassa fever, and hantavirus) that have long been a danger to populations in West Africa. The Ebola virus causes ruptures in small blood vessels throughout the body, leading to internal bleeding in the pleural cavity, around the lungs, and the pericardial cavity, around the heart, as well as external bleeding from orifices and through the skin. Blood loss results in coma and death: victims appear to "dissolve in their beds."[166] All such viruses require an animal reservoir, because they are so swiftly fatal as to die out in human populations—in the case of Ebola, the IFR can be as high as 80 to 90 percent. Long-established cultural practices, such as the consumption of bushmeat and the washing of bodies in funerary rituals, make outbreaks relatively common. Between 1976 and 2012, according to the WHO, there were twenty-four Ebola outbreaks, 2,387 cases, and 1,590 deaths. The biggest Ebola outbreak of modern times began in the remote Guinean village of Meliandou in December 2013, when a toddler named Emile Ouamouno fell ill after playing with bats known locally as *lolibelo* (probably Angolan free-tailed bats). Emile died on December 26. His grandmother died two days later. The disease spread rapidly from their village to Foya, in northern Liberia, and Conakry, the capital of Guinea. The puzzle in 2014 was why the WHO, which had been so effective against SARS, so badly mishandled the crisis.

Part of the reason was budget cuts that had followed the 2008–9 financial crisis, which had led to the redundancy of 130 staff members of GOARN. But there were also basic errors of judgment.[167] WHO press spokesman Gregory Hartl tweeted on March 23, "There has never been an Ebola outbreak larger than a couple of hundred cases." Two days later he insisted that "Ebola has always remained a localized event."[168] In April the WHO repeatedly referred to the outbreak as "improving," a view endorsed by the American CDC; in reality, by June the situation was "out of control," according to Médecins Sans Frontières.[169] Hans Rosling, the eminent statistician at Sweden's Karolinska Institute and a member of the WHO's expert panel, argued against diverting resources away from anti-malaria campaigns for the sake of a "small problem" like Ebola.[170] It was not until August 8 that the WHO declared a "public health emergency of international concern," by which time Guinea, Liberia, and Sierra Leone were descending into chaos, with sporadic attacks on health workers by fearful people. This was the moment when the CDC released its forecast predicting exponential growth to more than a million Ebola cases by February 2015 in the absence of major international intervention.[171] In reality, by the time the emergency was declared over, on March 29, 2016, there had been 28,646 cases and 11,323 deaths. This shift from complacency to panic is one we shall encounter again.

More than half a century separates the Asian flu of 1957–58 from the Ebola epidemic of 2014–16. Yet the ability of musicians to find inspiration even from contagious pathogens would appear to be a human constant. In the summer of 2014, Liberian musicians Samuel "Shadow" Morgan and Edwin "D-12" Tweh recorded an Ebola-inspired song that rapidly spread (no journalist could resist saying that it went viral) from Monrovia to the rest of the country:[172]

> *Ebola, Ebola in town*
> *Don't touch your friend!*
> *No touching*
> *No eating something*
> *It's dangerous!*

"Ebola in Town" inspired a dance in which dancers mimicked kissing and hugging from a distance. Anyone listening to it in 2014 was bound to conclude that the world had advanced a good deal less than had seemed achievable in the year of Sputnik.

8

THE FRACTAL GEOMETRY
OF DISASTER

Puisque de ma prison elle s'était évadée pour aller se tuer sur un che-
val que sans moi elle n'eût pas possédé . . . (Since from my prison
she had escaped, to go and kill herself upon a horse which but for me
she would not have owned . . .)

—Proust, *Albertine disparue*

ACCIDENTAL CATASTROPHES

There is a fractal geometry to disaster. Just as a snow crystal, at increasing
magnifications, is revealed to consist of multiple smaller versions of itself, so,
too, nested within a massive event like the collapse of an empire are multiple
smaller but similar disasters, each one, at each scale, a microcosm of the
whole. Thus far, this book has concerned itself mainly with large disasters of
every kind, to seek their common features. Yet we can also learn from the
smaller calamities, in which not many people die—dozens or hundreds rather
than thousands or millions—because, like Tolstoy's happy families, all disasters are fundamentally alike, even if (unlike families) they vary greatly in
their magnitude.

Accidents will happen. A banal error can have terrible consequences.
Since we began to build large structures out of wood or other flammable

materials, there have been accidental fires, from the Great Fire of London (1666) to Grenfell Tower (2017). Since we began digging under the earth's surface for gold, silver, lead, or coal, there have been mining disasters; the worst were the Courrières mine disaster, which killed more than a thousand French coal miners in 1906, and the explosion at Benxihu (Honkeiko) Colliery, which claimed the lives of 1,500 mostly Chinese miners in Japanese-controlled Manchuria in 1942. And since we began to manufacture explosives and toxic chemicals, there have been explosions and toxic leaks, from the Wang-gongchang gunpowder explosion in Beijing (1626) to the Union Carbide disaster in Bhopal (1984). Ships have been sinking since men began sailing. The world seems unlikely to forget the loss of the *Titanic* in 1912, which cost the lives of 1,504 passengers and crew. But who remembers the comparably lethal or even worse sinkings of the *Sultana,* in the Mississippi River in 1865, in which more than a thousand passengers drowned; the SS *Kiangya,* off Shanghai in 1948, when between 2,750 and 3,920 were lost; or the MV *Doña Paz,* which sank off the Philippine island of Marinduque in 1987, claiming more than 4,000 lives?

With each technological advance, it might seem, the potential scale of an individual disaster grows. Trains collide. Planes crash. Spaceships blow up. And nuclear power stations, as we have seen, have created a new and potentially catastrophic risk since the 1950s. In a society with financial markets, the rule of law, representative government, a competent bureaucracy, and a free press, the tendency should be for transportation and energy generation to become safer over time. Insurance, lawsuits, public inquiries, regulations, and investigative reporting—and of course competition—these are the institutional pressures on both private and public operators that incentivize effective safety procedures. Over time, things generally do get safer. Between the mid-1950s and the mid-1970s, as commercial travel boomed, the number of people who died each year in airliner accidents rose from around 750 to nearly 2,000, but the five-year average declined to around 1,250 in the 1980s and 1990s and dropped below 500 in 2016.[1] Relative to the total volume of air travel, the improvement since 1977 has been sustained and impressive, from more than four accidents per million flights to 0.3 in 2017.[2]

Still, accidents will keep happening, and the less frequent they become, the more inclined we are to attribute them to extraordinary circumstances. The popularity of Sebastian Junger's book *The Perfect Storm* illustrates this well: since its publication, few phrases have been used more often than its title to explain disasters of all kinds.[3] The fate of the crew of the *Andrea Gail* was indeed tragic. The seventy-two-foot fishing boat from Gloucester, Massachusetts, went down while fishing for swordfish around 162 miles east of Sable Island in the nor'easter that blew between October 28 and November 4, 1991. But were Frank W. "Billy" Tyne Jr. and his crew the unfortunate victims of a perfect storm, or were the crew the victims of Tyne's poor judgment? Bob Case, who was the deputy meteorologist at the National Weather Service's Boston forecast office at the time, told Junger that a high-pressure system, originating in northern Canada, had provided a large pool of cold air, the front of which pushed off the New England coast on October 27. The cold air behind this front and the warm air ahead of it caused a strong temperature contrast to form over a relatively small area. The result was an "extra-tropical cyclone," known in New England as a nor'easter because of the direction from which the wind is coming when it hits Massachusetts. In addition, there was abnormal moisture in the air, owing to the recent passage of Hurricane Grace. According to Junger, the storm created waves in excess of a hundred feet in height. Yet this storm was by no means the biggest nor'easter in recent history. There had been worse weather at sea during the 1962 Columbus Day Storm and would be during the 1993 "Superstorm."[4] Weather buoys in the vicinity of the *Andrea Gail*'s last known location recorded peak wave heights of just above sixty feet—big but not unprecedented. The loss of the *Andrea Gail* surely owed more to Tyne's error in risking being at sea in such conditions. Like hurricanes in Florida, nor'easters in New England are not by any stretch of the imagination black swans. Every year there are big storms, and generally fishermen react to adverse forecasts by not setting sail.

The psychologist James Reason has defined two types of errors: active and latent. Active errors are committed by people "in direct contact with the human-system interface" and are often referred to as human errors. Individuals who commit these errors are those at the "sharp end"—on the bridge, in the case of the *Andrea Gail*.[5] Active errors can be further subdivided into three categories of behavior: skill-based, rule-based, and knowledge-based.[6] By contrast, latent errors are the "delayed consequences of technical and organizational actions and decisions—such as reallocating resources, changing the scope of a position, or adjusting staffing. Individuals who commit these errors are at the 'blunt end'"—for example, the owners or managers of a vessel, back on land.[7] Because the *Titanic* is such a famous disaster, we can answer the question of which type of error led to its sinking and the heavy losses of those on board. The answer is both.

SINKING *TITANIC*

The iceberg the *Titanic* struck on April 15, 1912, was not to blame. It had every right to be where it was at that time of year. Nor was there fog in the vicinity: it was a clear but moonless night. Captain Edward Smith was an experienced sailor, but his record was not unblemished. He had been in command of the *Titanic*'s sister ship, the *Olympic,* when she collided with a British warship, HMS *Hawke,* just seven months before. When Smith was informed of an ice field ahead, he did not reduce his speed. (It is often alleged that Smith was under pressure from the *Titanic*'s owner, the White Star Line, to set a new record for the passage to New York, but this is untrue: the *Titanic*'s maximum speed under full steam was less than the record speed of 23.7 knots set by Cunard's *Mauretania* in 1907, and the *Titanic*'s average speed in the time prior to the collision was only 18 knots.) The ship's wireless officer, Jack Phillips, has also borne a share of the blame for the disaster: he allegedly attached more importance to sending out personal messages from wealthy passengers such as Madeleine Astor than to incoming warnings about icebergs. The lookout, Fred Fleet, spotted the iceberg ahead at five hundred yards, but if he had been using binoculars, which he could not locate, he would have seen it when it was a thousand yards away. The first officer, William Murdoch, who was in charge of the ship at the crucial moment, thus had at most thirty-seven seconds (more likely half that) before the collision.[8] On hearing the cry of "Iceberg, dead ahead"—or seeing it himself—he gave the helmsman the order

"Hard a-starboard" and the engine room the order to stop the engines. This was not an incorrect response, but it may have had the unintended consequence of exposing the *Titanic*'s starboard side for longer to the iceberg than if Murdoch had maintained full speed and tried to go around it or simply rammed it head-on. These were the active errors that caused the *Titanic* to strike the iceberg. A few seconds of different behavior by a handful of men and we might no more care about the *Titanic* than we do about her long-forgotten sister, the *Olympic*. But why, after the collision, did the *Titanic* sink so fast? And why were so many lives lost—two thirds of all those on board? Two latent errors provide the answer.

First, all three of the *Olympic*-class ships featured fifteen watertight bulkhead compartments equipped with electric watertight doors that could be operated individually or simultaneously by a switch on the bridge. If the ship were holed, the crew on the bridge could simply close the doors electronically, keeping the water confined to the damaged compartment. It was this system that inspired *The Shipbuilder* magazine to deem the *Titanic* "practically unsinkable."[9] However, although the individual bulkheads were watertight, the walls separating the bulkheads extended only a few feet above the waterline, so water could pour from one compartment into another if the ship began to list or pitch forward.[10] The marine architect responsible, Thomas Andrews, was on board when the ship hit the iceberg. As soon as he surveyed the damage with Captain Smith, he grasped the error he had made and predicted that the ship would sink in an hour and a half.[11] In fact, the *Titanic* did not go down until 2:20 a.m., having struck the iceberg at 11:40 p.m.—a relatively slow submersion compared with her sister ship the *Britannic,* which would vanish beneath the waves just fifty-five minutes after striking a German mine in the Aegean in 1916.

Smith, Phillips, Murdoch, and Andrews all went down with the *Titanic*. However, many more people could have been saved, it has been argued, if there had been enough lifeboats. In fact, there were just sixteen, plus four "collapsible" boats, enough to carry 1,178 people—roughly half the number of passengers and crew on board. This was partly because of defective regulation, as the Board of Trade lifeboat requirements were at that time based on the tonnage of the ship and not the number of people on board. A change to the regulation was under consideration, but it was opposed by the shipowners on grounds of cost. Assuming the owners would lose this argument, the *Titanic*'s designers had provided double davits to accommodate the extra lifeboats. However, the White Star chairman and managing director, J. Bruce Ismay, elected not to add the extra lifeboats, as they would have reduced the space on the first-class passengers' promenade deck. Ismay, who was also on board, survived the disaster but was reviled as a coward by the press and spent much of the rest of his life as a recluse at Cottesloe Lodge, the secluded country house overlooking the Atlantic that Edwin Lutyens had designed for him in County Galway, Ireland. As Ismay's granddaughter later recalled, "Having had the misfortune (one might say the misjudgment) to survive—a fact he recognised despairingly within hours—he withdrew into a silence in which his wife made herself complicit—imposing it on the family circle and thus ensuring that the subject of the *Titanic* was as effectively frozen as the bodies recovered from the sea."[12]

Yet an anonymous "officer on an Atlantic passenger steamer" came to Ismay's defense in 1913, contemptuously dismissing the argument for more boats. More lifeboats, especially if they were of inferior quality, such as rafts or collapsibles, would have done little good. First, without adequate space to launch them, extra boats might simply have slowed down the evacuation. Second, the crews of passenger liners were not well trained in launching lifeboats, nor were they well trained in how to keep them afloat. Third, in any case, crowded lifeboats were "helpless . . . in anything but a calm, if loaded according to law." Given the nature of the *Titanic*—a floating palace, commercially viable only because of the luxury it offered passengers, with a largely inexpert crew and a tiny number of "certificated" officers—it had been "giants' work . . . to save over seven hundred lives."[13] "Atlanticus" might have gone further. Compared with eighteen other ships that sank with heavy loss of life between 1852 and 2011, *Titanic* was exceptional in that women and children had significantly higher survival rates than crew and male passengers.[14] This was one of the rare occasions when the rule of "women and children first" was actually observed.

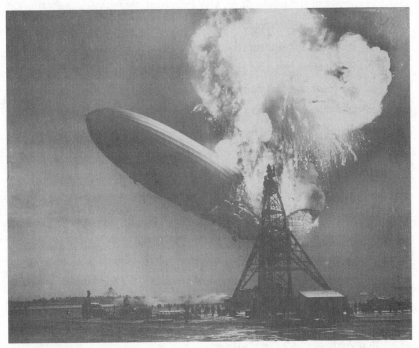

The *Hindenburg* on fire at the mooring mast in Lakehurst, New Jersey, May 6, 1937.

Most transport disasters have these same elements: adverse weather and active and latent errors. Compared with the *Titanic*, many fewer lives were lost when the eight-hundred-foot German passenger airship *Hindenburg* caught fire over Lakehurst, New Jersey, on May 6, 1937, as there were just thirty-six passengers and sixty-one crewmen on board. And compared with that of the *Titanic*, the weather doubtless played a bigger part in the *Hindenburg*'s destruction. Strong headwinds had slowed the airship's passage across the Atlantic. As the *Hindenburg* approached Lakehurst, there was lightning visible. The fatal fire was caused when a spark of static electricity ignited hydrogen that had leaked from one of the rear gas cells, which may have been torn by a broken length of wiring. (Each gas cell was made from a plastic film sandwiched between two layers of thick cotton, so it would have taken considerable force to rupture one.) The airship was about two hundred feet off the ground when the fire broke out. She burned from tail to nose in just thirty-four seconds.

The captain of the *Hindenburg*, Max Pruss, subsequently claimed that the disaster was a result of sabotage. It is now generally agreed that he was in fact to blame. Instead of opting for the more usual and less risky "low landing," which involved slowly bringing the airship low enough that it could be dragged along the ground to the mooring mast, Pruss opted for a "high landing," which involved throwing ropes from the airship so that ground staff could pull the airship down to the mast.[15] His motive appears to have been haste. The *Hindenburg* was running twelve hours late and was due to set off back to England the following day, carrying VIPs to attend George VI's coronation. Ernst Lehmann, the Zeppelin Company's director of operations, was in the cockpit with Pruss and appears to have urged the rapid landing.[16] The danger Lehmann and Pruss overlooked was that the mooring ropes, which quickly became soaked through with rain, allowed the electric charge from the airship's metal frame to flow to the ground as soon as they touched it. The voltage of the airframe instantly fell to zero, but the airship's outer fabric cover, which did not conduct electricity so easily, retained its charge, creating the conditions that generated the fatal spark. The hydrogen leak itself can only have occurred because a part of the airship's structure—perhaps a bracing cable—snapped. This probably happened when, with strong winds buffeting the *Hindenburg*, Pruss was forced to make a sharp left turn, which he then had to correct with a sharp right turn to line the airship up with the mooring mast.[17] Although Pruss and Lehmann were cleared of having wrecked the *Hindenburg*, Hugo Eckener—the chairman of the Zeppelin Company and an experienced airship pilot in his own right—blamed them for attempting the high landing in a thunderstorm.

AIRPLANE!

Despite Pruss's efforts to revive civilian passenger airships after the war—which cannot have been helped by the severe disfigurement he suffered in the *Hindenburg* disaster—the future lay with airplanes. As we have seen, these grew steadily safer after the 1970s. Indeed, the worst aircraft accident in history occurred on March 27, 1977, when two Boeing 747 passenger jets—KLM

Flight 4805, from Amsterdam, and Pan Am Flight 1736, from Los Angeles and New York—collided on the runway at Los Rodeos Airport, on the Spanish island of Tenerife. In all, 583 people were killed, including everyone on board the KLM flight. Sixty-one people on the Pan Am flight survived, including the pilot and copilot. Neither plane would normally have been at that airport. Both had been bound for Las Palmas de Gran Canaria but had been diverted because of a bomb planted at that airport by the Canary Islands Independence Movement. Los Rodeos was a very small, regional airport, not designed for the number of diverted planes it had to accommodate that day, nor for larger aircraft such as the 747. The airport quickly became congested, which meant that stationary aircraft had nowhere to wait except the airport's main taxiway, while departing aircraft had to taxi on the runway and do a 180-degree turn before taking off. There were four separate taxiways connecting the main taxiway and the runway, but these were designed for smaller aircraft, and some of the turns required would have been difficult for a bulky 747. It did not help that the entrances to the taxiways were not clearly marked. When the Las Palmas airport reopened, both planes were ready to depart but had to taxi up the runway, the KLM plane going first and making a 180-degree turn to prepare for takeoff. The collision occurred when the KLM plane initiated its takeoff run while the Pan Am plane was still on the runway.[18]

The weather played a part in the disaster but, as usual, not the leading role. Los Rodeos Airport is 2,080 feet above sea level, which creates a risk of patchy low clouds. While the planes were waiting, a heavy fog had rolled in, reducing visibility to around 1,000 feet, whereas the threshold for takeoff was 2,300 feet. The air traffic control tower was not equipped with ground radar, and the two operators could not actually see the planes through the fog. Nevertheless, the KLM plane, after refueling, restarted its engines and taxied out onto the runway. The Pan Am plane was instructed to follow. By now (5:02 p.m.) the two aircraft, moving at about ten miles per hour, could not see each other. According to the subsequent Air Line Pilots Association report, as the Pan Am aircraft taxied to the runway, the visibility was about 1,640 feet. After they turned onto the runway, it decreased to less than 330 feet. To make matters worse, the central lights on the runway were not working. However, at the other end of the runway, the KLM plane seemed to have adequate 3,000-foot visibility.[19]

Three distinct forms of active or "sharp-end" error caused the disaster. First, the air traffic controllers failed at their job, not least because they were being distracted by a soccer game on the radio. Second, the Pan Am crew became confused when they were told by the control tower operators to move off the runway by taking the third exit on their left, taxiway C-3. As there were no markings to identify the exits (a blunt-end error), the crew were unsure which exit was meant: C-3 or the third exit after the first one (which was C-4). The problem with C-3 was that it required a very sharp turn, whereas C-4 sloped at a 45-degree angle and therefore seemed the logical one to take. In a state of indecision, Pan Am 1736 therefore taxied past C-3 and hovered at C-4. By this point (5:05 p.m.), KLM 4805 had reached the end of the runway and was now turning around to point straight at Pan Am 1736, although neither plane was aware that the other was only half a mile away.

The third and crucial error was that the KLM captain, Jacob Veldhuyzen van Zanten, was a man in a hurry. He had enough fuel to get back to Amsterdam and he didn't want to be stranded on the island overnight. After lining up, van Zanten began to advance the plane's throttle for "spin-up," a test to verify that the engines were operating properly for takeoff. His copilot, surprised, said, "Wait a minute. We don't have ATC clearance." "I know that," replied van Zanten, flustered. "Go ahead, ask." The copilot did so, and the tower gave them permission to fly the route once airborne. This was not yet permission to take off, but van Zanten said simply, "We're going." The copilot, perhaps reluctant to question his captain a second time, remained silent as the plane moved forward. The air traffic controllers then asked the Pan Am crew if they were off the runway yet, to which the Americans replied that they were still on it. The controller then told van Zanten, "Stand by for takeoff, I will call you." He had not heard the captain's intention to go ahead, as van Zanten had said "We're going" to his crew, not into the radio. A simultaneous call from the Pan Am crew caused interference, and the KLM crew did not hear the Pan Am crew say that they were still on the runway. Just after the KLM plane began to take off, the tower told the Pan Am crew to report when the runway was clear. Hearing this, the KLM flight engineer asked van Zanten, "Is he not clear, that Pan American?" Van Zanten merely replied, "Oh, yes," and continued throttling up to speed. At this point (5:06 p.m.), the Pan Am captain, Victor Grubbs, saw the KLM approaching, shouted, "Goddamn, damn, that son of a bitch is coming straight at us!" and opened the throttle to try to get out of the way. At the same time, van Zanten, sighting the Pan Am, tried to take evasive action by lifting off early, tilting the plane back so sharply that its tail hit the runway. It was too late. Weighed down with fifty-five tons of fuel, KLM 4805 hit the top of Pan Am 1736 at a right angle, shearing off the entire roof of its fuselage. The number-one engine of the KLM, which was now moving at 160 miles per hour, broke off in the collision, and after rising a hundred feet in the air, the plane smashed into the runway. The plane's heavy fuel load exploded almost at once, killing everyone on board. The Pan Am 747 also caught fire, though some passengers had time to escape.

It has been suggested that Captain van Zanten might have been suffering from "technological fatigue" or "closed-circuit machinic symbiosis," meaning that he had become "an extension of the tightly mechanized world within which he was embedded and constrained. His thinking had shifted *out* of the human world and its concerns, and . . . [had become] an extension of the machine itself."[20] Another psychological theory is that, as a pilot much more accustomed to simulated training flights than to regular passenger flights—van Zanten was head of the KLM flight training department—he was "regressing to more habituated ways of responding," as people often do when they are under stress. (On a simulated flight, the instructor acts as flight controller, giving himself permission to take off.) The precise nature of his psychological lapse need not concern us, however. For the crash also exposed two systemic problems distinct from the three sharp-end errors described above. Nowadays, a pilot cannot take off without a cockpit consensus. That was not true in 1977. Second, the reason van Zanten was in such a hurry was that he and his colleagues were subject to new "Work and Rest Regulations for Flight Crews" that the Netherlands had enacted the previous year. These imposed strict limits on flying hours, mandating fines, imprisonment, and even the loss of pilots' licenses if monthly limits were exceeded.[21] The fact that the accident occurred near the end of the month was therefore not insignificant. Ironically, a regulation intended to prevent fatigued pilots from making lethal mistakes had made such a lethal mistake more likely.

According to one study, "eleven separate coincidences and mistakes, most of them minor . . . had to fall precisely into place" for the Tenerife runway crash to happen.[22] This smacks of "perfect storm" reasoning. Another systems-based analysis concludes that there were four things that went wrong that could go wrong again in comparable situations: first, "the interruption of important routines among and within interdependent systems"; second, "interdependencies that became tighter" in a crisis; third, "a loss of cognitive efficiency due to autonomic arousal"; and, fourth, "a loss of communication accuracy due to increased hierarchical distortion." Together, these led to the "occurrence and rapid diffusion of multiple errors by creating a feedback loop" that magnified "minor errors into major problems."[23] All this tends to overcomplicate a story of two planes and a control tower on a foggy day. Perhaps the key point is simply that the Tenerife plane crash happened very fast indeed. The time that elapsed between the KLM plane's entering the runway and the collision was precisely seven minutes and thirty-nine seconds. The time after the Pan Am plane entered the runway was just four minutes and forty-one seconds.

FEYNMAN'S LAW

The disaster that happened less than nine years later, on January 28, 1986, when the space shuttle *Challenger* blew up high above Cape Canaveral, Florida, was even faster. Between liftoff and the disintegration of the spacecraft, just over seventy-three seconds elapsed. Although only seven people died, the *Challenger* disaster is among the most famous in American history, far better known than the much deadlier but long-forgotten Tenerife plane collision. This is partly because one of the astronauts was a high school teacher from Concord, New Hampshire, named Christa McAuliffe. Media interest in her voyage meant that approximately 17 percent of the U.S. population witnessed the spectacular explosion on live television, and 85 percent of Americans had heard the news of the disaster within an hour of its happening.

In this case, unlike in the other disasters discussed in this chapter, the errors were all latent, not active; the flight crew, all of whom perished, were entirely blameless. But what exactly had gone wrong? Two months after *Challenger*'s destruction, a story surfaced that the White House had been applying pressure on NASA to ensure that the launch happen before President Reagan's State of the Union address, originally scheduled for later the same day.[24] This illustrates the ingrained compulsion of the Washington press corps to attribute blame, wherever possible, to the occupant of the Oval Office. In reality, a proposed draft of the speech that mentioned Christa McAuliffe had been discarded before it even reached Reagan's desk. Pressure from the top was most certainly not the reason *Challenger* blew up. Nor was the weather more than an accessory to the deed, though the morning of the launch was indeed unusually cold for Florida—"a hundred-year cold"—perhaps as low as 18 degrees Fahrenheit, with ambient air temperature at the planned liftoff time forecast to be 26 to 29 degrees (though it turned out slightly warmer).[25]

Another explanation for the disaster that gained currency at the time was that those responsible for the launch of *Challenger* had succumbed to "groupthink," a term coined in 1972 by the Yale psychologist Irving L. Janis. Groupthink, he argued, was "a mode of thinking that people engage in when they are deeply involved in a cohesive in-group, when the members' strivings for unanimity override their motivation to realistically appraise alternative courses of action." This, he suggested after the *Challenger* disaster, had been the problem at NASA.[26] Subsequent revelations have shown that this, too, was a misleading explanation.

The *Challenger* disaster can be traced back to a flaw in the original design of the solid rocket boosters used to launch the space shuttle into orbit. Morton Thiokol, the company that had won the contract to build the boosters, had based its design on the Titan III rocket. The cylindrical booster sections were manufactured separately, then mounted end-to-end, the joints between them sealed with two flexible and snugly fitting O-rings made from Viton, a rubber-like material. Putty was laid inside at the joints to provide further protection. However, Morton Thiokol had made a number of changes to the Titan III design to simplify the manufacturing process and to cut costs. During initial testing and even after space shuttles started flying, engineers at Morton Thiokol and at NASA noticed with alarm that hot combustion gases were burning through the putty, leaking into the joints, and burning the O-rings.[27] In the shuttle launch on January 24, 1985, for example, the primary O-rings on two of the joints had been compromised by fuel "blowing by" and eroding them. Only the secondary O-ring was left, and even it had been damaged. There had in fact been seven problematic launches (out of twenty-four) prior to *Challenger,* though in two of these the issues were unrelated to the O-rings. After the January 1985 launch saw worse-than-usual damage to the primary O-ring, Morton Thiokol engineer Roger Boisjoly began to suspect that cold weather had affected the resiliency of the O-ring.[28] In a memo, he warned that "If the same scenario should occur in a field joint (and it could), then it is a jump ball as to the success or failure of the joint. . . . The result would be a catastrophe of the highest order—loss of human life."[29] In January 1986, the Morton Thiokol management therefore accepted the recommendation of their engineers not to launch *Challenger* and sent that recommendation on to NASA.[30] Morton Thiokol also advised NASA not to launch the shuttle in temperatures below 53 degrees Fahrenheit, the temperature at the previous coldest launch, one year earlier. And yet, despite all this, the launch went ahead, with precisely the catastrophic consequences Boisjoly had foreseen.

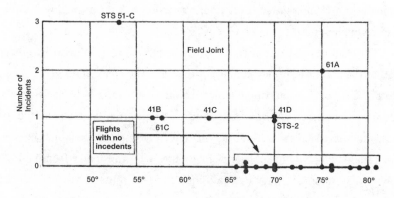

The correlation between space shuttle O-ring incidents and temperatures at launch.

The day after the *Challenger* disaster, Allan "Al" McDonald, the director of the Space Shuttle Solid Rocket Motor Project at Morton Thiokol, went to Huntsville, Alabama, to join the failure review team. At that point, he believed that either engine failure or a problem with the fuel tank structure was to blame. However, video footage he saw in Huntsville persuaded him that "an O-ring seal had failed at launch, but the hole was quickly resealed by aluminum oxides before any flames could escape and cause an explosion. Strong wind shear that began 37 seconds into flight then tore the seal back open, resulting in the catastrophic breakup."[31] At the first hearing of the presidential commission set up to investigate the cause of the disaster, under the chairmanship of former secretary of state William P. Rogers, McDonald dropped his bombshell: "We recommended not to launch." However, it took the seemingly unworldly figure of the Caltech physicist Richard Feynman—ably assisted by Air Force general Donald Kutyna and NASA astronaut Sally Ride, also members of the Rogers Commission—to establish beyond reasonable doubt that the O-rings (to be precise, the effect of low temperatures on their soundness as seals) were the cause of the failure and that NASA had been explicitly warned of this risk.[32]

Feynman's account of his role in the Rogers Commission is a classic—a kind of academic version of *Mr. Smith Goes to Washington*.[33] For Feynman, the culprits were the midlevel NASA bureaucrats who chose to disregard the engineers. "If all the seals had leaked, it would have been obvious even to NASA that the problem was serious," Feynman wrote. "But only a few of the seals leaked on only some of the flights. So NASA had developed a peculiar kind of attitude: if one of the seals leaks a little and the flight is successful, the problem isn't so serious. Try playing Russian roulette that way."[34] The more he explored the way NASA worked, the more Feynman was appalled: a hierarchical command structure, a formalistic insistence on doing things by the book, even if the book was wrong, and above all a refusal to accept warnings about the risk of a disaster. At the heart of the matter, for Feynman, was the refusal of NASA managers to listen when they were told that the probability of a disaster was 1 in 100:

As range safety officer at Kennedy, Mr. [Louis] Ullian had to decide whether to put destruct charges on the shuttle. . . .

Every unmanned rocket has these charges. Mr. Ullian told us that 5 out of 127 rockets that he looked at had failed—a rate of about 4 percent. He took that 4 percent and divided it by 4, because he assumed a manned flight would be safer than an unmanned one. He came out with about a 1 percent chance of failure, and that was enough to warrant the destruct charges.

But NASA told Mr. Ullian that the probability of failure was more like 1 in 10^5.

I tried to make sense out of that number. "Did you say 1 in 10^5?"

"That's right; 1 in 100,000."

"That means you could fly the shuttle *every day* for an average of *300 years* between accidents—every day, one flight, for 300 years—which is obviously crazy!"

"Yes, I know," said Mr. Ullian. "I moved my number up to 1 in 1000 to answer all of NASA's claims." . . . [But] the argument continued: NASA kept saying 1 in 100,000 and Mr. Ullian kept saying 1 in 1000, at best.

Mr. Ullian also told us about the problems he had in trying to talk to the man in charge, Mr. Kingsbury: he could get appointments with underlings, but he never could get through to Kingsbury and find out how NASA got its figure of 1 in 100,000.[35]

Feynman encountered the same gap between engineers and management in other contexts, too—for example, the probability of engine failure: "I had the definite impression that I had found the same game as with the seals: management reducing criteria and accepting more and more errors that weren't designed into the device, while the engineers are screaming from below, 'HELP!' and 'This is a RED ALERT!'"[36]

Feynman's findings had implications that were not congenial to William Rogers, the personification of the legally trained, worldly-wise Washington establishment. Feynman therefore insisted on his own addendum to the final report, in which he castigated the NASA management for "playing Russian roulette" when the evidence of O-ring erosion clearly indicated that "something was wrong":

Subtly, and often with apparently logical arguments, the criteria are altered so that flights may still be certified in time. They therefore fly in a relatively unsafe condition, with a chance of failure of the order of a percent (it is difficult to be more accurate).

Official management, on the other hand, claims to believe the probability of failure is a thousand times less. One reason for this may be an attempt to assure the government of NASA perfection and success in order to ensure the supply of funds. The other may be that they sincerely believed it to be true, demonstrating an almost incredible lack of communication between themselves and their working engineers. . . .

For a successful technology, reality must take precedence over public relations, for nature cannot be fooled.[37]

In his subsequent memoir of the experience, Feynman went further. "It struck me," he wrote, "that there were several fishinesses associated with the big cheeses at NASA. Every time we talked to higher level managers, they kept saying they didn't know anything about the problems below them. . . . Either the guys at the top didn't know, in which case they should have known, or they did know, in which case they're lying to us."[38] Feynman astutely inferred that NASA's management had fallen victim to its own version of mission creep:

When the moon project was over, NASA had all these people together. . . . You don't want to fire people and send them out in the street when you're done with a big project, so the problem is, what to do?

You have to convince Congress that there exists a project that only NASA can do. In order to do so, it is necessary . . . to exaggerate: to exaggerate how economical the shuttle would be, to exaggerate how often it could fly, to exaggerate how safe it would be, to exaggerate the big scientific facts that would be discovered. "The shuttle can make so-and-so many flights and it'll cost such-and-such; we went to the moon, so we can *do* it!"

Meanwhile, I would guess, the engineers at the bottom are saying, "No, no! We can't make that many flights." . . .

Well, the guys who are trying to get Congress to okay their projects
don't want to hear such talk. It's better if they don't hear, so they can be
more "honest"—they don't want to be in the position of lying to Congress! So pretty soon the attitudes begin to change: information from the
bottom which is disagreeable—"We're having a problem with the seals;
we should fix it before we fly again"—is suppressed.[39]

This was nearly the whole story—but not quite. Certainly, NASA's leadership felt compelled to keep expanding the space shuttle program, ultimately
aiming for twenty-four shuttle flights per year.[40] But the division between engineers and management existed not only at NASA but also at the manufacturer Morton Thiokol. On a teleconference call the day before the disaster,
Lawrence Mulloy of NASA asked Joe Kilminster, vice president of the solid
rocket booster program at Morton Thiokol,

what the program office recommendation was, and Kilminster said that
he would not recommend launch based upon the engineering position
that was just presented. Mulloy then challenged the engineering position based upon his own assessment that the engineering data was in-
conclusive. He mentioned that we had presented data that observed
blowby on cold motors and warm motors, and he wanted more quantitative data that the temperature really affected the ability of the joint
to seal.

This puzzled Al McDonald, as he was much more used to NASA "challenging
our rationale on why it was *safe* to fly. . . . For some strange reason, we found
ourselves being challenged to prove quantitatively that it would definitely
fail, and we couldn't do that." As McDonald recalled, Mulloy snapped: "Well,
then, Thiokol, when the hell do you want me to launch, next April? . . . You
know, the eve of the launch is a hell of a time to change the launch commit
criteria." The general manager of Morton Thiokol, Jerry Mason, then intervened, on the side of NASA. "Am I the only one here that thinks it's okay to

go ahead with the launch as planned?" he asked. Only two engineers—Roger Boisjoly and Arnie Thompson—spoke up. Thompson "walked over to the table where the senior managers were sitting and laid out sketches of the joint design along with copies of the data" showing the effect of low temperatures. The response from Mason and Cal Wiggins, vice president and general manager of the company's space division, was a "cold stare." Boisjoly then showed them the photographs of the jet-black soot that had been observed between the primary and secondary O-rings on the January 1985 launch. "Look carefully at these photographs!" he exclaimed. "Don't ignore what they are telling us, namely, that low temperature causes more blowby in the joint!" It was useless. Mason was able to browbeat the other managers, including Bob Lund, the vice president of engineering, into overruling the engineers and changing Morton Thiokol's recommendation from "don't launch" to "launch." But when George Hardy, of NASA's Marshall Space Flight Center, asked for the new recommendation to be put into writing, McDonald refused.[41] In the end, Kilminster had to sign.[42]

The difference between the Morton Thiokol managers and the company's engineers was clear. For the engineers, avoiding a catastrophic failure was paramount. For management, the long-term relationship with NASA was paramount. As McDonald recalled,

Mulloy knew that he had leverage with Kilminster, because Kilminster essentially worked for him. . . . I wanted this to be an engineering recommendation only, because I knew all about the schedule pressures and other pressures weighing down on our management team as a result of NASA's continued interest in possibly second-sourcing some of the SRB [solid rocket booster] production. Our behind-schedule position on the current program and lack of a signed contract from NASA for the next sole-source procurement for sixty-six more flight sets of motors were tremendous leverage for NASA. . . . It was just not good politics— and not good business—to go against your most important customer's wishes when you are as vulnerable as Morton Thiokol thought it was relative to second-source issues—especially with an unsigned contract from the customer for the next, and probably last, noncompetitive buy of solid rocket motors.[43]

Anyone who has studied defense procurement—which Richard Feynman had not—will recognize the pathology. Morton Thiokol was the sole supplier of rocket boosters to a program that was aiming for two shuttle launches a month. If it did not meet the needs of NASA management, then NASA would look to the company's competitors. If NASA wanted to play Russian roulette, Morton Thiokol's managers were willing to load the gun, ignoring their engineers just as their NASA counterparts ignored theirs.

The true point of failure in the *Challenger* disaster was not therefore the O-rings themselves, any more than it was bad weather, Ronald Reagan, or groupthink. It was the way, on that crucial conference call, Mulloy bullied Kilminster, and the way Mason and Wiggins then shut down the engineers' objections. The politics of a catastrophe can turn out to hinge on such obscure deliberations, far from the presidential conferences and cabinet meetings that historians tend to study—somewhere between the blunt end and the sharp, in the crepuscular realm of middle management.

CHERNOBYL REVISITED

It is a delusion, though no doubt a comforting one, to imagine that a disaster such as Chernobyl could happen only in an authoritarian, one-party state like the Soviet Union.

What is the cost of lies? It's not that we'll mistake them for the truth. The real danger is that if we hear enough lies, then we no longer recognize the truth at all. What can we do then? What else is left but to abandon even the hope of truth and content ourselves instead with stories? In these stories, it doesn't matter who the heroes are. All we want to know is: "Who is to blame?"

At the beginning of Craig Mazin's gripping five-part drama *Chernobyl*, these words are spoken by Jared Harris, in the role of Valery Legasov, the chemist who led the Soviet government commission to investigate the disaster. In a later scene, he exclaims:

> Our secrets and our lies . . . are practically what define us. When the truth offends, we—we lie and lie until we can no longer remember it is even there. But it is . . . still there. Every lie we tell incurs a debt to the truth. Sooner or later, that debt is paid. That is how . . . an RBMK [nuclear] reactor core explodes: lies. . . . The truth doesn't care about our needs or wants. It doesn't care about our governments, our ideologies, our religions. It will lie in wait for all time. And this, at last, is the gift of Chernobyl. Where I once would fear the cost of truth, now I only ask: What is the cost of lies?

As far as I can establish, the real Valery Legasov never uttered those words—and yet they are the most memorable lines in the series. What makes them memorable is that they tell us what we are predisposed to believe, namely that Chernobyl was a microcosm of the decline and fall of the Soviet Union, as surely as the fall of Singapore was a microcosm of the decline and fall of the British Empire.

In some respects, of course, it was just that. The immediate reaction of the Soviet authorities was to try to cover up what had happened. The evacuation of Pripyat's inhabitants did not start until April 27, 1986, some thirty-six hours after the explosion that exposed the core of reactor number 4. Not for another day and a half after the evacuation did the Soviet government publicly acknowledge that there had been an accident, and then only because the Swedish nuclear authorities had detected it. The evacuation zone was not established (with an arbitrary radius of nineteen miles) until six days after the disaster. The local population was lied to about the dangerous level of radiation it had been exposed to; Soviet citizens as a whole had no inkling of how perilous the situation was in the days after the disaster. In the words of the

leading historian of modern Ukraine, the attempt to censor the disaster out
of existence "endanger[ed] millions of people at home and abroad and [led]
to innumerable cases of radiation poisoning that could otherwise have been
avoided."[44] Firemen like Volodymyr Pravyk were sent to their deaths in the effort to prevent the fire from spreading to the other reactors. Soldiers like Nikolai Kaplin were later deployed into the contaminated area as "liquidators" or
"bio-robots," with minimal protection against the immense doses of radiation
to which they were exposed. They, like the pilots who flew the helicopters to
dump tons of boron, lead, and dolomite on top of the exposed reactor core,
and the miners who dug a tunnel underneath the reactor for a cooling layer
thought necessary to prevent a "China syndrome," were worthy heirs of the
selfless cannon fodder of the "Great Patriotic War"—especially as both these
efforts proved to be futile.[45] The disaster had both active and latent causes,
some of which were undoubtedly of a uniquely Soviet nature. The reactor's
operators took excessive risks in a way that exemplified the "We can do it no
matter what" mentality instilled by Soviet propaganda since 1917, and especially in the late Stalin and Khrushchev eras, the formative years of the key
actors. The design flaws of the reactor itself, and the operators' unawareness
of its potential instability, were also consequences of the peculiar political
economy of the planned economy.[46] Yet in some respects, as we shall see,
Chernobyl could have happened anywhere.

The proximate cause of the disaster was clearly simple operator error, as
the official Soviet report concluded, the principal culprit being Anatoly Dyatlov, the deputy chief engineer. (In 1987, he and five other senior personnel
were sentenced to terms of between two and ten years in labor camps.) Dyatlov wanted to simulate an electrical power outage to see if the residual rota-
tional energy in a turbine generator would suffice to maintain water coolant
circulation until the backup electrical generators kicked in (after around a
minute). Three such tests—each of which involved disabling some safety systems, including the emergency core-cooling system—had been conducted since
1982, but they had not been conclusive. On the fourth attempt, which was
timed to coincide with a maintenance shutdown of Chernobyl's number 4
reactor, an unexpected ten-hour delay, requested by the Kiev electrical grid,

meant that the night shift was on duty for the test, which they had not expected to have to run. Moreover, during the planned reduction of reactor power in preparation for the test, the power unexpectedly plunged to almost zero, possibly because of a reactor's production of a fission by-product, xenon-135, a reaction-inhibiting neutron absorber (the process known as reactor poisoning), possibly because of another unidentified equipment failure or operator error. To get the power back up, the operators disconnected the reactor control rods from the automatic regulation system and manually extracted nearly all of them. Ignoring emergency alarms about the levels in the steam/water separator drums and variations in the flow rate of coolant water, they went ahead with the test at 1:23:04 a.m. Thirty-six seconds later, an emergency shutdown of the reactor was initiated when someone—it is not clear who—pressed the AZ-5 button, which inserted all the control rods that had been withdrawn. Instead of shutting down the reactor (for reasons to be discussed below), this led to a power surge so great that it caused the fuel cladding to fail, releasing uranium fuel into the coolant, which in turn caused an enormous steam explosion that blew off the reactor casing, including its steel roof. A second explosion filled the air with flying lumps of the graphite moderator, which caught fire as they fell to the ground. These explosions and the subsequent ten-day fire sent a plume of uranium particles and much more hazardous radioactive isotopes such as cesium-137, iodine-131, and strontium-90 into the night sky.

The initial *Summary Report on the Post-Accident Review Meeting on the Chernobyl Accident,* produced in 1986 by the International Atomic Energy Agency (IAEA) International Nuclear Safety Advisory Group, accepted the Soviet view that "the accident was caused by a remarkable range of human errors and violations of operating rules in combination with specific reactor features which compounded and amplified the effects of the errors." In particular, "the operators deliberately and in violation of rules withdrew most control and safety rods from the core and switched off some important safety systems."[47] However, in November 1991, a commission of Soviet nuclear scientists led by Yevgeny Velikhov concluded that both the design and the construction of the reactor had been at fault.[48] The IAEA's updated 1992 report

accordingly laid much more emphasis on "the contributions of particular design features, including the design of the control rods and safety systems, and
arrangements for presenting important safety information to the operators":

> The operators placed the reactor in a dangerous condition, in partic-
> ular by removing too many of the control rods, resulting in the lowering
> of the reactor's operating reactivity margin [ORM]. . . . However, the
> operating procedures did not emphasise the vital safety significance
> of the ORM but rather treated the ORM as a way of controlling reactor
> power. It could therefore be argued that the actions of the operators were
> more a symptom of the prevailing safety culture of the Soviet era rather
> than the result of recklessness or a lack of competence on the part of the
> operators.[49]

The Chernobyl plant was known as an RBMK-1000: *reaktor bolshoy
moshchnosty kanalny,* a high-power channel reactor. This design was preferred by Soviet planners to the water-water energetic reactor, the equivalent
of the U.S. pressurized water reactor, which had been developed in the 1950s
with technology originally intended for nuclear submarines. In the water-
water reactors, energy was produced by placing fuel rods, which generate
heat through the fission of uranium atoms, into pressurized water. Water
acted as both a moderator, controlling the fission, and a coolant. The RBMK
used water as a coolant, too, but it used graphite to moderate the reaction.
This combination of graphite moderator and water coolant was and is unique:
the RBMK is the only kind of power reactor in the world to use it. It was favored in Moscow not only because its output of electrical energy was twice
that of the water-water reactor; it was also cheaper to build and operate.
Water-water reactors required enriched uranium-235; RBMKs could run on
almost natural uranium-238. Moreover, the RBMK reactors could be built
on location with prefabricated components produced by regular machine-
building plants. Anatoly Aleksandrov, the director of the Igor Kurchatov Institute of Atomic Energy, declared the RBMK "as safe as a samovar." Indeed, the
RBMKs were said to be so safe that they could be built without the concrete

superstructure that encased Western reactors to contain radiation in the event of a reactor failure. Significantly, Nikolai Dollezhal, the chief designer of the RBMK, argued against building such power stations in the European part of the Soviet Union. But he was overruled.[50]

Construction of the Chernobyl power plant began in 1977. By 1983 four reactors had been completed, and the addition of two more reactors was planned in subsequent years. But the process was rushed, under the usual pressure from party officials to beat deadlines and exceed quotas, and the quality of the work was inferior. Earlier reactors had been built under the auspices of the formidable Yefim Slavsky, the head of the Ministry of Medium Machine Building, who ran the early Soviet nuclear program as a military-industrial fiefdom. But Chernobyl was a project of the less powerful Ministry of Energy and Electrification, which essentially left construction to the locals. At the heart of Dyatlov's defense of his own role was his complaint that the reactor had been built by second-rate factories.[51]

Far from being as safe as a samovar, as Dollezhal well knew, the RBMK had a number of design defects that made it anything but safe, regardless of how well it was built. The reactor works (present tense, as ten of them are still in operation) as follows. Pellets of slightly enriched uranium oxide are enclosed in zirconium alloy tubes twelve feet long: these are the fuel rods. Eighteen of the rods, arranged cylindrically, form a fuel assembly, and each fuel assembly is placed in its own vertical pressure tube, through which flows pressurized water that cools the assembly, emerging at about 550 degrees Fahrenheit. The pressure tubes, in turn, are surrounded by graphite blocks that act as the moderator to slow down the neutrons released during fission, ensuring a continuous and stable chain reaction. To control the rate of fission automatically or manually, boron carbide control rods can be inserted either upward from the bottom of the core or from the top down. A number of these control rods always remain in the core during operation. The two water coolant loops that circulate water through the pressure tubes each have steam drums, or separators, where steam from the heated coolant is fed to a turbine to produce the electricity through a turbogenerator. The steam is then condensed and fed back into the circulating coolant. The reactor core is housed in a reinforced concrete-lined cavity. It sits on a heavy steel plate, with another steel cover plate on the top as a lid.[52]

This design had at least two fatal flaws that the operators did not fully understand.

Because water is both a more efficient coolant and a more effective neutron absorber than steam, a change in the proportion of steam bubbles ("voids") in the coolant would result in a change in core reactivity. The ratio of these changes was termed the "void coefficient" of reactivity. When the void coefficient was negative, an increase in steam would lead to a decrease in reactivity. In water-water reactors, where water acts as both moderator and coolant, excess steam generation slows the nuclear chain reaction—a built-in safety feature. This is not the case in a reactor that uses graphite as the moderator. In an RBMK, the reduction in neutron absorption as a result of increased steam production can increase the reactivity of the system if the void coefficient is positive. When the Chernobyl reactor's power began to increase, more steam was produced, which in turn led to an increase in power, which raised the temperature in the cooling circuit, which produced more steam. This led to the surge in power that caused the first explosion.

The second fatal flaw was that the operators had less control than they assumed over the RBMK's operating reactivity margin, defined as the number of equivalent control rods in the reactor core. Dyatlov and his colleagues believed that safety criteria were being met so long as they did not go below an operating reactivity margin of fifteen equivalent rods. They did not realize that reinserting all the control rods in an emergency would initially add to, rather than reduce, the reactivity of the core, because of the rods' graphite tips. The Soviet nuclear *nomenklatura* were in fact aware of this problem, because of a smaller mishap at another RBMK in Lithuania in 1983, but they did not think to inform the lesser mortals running Chernobyl.

The exact death toll of Chernobyl is uncertain and controversial, but it was smaller than might be imagined. Of the 237 power station staff and firemen hospitalized after the blast, twenty-eight died of acute radiation sickness soon afterward, and fifteen of radiation-induced cancer in the subsequent ten years. The United Nations Scientific Committee on the Effects of Atomic Radiation concluded that fewer than a hundred deaths could be conclusively attributed to increased exposure to radiation. Around six thousand cases of thyroid cancer, mainly in people who were children and adolescents at the time of the accident, might be attributed to their drinking contaminated milk, but only nine of these resulted in death.[53] Remarkably, the three men who heroically entered the flooded basement area to drain the water reservoir beneath the reactor all survived. According to a 2006 report of the International Atomic Energy Agency's Chernobyl Forum, exposure to radiation caused by the disaster "might eventually represent up to several thousand fatal cancers in addition to perhaps one hundred thousand cancer deaths expected in these populations from all other causes," a modest rise in percentage terms.[54] Antinuclear groups such as the Union of Concerned Scientists and Greenpeace challenged this estimate as much too low. But the fact that by 2000 there were 3.5 million Ukrainians who claimed to be radiation "sufferers" might better be explained by the more generous state benefits that status conferred. Evidence of fetal abnormalities explained by radiation exposure has not been found; it seems that many more lives were lost due to precautionary abortions requested by pregnant women fearful of such abnormalities than from the direct effects of the explosion itself.[55]

The Chernobyl cleanup operation is supposed to be complete by 2065. However, the area around Chernobyl will be uninhabitable for a very long time—for hundreds, thousands, or even tens of thousands of years.[56] This will likely be the Soviet Union's most enduring legacy in Ukraine, an independent country since 1991, though it should be remembered that the two thousand square miles that saw the worst contamination (in terms of concentrations of cesium-137, which has a half-life of thirty years) extended well into Russia and Belarus and as far as the Balkans and Scandinavia.[57] In what is referred to as his "Testament," which was published following his suicide, two years after the accident, Valery Legasov did indeed indict the Soviet system, even if less eloquently than Craig Mazin would have liked:

> After I had visited Chernobyl . . . I came to the conclusion that the
> accident was the inevitable apotheosis of the economic system which had

been developed in the USSR over many decades. Neglect by the scientific management and the designers was everywhere with no attention being paid to the condition of instruments or of equipment. . . .

When one considers the chain of events leading up to the Chernobyl accident, why one person behaved in such a way and why another person behaved in another etc., it is impossible to find a single culprit, a single initiator of events, because it was like a closed circle.[58]

Yet it should have occurred to the reader by now that something not entirely different had been true of NASA at the time of the *Challenger* disaster, three months before. At NASA and at Morton Thiokol, the engineers knew there was a problem with the O-rings. It was middle management that ignored their warnings and went ahead with the launch. At Chernobyl, by contrast, the operators were unaware of the key vulnerabilities of the RBMK. It was senior Soviet officials who knew but opted to keep quiet. Paradoxically, perhaps, the first impulse of the American media in 1986 was to blame the president; the first impulse of the Soviet government was to blame the workers.

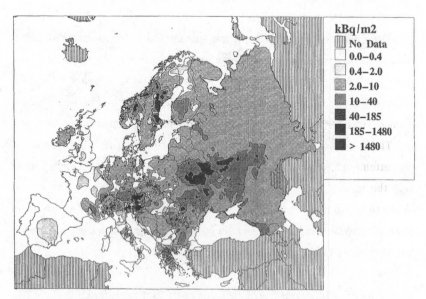

Cesium-137 deposition levels across Europe following the Chernobyl nuclear disaster, kilobecquerels per square meter, May 10, 1986.

In reality, the point of failure was not at the top, nor at the bottom, but in the middle. Clearly, the incentive structures were quite different in the two systems. For the managers at Morton Thiokol, the principal preoccupation was to keep the NASA orders coming. For the Soviet apparatchiks, the default setting was to keep knowledge of any problem to the smallest circle possible. Yet in both cases, concerns about cost played a key role. The reliance on O-rings and putty was an improvisation to avoid addressing a fundamental structural flaw with the rocket boosters. The decision to build the Chernobyl reactors on the cheap, without sufficient concrete outer cladding, sprang from the same kind of false economy.

IT CAN'T HAPPEN HERE

Nothing illustrates better how little separated the Soviet and American nuclear programs than the partial meltdown of reactor number 2 at Three Mile Island, near Middletown, Pennsylvania, on March 28, 1979. Unlike Chernobyl, it is true, the Three Mile Island disaster killed no one. There was minimal leakage of radioactive material beyond the power station site. But the conclusion of the Nuclear Regulatory Commission's summary of the incident was damning: "A combination of equipment malfunctions, design-related problems and worker error led to TMI-2's partial meltdown."[59] The producers of the film *The China Syndrome*—about an American nuclear power plant that comes close to meltdown—could hardly believe their luck. The movie had opened in theaters just twelve days before the accident.

The proximate cause of the Three Mile Island near disaster was a bungled attempt to fix a blockage in one of the eight condensate polishers, which kept the reactor's secondary-loop water free of impurities. By using water rather than condensed air to clear an accumulation of resin, the operators inadvertently caused the feedwater pumps, condensate booster pumps, and condensate pumps to turn off at around 4:00 a.m., cutting off the flow of water to the steam generators that removed heat from the reactor core. This caused an automatic emergency shutdown of the reactor, but because the valves of three auxiliary pumps had been closed for routine maintenance, no water at all could reach the reactor to offset its rapidly rising decay heat. To control the rising pressure, the manually operated relief valve on top of one of the pressure tanks was opened. The relief valve should have closed when the pressure returned to normal levels, but—in another malfunction—it became stuck open. A light on the control room panel, however, seemed to indicate that the valve was closed—this was not a malfunction but a design flaw. As a result, the operators had no idea that cooling water in the form of steam was still pouring out of the defective valve. They also wrongly believed that the water level was rising in the core, not realizing that it was steam, not water, that was accumulating. This misapprehension led them to turn off the emergency core-cooling pumps, which had automatically started after the relief valve failed to close. At 4:15 a.m., radioactive coolant began to leak out into the general containment building and was then pumped to an auxiliary building outside the containment boundary until the pumps were stopped, at 4:39 a.m. Soon after 6:00 a.m., the top of the reactor core was exposed and the intense heat caused a reaction to occur between the steam in the core and the zircaloy nuclear fuel rod cladding. This reaction melted the cladding and damaged the fuel pellets, which released radioactive isotopes into the reactor coolant and also produced flammable hydrogen gas, some of which may have exploded. At 6:45 a.m., radiation alarms were activated as contaminated water reached detectors. For a time, on the third day following the accident, there seemed to be a risk that a hydrogen bubble in the dome of the reactor would trigger an explosion. Had oxygen been present in the dome, that might well have happened. As it was, half the uranium fuel melted down and nearly all the cladding failed, but, crucially, the reactor vessel—the second level of containment after the cladding—held, containing the damaged fuel with nearly all the radioactive isotopes in the core. The amount of radioactive material that leaked was therefore minimal, and adverse health consequences for the local population barely detectable. The principal damage, which was only reinforced by the subsequent Chernobyl disaster, was to the American nuclear industry, the rapid expansion of which now slowed. At the time of the Three Mile Island accident, 129 nuclear power plants had been approved; only 53 of them were ever completed.

The President's Commission on the Accident at Three Mile Island, chaired by John G. Kemeny, was unsparing in its criticism of the responsible institutions: the manufacturer, Babcock & Wilcox; Metropolitan Edison (Met-Ed), which operated the power plant; and the Nuclear Regulatory Commission (NRC). It emerged, for example, that a similar incident had occurred eighteen months earlier at another Babcock & Wilcox plant; the problem with the defective relief valve had been an unknown known, not so different from the problem with the graphite-tipped rods at Chernobyl. By contrast, the operators themselves got off lightly. The NRC's Three Mile Island Special Inquiry Group concluded that the human errors were due not to simple "operator deficiencies" but rather to inadequacies in equipment design, information presentation, emergency procedures, and training. The reactor had been "designed and built without a central concept or philosophy for man-machine integration," so the role of operators in an emergency was not clearly defined. They had too much unnecessary information, and at the same time "some critical parameters were not displayed" or were not immediately available to them. The control room panel was poorly designed, resulting in "excessive operator motion, workload, error probability, and response time." The operators had not been given "a systematic method of problem diagnosis," nor had they been equipped by their training with "the skills necessary to diagnose the incident and take appropriate action."[60] How much better off were the Three Mile Island operators than their Chernobyl counterparts? Both sets of workers were to some extent laboring in the dark. Were the Americans merely lucky that a big explosion did not happen?

Nor did the U.S. authorities deal with the local population much more effectively and candidly than their Soviet counterparts would seven years later. From the moment a general emergency was announced by station manager Gary Miller, confusion reigned. Met-Ed at first denied that radiation had been released. Lieutenant Governor William Scranton III at first said the same, then seemed to have second thoughts. On March 30—that is, two days after the initial accident—the NRC advised everyone within ten miles of the power plant to stay inside. A few hours later, Governor Dick Thornburgh, on the advice of NRC chairman Joseph Hendrie, advised the evacuation "of pregnant

women and pre-school age children . . . within a five-mile radius." That evening, as the risk of an explosion seemed to rise, officials came to realize that
they might need to evacuate everyone within a ten- or even a twenty-mile
radius—in which case more than 600,000 people in the six surrounding counties might have to move. No plan for such an evacuation existed: the only contingency plan was to evacuate those within a five-mile radius. The result was
chaotic. About 40 percent of those who lived within fifteen miles of Three
Mile Island opted to evacuate, precipitating a bank run as they withdrew cash
before driving off. Local priests began granting "general absolution," which
was not calculated to reassure remaining residents. Three hundred journalists swarmed around the scene. Only a week after the initial accident were officials able to announce that the hydrogen bubble would not explode. Five
days later, the evacuation advisory was rescinded.[61]

In the Soviet Union, the central government had too much power. In the
United States, power is distributed to too many federal, state, and local agencies. More than 150 different agencies were involved in the Three Mile Island
emergency and the public communications about it. To say that their efforts
were poorly coordinated would be an understatement.[62] Reviewing the coverage of the crisis on the three television networks, President Jimmy Carter—
who had studied nuclear energy as a naval officer and who had been directly
involved in the cleanup after the 1952 accident at the Chalk River reactor, in
Canada—grew impatient: "There are too many people talking," he complained to Jody Powell, his press secretary. "And my impression is that half of
them don't know what they are talking about. . . . Get those people to speak
with one voice." Sending the Nuclear Regulatory Commission's Harold R. Den-
ton to the scene had not sufficed. On April 1, Carter himself flew to Three Mile
Island in an attempt to reassure the public that the situation was under
control.[63]

Complexity is once again the crucial concept, a point popularized at the
time by the Yale sociologist Charles Perrow's idea of the "normal accident,"
i.e., accidents made normal by ubiquitous complexity.[64] The Three Mile Island
reactor was itself highly complex, but the interface between the people working there and the technology of the reactor was so inadequate that a simple

stuck valve and a misleading light on a control panel caused a partial melt-down and very nearly a much larger disaster. In the face of an emergency, scores of government agencies sought to lead or at least contribute to the response, but no plan for a large-scale evacuation existed. Had the hydrogen bubble exploded, no doubt the media would have found a way to pin responsibility on President Carter, though this would have been harder if he had been close to the explosion. Yet, as we saw in chapter 6, it is usually a version of Tolstoy's Napoleon fallacy to attribute a crucial role to a leader in a disaster, unless it is one of those leaders like Stalin, Hitler, or Mao who purposefully sets out to cause a disaster. Most disasters occur when a complex system goes critical, usually as a result of some small perturbation. The extent to which the exogenous shock causes a disaster is generally a function of the social network structure that comes under stress. The point of failure, if it can be located at all, is more likely to be in the middle layer than at the top of the organization chart.*[65] When failure occurs, however, society as a whole, and the different interest groups within it, will draw much larger inferences about future risk than are warranted[66]—hence the widespread conclusion from a small number of accidents that nuclear power was chronically unsafe. This is the framework we should have in mind as we endeavor to understand the much larger disaster—or disasters—of 2020.

---

*That is why, for example, the attempt by some newspapers to make a Conservative councillor the villain of the piece in England's Grenfell Tower disaster deserves to fail. Although the public inquiry continues at the time of writing, it was already clear soon after the fire that the building's vulnerability was a consequence of overly complex regulation, overlapping jurisdictions, and unclear responsibilities.

9

THE PLAGUES

Briefly, he enlightened me that the plague was spread by the creatures of the Moon. The Moon, our Lady of Ill-aspect, was the offender.

—Rudyard Kipling, "A Doctor of Medicine"

ANTHROPAUSE

To write the history of a disaster that is not yet over is, on the face of it, impossible. And yet the act of thinking historically about an unfolding event is not without its value. Indeed, it is an essential part of any effort to apply history to present predicaments in a systematic way. This chapter was written in the first week of August 2020 and revised a month later, when much that is now known to the reader was unknown. Some of its judgments may already prove to have been wrong at the time of publication. It should therefore be read rather as a diary of the plague half year—which is indeed how it took shape, as a weekly slide deck that was born on January 29, shortly after I attended the World Economic Forum at Davos. It was updated every week until the time came to write this book.

As I saw it then, the world's economic and political leaders were focused on the wrong worry. Even as a global pandemic was getting under way—as flights carrying infected passengers were leaving Wuhan for destinations all over the world—the discussions at the World Economic Forum were focused almost exclusively on the problem of climate change. Questions of environmental responsibility, social justice, and governance (ESG) dominated discussions on corporate boards. On January 23, the atomic scientists advanced the hands on their Doomsday Clock "closer to apocalypse than ever," but not because they foresaw a pandemic: their worries were nuclear war, climate change, "cyber-enabled information warfare," and "erosion" of the "international political infrastructure."[1] People all over the Western world missed, until it was too late, the significance of the "novel coronavirus" belatedly disclosed by the Chinese government to the World Health Organization on the last day of 2019. By a rich irony, COVID-19 granted the wish of Greta Thunberg, the child saint of the twenty-first-century millennialist movement. "Our emissions have to stop," she had declared at Davos. "Any plan or policy of yours that doesn't include radical emission cuts at the source, starting today, is completely insufficient."[2] Within a matter of weeks, satellite observations showed dramatic declines of nitrogen dioxide emissions above China (down 40 percent relative to the same period in 2019), the United States (down 38 percent), and Europe (down 20 percent).[3] These were, of course, direct consequences of the suspension of economic activity thought necessary to limit the spread of the new virus. Conservationists were also able to celebrate the "anthropause" as hundreds of millions of birds and millions of animals were spared their usual massacre at the hands of human motorists.[4] Nothing, it turned out, could be more beneficial to the rest of the planet than to lock up humans in their homes for a few months.

This is not to dismiss the potential risks that may arise from rising global temperatures, but simply to suggest that obsessive discussion of those risks in 2019 and early 2020 led to myopia. For the average American on the eve of the pandemic, the chance of dying from an overdose was two hundred times greater than the chance of being killed by a cataclysmic storm, and the chance of dying in a motor vehicle accident was fifteen hundred times higher than the chance of being killed by a flood.[5] The threat of climate-related disaster lay in the future; the threat of pandemic was proximate. In 2018, the number of Americans killed by influenza and pneumonia (59,120) was substantially higher than the number who died in car crashes (39,404).[6] Just a century earlier, the 1918–19 influenza pandemic had demonstrated just how lethal a new virus that targets the respiratory system could be. Despite repeated warnings, policymakers' attention had drifted away from this risk.

The initial outbreak of the new virus SARS-CoV-2 could be traced back to China's dysfunctional one-party state. However, we need the insights of network science to explain how exactly the virus spread. Governments in the United States, the United Kingdom, and the European Union failed in their different ways to respond swiftly and effectively to the threat. The failure in Latin America was even more lamentable. But this was not just the fault of populist leaders, as was often claimed; it was also a systemic failure, and Taiwan, South Korea, and other smaller, better-prepared states showed that this failure was not inevitable. However, matters were made much worse by misinformation and disinformation about the virus that also went viral on the internet, leading to widespread confusion about how seriously to treat the contagion. While social distancing was the correct response, the economic consequences of belated measures to "lock down" economies were historically unprecedented and—as the true infection fatality rate of COVID-19 became clearer—may have exceeded the public health benefits. As I argue in chapter 10, monetary and fiscal measures were palliatives, not stimulus. Their principal effect was to decouple asset prices from economic reality and (perhaps) sow the seeds of future financial instability and inflation. By the summer of 2020 it was clear that there was a path forward—but it was not a path straight back to an old normality that might take years to recover, if it could be recovered at all. The danger, my final chapter suggests, was that this path might lead to political crisis and geopolitical confrontation—potentially even to war.

THE WUHAN EXHALATION

The COVID-19 pandemic *might* have been as bad as the Imperial College London epidemiological models projected in mid-March. It was impossible to be certain at that stage. The epidemiologist Neil Ferguson and his colleagues implied that the world faced a pandemic as severe as the Spanish influenza of 1918–19, with up to 2.2 million American lives at risk if drastic measures such as lockdowns were not taken. But that assumed a higher infection fatality rate (0.9 percent) than seemed probable even at that relatively early stage. By August, the pandemic of 2020 seemed more likely to end up closer to the 1957–58 Asian flu in terms of excess mortality. (As we saw in chapter 7, the Asian flu killed up to 115,700 Americans, the equivalent of 215,000 in 2020, and between 700,000 and 1.5 million people worldwide, equivalent to 2 to 4 million dead today.) That meant that in August 2020, COVID-19 was still capable of killing many more people.

At the end of January 2020, there had been just under 10,000 confirmed cases and 212 deaths attributed to the new disease, nearly all of them in China's Hubei Province.[7] By that time, however, untold numbers of infected travelers had left Wuhan for cities all over the world, because of obfuscation and foot-dragging by the Chinese authorities. By the end of February, total confirmed cases worldwide were 86,000; by the end of March, 872,000; by the end of April, 3.2 million; by the end of May, 6.2 million; by the end of June, 10.4 million. By August 3, 2020, there had been a total of 18.1 million confirmed COVID-19 cases around the world, with just over 690,000 deaths. Slightly less than a quarter (23 percent) of all the deaths had occurred in the United States. And just under a third (31 percent) of those deaths had been in just two states: New York and New Jersey.[8] How many more people would ultimately die of COVID-19? At the time of writing, the seven-day weekly average of deaths attributed to the disease around the world was rising. After peaking on April 18 at more than 7,000, it had declined to around 4,000 in late May, only to rise again to 6,000 in early August. Unless this trend improved, the global death toll could be 1 million by October and 2 million by the end of the year. Epidemiological models for the United States varied in their projections, ranging from 230,822 deaths by November 1 to 272,000 by November 23.[9] In May, based on historical experience, I estimated a U.S. death toll of around 250,000 by the end of the year. That still seemed plausible in August. However, it would be historically unusual for a pandemic on this scale to confine itself to one calendar year. Among the many known unknowns were how much higher the death toll would rise in the southern hemisphere and how significant the return of colder weather or the reopening of schools would be in the northern. One survey concluded that around 349 million people (4.5 percent of the global population) were "at high risk of severe COVID-19 and would require hospital admission if infected," but clearly only some fraction of these actually would become infected, of whom only a smaller fraction would die.[10] This was a global disaster, then, but in terms of mortality (whether excess mortality or quality-adjusted life years) on the scale of 1957–58, not 1918–19, assuming that the virus did not mutate in a way that made it more contagious or more lethal or both.

There was nothing surprising about its location of origin. As we have seen, a significant number of history's pandemics have originated in Asia, and especially in China. What exactly happened in Wuhan was not yet clear in August 2020. According to Western press reports, in 2018 U.S. diplomats had raised concerns about safety at the Wuhan Institute of Virology, where Shi Zhengli had for several years been engaged in research on coronaviruses in bats, as well as at the nearby Wuhan Center for Disease Control and Prevention.[11] The Chinese government, however, stuck to the story that the initial outbreak was at the Huanan "seafood" market, where all kinds of live wild animals were in fact for sale.[12] Either way, there was no evidence to suggest the virus was engineered. It was just the latest case in a history of zoonotic transfer from animals to humans. Probably the *Rhinolophus affinis* horseshoe bat was the reservoir host; possibly imported Malayan pangolins acted as a stepping-stone. The virus may have mutated further in early human-to-human transmission.[13]

Had the Chinese authorities acted with speed and candor, the disaster might have been averted.[14] The earliest Wuhan case (who had no connection to the Huanan market) had symptoms on December 1. Five days after a man linked to the market presented pneumonia-like symptoms, his wife fell similarly ill, suggesting human-to-human transmission. It later emerged that there were 104 cases and fifteen deaths during the month of December; of the first forty-one cases, six died.[15] Yet the Wuhan Health Commission (WHC) dragged its feet for an entire month. Local doctors such as Zhang Jixian and Li Wenliang noticed something amiss in the spate of abnormal pneumonia cases they were seeing, but Li (who suggested on WeChat that the illness might be SARS) was admonished for spreading "false rumors" and forced to retract what he had said. (He died of COVID-19 on February 7.) The official Chinese report to the World Health Organization on December 31 acknowledged a cluster of viral pneumonia cases of unknown etiology in Wuhan but stated that there was "no clear evidence" of human-to-human transmission. "The disease is preventable and controllable," the government said. The cover-up continued into January, even after the first death from the new virus was announced on the eleventh (a sixty-one-year-old man who had died two days before). Doctors were silenced, social media censored. On January 10, a respected Beijing physician, Wang Guangfa, said the outbreak was "under control" and mostly a "mild condition." As Wuhan and Hubei political leaders gathered in Wuhan for annual meetings, the WHC kept the number of the infected artificially low and repeatedly downplayed the risks of contagion. Wuhan officials also allowed large public gatherings ahead of the Lunar New Year.

Chinese scientists did what they could. By January 2, Shi Zhengli had decoded the entire genome of the virus, but the next day the National Health Commission (NHC) prohibited Chinese laboratories from publishing information about the virus without government authorization. By January 3, the Chinese Center for Disease Control had also sequenced the virus. By January 5, so had Zhang Yongzhen's team at the Shanghai Public Health Clinical Center. But the government sat on all these findings. On January 11, Zhang went ahead and posted the virus's genome on the website virological.org. The next day his lab was ordered to close for "rectification," but the cat was out of the bag.[16] In a confidential teleconference on January 14, National Health Commission chief Ma Xiaowei privately warned other Chinese officials that the Wuhan outbreak was "likely to develop into a major public-health event" and that "clustered cases" suggested "human-to-human transmission." Around the same time, according to a Canadian report, the regime issued urgent worldwide guidance to Chinese consulates "to prepare for and respond to a pandemic" by importing, on a massive scale, supplies of personal protective equipment. Not until January 20—following a report from Wuhan by a team of experts sent by the NHC—did the Chinese government confirm the first cases of human-to-human transmission and acknowledge publicly that (in Xi Jinping's words) the "outbreak must be taken seriously." At the very least, then, China wasted weeks— and it may have been longer. According to a Harvard study based on satellite photography and internet data, there was a noticeable rise in vehicles parking outside six hospitals in Wuhan from late August to December 1, 2019, as well as an increase in online searches for terms such as "cough" and "diarrhea."[17]

The conduct of the Chinese authorities was much as it had been at the beginning of the SARS epidemic. The difference was that this time the World Health Organization, under its director general, Tedros Adhanom Ghebreyesus, was supine, if not sycophantic. China had strongly backed his candidacy for the job; Tedros reciprocated by endorsing the Chinese scheme for a "Health Silk Road." In the early phase of the crisis, Tedros echoed Beijing's line ("the Chinese authorities have found no clear evidence of human-to-human transmission," on January 14), failed to declare a global public health emergency until a week after Wuhan was locked down, and waited until March 11 to acknowledge that there was a pandemic. One country was setting a shining example of contagion containment without lockdowns that others might have followed: Taiwan. Deferential to the People's Republic of China, WHO officials acted as if it did not exist.[18]

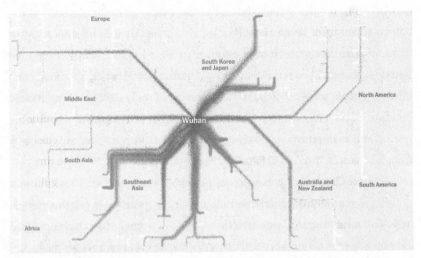

Passenger flows from Wuhan before the January 23 lockdown of the city. Nineteen flights departed Wuhan for John F. Kennedy Airport or San Francisco in January. The flights were largely full, according to VariFlight. About 85 percent of infected passengers went undetected.

On the morning of January 23, Wuhan was placed under quarantine, followed two days later by fifteen other cities in Hubei. The next day, an order was issued suspending group travel within China. However, in a blunder that would have far-reaching consequences, China did not issue an order suspending group travel to foreign countries until three days later, on January 27, and did nothing to prevent individuals from traveling overseas.[19] In all, about seven million people left Wuhan in January, before travel was restricted.[20] In the days leading up to the Lunar New Year holiday, an unknown number of infected people—because at this point 86 percent of infections were undocumented[21]—traveled all over China and the world to see relatives and close friends.[22] By bus, train, and plane, the virus spread.[23] Yet in no province of China other than Hubei did COVID-19 spread exponentially,[24] whereas in the rest of the world—in Europe, North America, and Latin America—it did. Why was this? The answer was not that travel restrictions were much more rigorously enforced between Wuhan and the rest of China than between Wuhan and the rest of the world, though they were. The answer was that the rest of China imposed non-pharmaceutical interventions (NPIs)—suspending intra-city public transport, closing schools, closing entertainment venues, and banning public gatherings, as well as quarantining suspected and confirmed patients—more quickly than the rest of the world.[25] The significance of the ban on travel from Wuhan was that it gave the authorities in other Chinese cities at most two or three days to put their NPIs in place. These were then strictly enforced all over the country by Communist Party neighborhood committees. People were confined to their homes, in some cases with apartment building doors welded shut. A nationwide system of temperature and other testing and manual contact tracing was hastily built out. This explains why Chinese cases leveled off in February.[26]

At first, in January and much of February, cases outside China did not grow exponentially. But then they did, first in Europe, then in North America. This was surprising. According to the WHO, the United States was supposed to be among the "better prepared" countries for the eventuality of a pandemic.[27] The 2019 Global Health Security Index ranked the United States along with Canada, the United Kingdom, and a handful of other countries as "most prepared."[28] But the WHO and GHS ratings turned out to count for nothing: they were in fact negatively correlated with pandemic containment. Having a system of universal healthcare also turned out not to be a statistically significant advantage: numerous countries with such systems fared badly.[29] An initial ranking of pandemic responses in April put Israel, Singapore, New Zealand, Hong Kong, and Taiwan at the top, closely followed by Japan, Hungary, Austria, Germany, and South Korea.[30]

The first case of COVID-19 in the U.S. was reported on January 20, 2020, in Snohomish County, Washington—a thirty-five-year-old man who had just returned from Wuhan—though he appears not to have infected anyone. The virus arrived directly from China and indirectly from Europe and Iran.[31] The number of cases grew exponentially across the United States throughout March, though with a heavy concentration in the Northeast, especially in and around New York City. After March, the curves of cases and deaths flattened, but new infections and new deaths continued to occur at higher rates than in other developed countries. Within four months the virus had spread to every state and to more than 90 percent of all counties.[32] By June, the United States was clearly faring worse than Italy had, even in per capita terms, and Italy was among the hardest-hit European countries.[33]

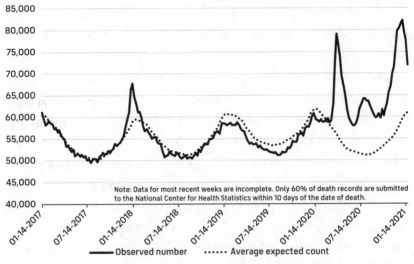

Observed and expected weekly excess mortality in the United States (all causes), 2017–20.

The most illuminating measures of a pandemic's impact are deaths relative to population and excess deaths above recent seasonal averages. On the
basis of the former measure, the United States (469 COVID-19 deaths per million by August 4) did significantly worse than Ireland (357), Canada (237),
Australia (9), and New Zealand (5), but better than the United Kingdom (680).
Also harder hit than the United States were Belgium (850), Spain (609), Italy
(582), and Sweden (569), with the difference that European case numbers
had largely (if only temporarily) leveled off by that time. Increasingly, the
path of COVID-19 mortality in the United States resembled that of Brazil (445)
or Mexico (372). By mid-July 2020, the United States had suffered around
149,000 excess deaths, 23 percent above historical averages, similar to the figures for Brazil, the Netherlands, Sweden, and Switzerland. (According to *The
New York Times,* estimated deaths above normal between March 1 and July
25 totaled 219,000.[34] However, CDC data suggest 205,985 excess deaths from
all causes for January 1 to August 1, 12 percent above total expected deaths
in that period.)[35] The rates for Chile (46 percent), the UK (45), Italy (44), Belgium (40), and Spain (56) were all substantially higher, with the UK faring
worse than all EU countries.[36] Peru (149 percent) and Ecuador (117) had the
highest excess mortality. Yet some countries (Iceland, Israel, and Norway) suffered no excess deaths. Germany's excess death rate was 5 percent.[37]

The problem in the summer of 2020 was that Americans all over the
country acted in ways that simply ignored what was known by that time about
the virus and the disease. Only in Vermont was the disease truly contained.
(Alaska, Hawaii, and Montana had been in that category in June, but case
numbers rose as vacationers arrived from states with higher infection numbers.) The situation had greatly improved in locked-down New England, New
Jersey, and New York, which had borne the brunt of the first wave in the
spring. But in a clear majority of states, notably in the South and the West,
cases of COVID-19 had continued to rise since Memorial Day (May 25). In
around a dozen there were second waves after a period when the disease
seemed to have been contained. In a number of important states—notably
California, Florida, and Texas—the initial wave had only just begun to crest
in early August.[38]

We knew a lot more in August about SARS-CoV-2 and COVID-19 than we had known in January, when the rational response to the unreliable information coming from China was to prepare for the worst by minimizing incoming traffic from China, ramping up testing for the new virus, and creating a system of contact tracing. (This was what Taiwan and South Korea did.) Its genetic code was extremely close to the bat coronavirus RaTG13. It was obvious even to amateur epidemiologists that the new disease was at least as infectious as seasonal influenza and significantly more lethal.[39] It was not as deadly as SARS, MERS, Ebola, or the 1918 Spanish flu, all of which had higher infection fatality rates. It was not as contagious as measles, which has the highest reproduction numbers of any disease. It was in what might be called the bitter (as opposed to sweet) spot: contagious enough to spread rapidly, but not so lethal as to remain geographically contained. Early estimates of the reproduction number (R_0, the number of other people infected by one virus carrier) varied widely—from 6 to 15—but they were high enough to be alarming.[40] The consensus by the summer was between 1.8 and 3.6.[41] Crucially, it was clear that a significant proportion of virus carriers—somewhere around 40 percent—had no symptoms when infectious; some, especially children, never developed symptoms at all.[42] In guidelines published on July 10, the CDC estimated R_0 at 2.5 and the percentage of transmission occurring prior to symptom onset at 50 percent.[43]

Scientists quite quickly established that the virus's spike protein binds to a protein on the surface of human cells (known as ACE2) and then, once inside the cell, releases its RNA and begins reproducing itself, beginning in the upper respiratory area. By July 2020 we knew that SARS-CoV-2 viruses could be spread in fine-particle aerosol, or Flügge, droplets.[44] That meant it was transmitted most readily by coughing, sneezing, shouting, or singing in relatively crowded indoor, air-conditioned locations.[45] In such situations, being six feet apart was insufficient protection.[46] This clinched the argument for wearing masks in any crowded place.[47] It was much rarer to catch the disease outside.[48] The virus was present in feces as well as breath and saliva, but there was no evidence of spread by this route, though in theory even the flushing of a toilet could propel viral particles through the air.[49] All this suggested that changes in average seasonal temperatures would have a limited impact on the rate of contagion; the role of heating, air-conditioning, and indoor spread made outside temperatures of trivial importance.[50] It was also clear that the most distinctive symptom of infection was anosmia (loss of sense of smell).[51]

But just how deadly was the disease? There was the rub. By the spring, it seemed likely, though not certain, that the overall infection fatality rate was going to land somewhere between 0.3 and 0.7 percent, not the 0.9 to 1.0 percent assumed in some early models. Many people infected had no symptoms; many had relatively minor ones, lasting a matter of days; a proportion had protracted illness, some of whom (in France just under 4 percent)[52] required hospitalization. Of those requiring intensive care, a high proportion died— roughly half in Britain—most commonly of acute respiratory distress syndrome accompanied by hypoxemia (low oxygen in arterial blood) and culminating in a fatal cytokine "storm."[53] The time between symptom onset and death was just two weeks on average.[54] Autopsies revealed distinctive forms of lung damage: severe endothelial injury associated with the presence of intracellular virus and disrupted cell membranes, and widespread thrombosis with microangiopathy.[55]

It was clear from a very early stage of the Wuhan epidemic that the elderly were the most vulnerable group, with case fatality rates (CFRs) around 8 percent in patients in their seventies and 15 percent among octogenarians.[56] In Europe, 80 percent of deaths linked to COVID-19 were of people over seventy-five.[57] The skew partly reflected the fact that elderly people have a variety of preexisting conditions, such as ischemic heart disease, diabetes, cancer, atrial fibrillation, and dementia, which made them more vulnerable.[58] In addition, British data showed that infected men were more likely to die than women and that obese people were more likely to die than those with normal body mass. Asthma emerged as another risk factor in the UK.[59] The picture in the United States was similar: COVID-19 CFRs rose from below 1 percent (for people aged twenty to fifty-four) to 1 to 5 percent (fifty-five to sixty-four) to 3 to 11 percent (sixty-five to eighty-four) to 10 to 27 percent (eighty-five and older).[60] Septuagenarians accounted for 9 percent of the population of New York State but 64 percent of the COVID-19 fatalities.[61] This was not to say that prime-age adults were safe. A higher proportion of American than European deaths were of people in their fifties, almost certainly reflecting higher rates of obesity and associated health issues in the U.S. population.[62] Strokes, abnormal blood clotting, and cases of acute limb ischemia

COVID-19 IN COMPARATIVE PERSPECTIVE

	Influenza 1918	Influenza 1957	Influenza 2009[a]	Influenza 2009[b]	SARS-CoV	SARS-CoV-2
Transmissibility, R_0	2.0		1.7		2.4	2.5
Incubation period, days	Unknown		2		2–7	4–12
Interval between symptom onset and maximum infectivity, days	2		2		5–7	0
Proportion of patients with mild illness	High		High		Low	High
Proportion of patients requiring hospitalization	Few		Few		Most (>70%)	Few (20%)
Proportion of patients requiring intensive care	Unknown		1/104,000		Most (40%)	1/16,000
Proportion of deaths in people younger than 65	95%		80%		Unknown	0.6–2.8%
Number of U.S. deaths (adjusted to year 2000 population)	1,272,300*	150,600*	7,500–44,100	8,500–17,600	0	164,037[†]
Mean age at death (years)	27.2	64.6	37.4		Unknown	Unknown
Years of life lost (adjusted to year 2000 population)	63,718,000	2,698,000	334,000–1,973,000	328,900–680,300	Unknown	3,730,530

Source: Petersen, "Comparing SARS-CoV-2," tables 1 and 3.

Notes:

[a] Range based on estimates of excess pneumonia and influenza deaths (lower-range number) and all-cause deaths (upper-range number); estimated from projections of mortality surveillance from 122 cities.

[b] Estimates from the Centers for Disease Control and Prevention using 2009 pandemic survey data.

*Estimates based on the excess mortality approach applied to final national vital statistics.

†For SARS-CoV-2 to September 11, 2020.

were reported among a number of otherwise healthy COVID carriers in their thirties and forties.[63] Evidence accumulated that many patients who had recovered from the disease had suffered lasting lung damage,[64] while others reported persistent symptoms such as fatigue, breathlessness, and aches.[65] In Italy and New York State, there were cases of children falling seriously ill, including a number with symptoms of inflammation similar to those in Kawasaki syndrome.[66] Four out of 582 COVID-positive children in a European study died.[67] It was also clear from quite early on that people of African heritage were more liable to die of COVID-19 than their white counterparts;[68] in the United Kingdom it was people of Caribbean and South Asian heritage.[69] In Chicago, for example, African Americans were 30 percent of the population but 52 percent of the COVID-19 deaths; overall, the fatality rate for black Americans was 2.5 times higher.[70] American Latinos and Native Americans were also getting infected at much higher rates than white Americans, especially after accounting for age.[71] How far this reflected socioeconomic disadvantages (e.g., poor healthcare, crowded accommodations, or exposed occupations), higher prevalence of conditions that increased vulnerability (e.g., obesity and diabetes), or genetic factors remained a matter for further research and debate, though there were those who wished to rule out the last of these *ex ante*.[72]

All of this was quite bad enough to make a simplistic strategy of herd immunity seem imprudent. On the basis of a standard epidemiological model, that could be achieved only if around 70 percent of the population caught the virus,* which would mean an unacceptably large number of deaths and serious illnesses even on the assumption of a relatively low IFR—nearly 1.4 million deaths in the United States, assuming an IFR of 0.6 percent.[73] Yet, even as the summer approached, there was still a lot that we did not know about the virus and the disease, and presumably a significant amount that we did not know we did not know. We did not know how long immunity lasted for those who got infected and recovered, though we knew they had immunity.[74] (Or did we? The theory that one could recover and then catch the disease

_____

*In the case of a pathogen with an R_0 of 4, on average, one infected person will infect four other people. Mathematically, the herd immunity threshold is defined by 1 minus $1/R_0$, so if $R_0 = 4$ then the corresponding herd immunity threshold is 75 percent of the population.

again appeared not to hold water, until a handful of asymptomatic cases proved otherwise.)[75] We did not know how long people who had recovered from COVID-19 but still felt unwell would remain impaired, and how seriously. We did not really understand well why, for example, the experiences of Germany and Japan had been so different from those of Belgium and the United States, or why the experience of Britain had been rather similar to that of Sweden, despite the two countries' adopting radically different public health policies, or why Portugal had fared better than neighboring and very similar Spain, or why Swiss Italians had fared so much worse than Swiss Germans. Was the Bacillus Calmette-Guérin (BCG) tuberculosis vaccine, mandatory in some countries but not in others, in some way protective against COVID-19?[76] Were blood groups relevant, with type A being more susceptible than type B?[77] What was the role of memory T cells or antibodies generated by exposure to other coronaviruses?[78] There was still, in short, a lot of unexplained "dark matter," to use the neuroscientist Karl Friston's term.[79] And what were the chances that the virus would mutate further in ways that would make it more contagious or more lethal or simply more resistant to a vaccine?[80]

Meanwhile, effective therapies for COVID-19 were proving elusive. Remdesivir, baricitinib, carmofur, and dexamethasone had some efficacy, but none could be described as a cure. Hydroxychloroquine, despite repeated presidential endorsement, did not work.[81] A vaccine looked likely to be found—202 were in development, twenty-four in clinical testing, and five in phase III trials,[82] with encouraging results from the Phase II trials at Moderna (mRNA-1273) and Oxford (ChAdOx1 nCoV-19)—but it would clearly be months before one was generally available, even in an optimistic scenario that would defy the recent history of vaccine development, in which new vaccines took a decade or more to develop.[83] As for tests, it was apparent by the summer of 2020 that there were limits to the reliability of most of those available: tests with high sensitivity produced false positives, while those with high specificity produced false negatives.[84] Until there was significant progress in these areas, limiting the spread of the virus would therefore depend on NPIs, such as mask wearing, sustained social distancing, widespread and regular testing, and systematic contact tracing, as well as effective quarantining of people known or suspected to be infected. Where governments and people did not grasp that, case and fatality numbers would remain elevated or, at best, would decline only slowly.

THE NETWORKED PANDEMIC

The COVID-19 pandemic crisis could be understood only through the lenses of history and network science. The former provided some sense of its potential scale and likely consequences. The latter explained why the virus spread so much farther and faster in some places and some populations than in others. Network science also explained why taking Hubei offline sent a shock wave through global supply chains. It explained why failure to contain the virus in Europe led to the extreme measure of lockdowns and why those triggered a global financial crisis. Above all, it explained why fake news about COVID-19, which spread virally through social media, encouraged inconsistent and often counterproductive behavior by so many people.

As we have seen (chapter 4), standard epidemiological models tend to omit network topology, assuming that any individual can come into contact with any other individual and that all individuals have a similar number of contacts. Such a homogeneous society does not exist. In the theoretical world of a randomly networked population, such models may suffice. But in a population with a scale-free network topology, as Albert-László Barabási has written, "the hubs are the first to be infected, as through the many links they have, they are very likely to be in contact with an infected node. Once a hub becomes infected, it 'broadcasts' the disease to the rest of the network, turning into a super-spreader. . . . This implies a faster spread of the pathogen than predicted by the traditional epidemic models."[85] Standard immunization strategies and herd immunity models break down in such cases.[86] Broadly speaking, social networks can be characterized in terms of their frailty (heterogeneity in susceptibility, exposure, or mortality) and interference (the extent to which connectivity can be reduced in the event of contagion). A pandemic exposes frailty and incentivizes interference.[87] Successful, targeted responses that take account of the population's heterogeneity therefore ought to be able to contain a pandemic with a much lower overall rate of infection than implied by standard notions of herd immunity.[88]

The history of COVID-19 was like a case study designed to illustrate the insights of Barabási and his collaborators. The virus spread at the speed of a jet plane through the scale-free network of international passenger airports, expedited by the unprecedented volume of journeys in December 2019 and January 2020, more than double the level of fifteen years before.[89] How far it spread on board the planes themselves did not much matter.[90] All that mattered in the first phase of the pandemic was effective (not geographic) distance from Wuhan. Between December 1, 2019, and January 23, 2020, forty-six direct flights flew from Wuhan to Europe (Paris, London, Rome, and Moscow) and nineteen to the United States (either New York or San Francisco). The flights were largely full, according to VariFlight; unfortunately, January is a peak month for Chinese air travel.[91] Data from FlightStats also showed a China Southern flight landed at San Francisco International Airport on February 1, though that turned out to have flown directly from Guangzhou.[92] Other flights that appeared to leave Wuhan for Asian destinations after the twenty-third proved to be empty apart from crew.[93] As we have seen, the January 23 quarantine of Wuhan slowed the spread of the virus only slightly in China; the effect may have been larger abroad.[94] But because international flights continued to depart from other Chinese airports, the virus continued to spread. President Trump's ban on Chinese passengers entering the United States that was announced on January 31 came too late and was too full of holes (U.S. citizens and permanent residents were exempt) to be effective.[95] In the first half of 2020, most countries closed their borders to foreign travelers entirely, and the remainder did so partially.[96] Never have so many stable doors been shut after the horses had bolted.

The United States was effectively much closer to Wuhan than a map of the world suggested. But other countries were closer. According to one network analysis, it was the fifth most likely country to import COVID-19 from China, after Thailand, Japan, Taiwan, and South Korea. Another ranked Cambodia, Malaysia, and Canada as more at risk than the United States.[97] To explain why all these countries suffered fewer COVID-19 cases and deaths than the United States in relative terms, we need to understand the next part of the contagion network. National, regional, and local transport networks are also a vital part of the story, because they are what most passengers use when they arrive at an airport. Buses were virus spreaders: one woman infected twenty-three people on a two-way trip.[98] Subways in London and New York (especially the Flushing local line) were, too.[99]

Beyond public transit, what other contexts furthered spread? Homes, obviously, where a single carrier was very likely to infect other family members.[100] For health outcomes, the extent of generational cohabitation was important: that may explain northern Italy's bad experience relative to Sweden's.[101] Apartment blocks with communal elevators were also hot spots: one woman who returned to China from abroad infected a total of seventy people simply by using the elevator.[102] Children might be less likely to catch the virus than adults, and children with the virus might not have symptoms, but (as a Berlin study showed) they could still spread it. Schools were therefore the next obvious hub in the COVID-19 network.[103] They could remain open only with elaborate and strictly enforced precautions, as in Taiwan.[104] A single outbreak at a Jerusalem school blotted Israel's initially outstanding record of pandemic containment.[105] Colleges were even more likely to spread the virus, because students come from farther afield and often live in crowded residence halls. (Few things were easier to predict in 2020 than that the return of students to campuses would trigger a new wave of contagion.) Even more crowded dormitories for migrant laborers were otherwise impeccable Singapore's downfall.[106] Restaurants, too, favored the contagion. One individual infected nine other people at three tables in a Korean diner.[107] Karaoke bars were best avoided.[108] More than two fifths of the employees on one floor of a Korean office building tested positive.[109] And, as in previous coronavirus epidemics, hospitals were themselves a major source of infection, though they lagged some way behind cruise ships, prisons, food-processing plants, and weddings in the ranking of superspreader locations.[110] No institutions, however, were more fatal in the plague year 2020 than eldercare homes.

The word "genocide"—meaning the murder of a tribe or people—was coined in 1944 by Raphael Lemkin, a Polish Jewish refugee from Nazism, whose family was all but obliterated in the Holocaust. The word "senicide"—meaning the deliberate murder of the elderly—is less well known, though of older provenance. According to the *Oxford English Dictionary,* it was first used by the Victorian explorer Sir Henry Hamilton Johnston. Lemkin's word caught on. Not so "senicide." There are just two books on that subject on Amazon's site, and a cacophonous song called "Senicide" by a Californian heavy metal band. A few older books used the word, nearly all in connection with the alleged practices of ancient or obscure tribes (the Padaeans of India, the Votyaks of Russia, the early American Hopi, the Netsilik Inuit of Canada, South Africa's San people, and the Amazonian Bororos). But "senicide" is so rare a word that Microsoft Word's spellchecker underlines it in red, itching to autocorrect it to "suicide." All that may change when the general public grasps what happened in the first half of 2020. In the UK, nearly twenty thousand excess deaths had been recorded in care homes by May 1, the paradoxical result of fetishizing the National Health Service at the expense of institutions beyond its aegis.[111] In the United States, 45 percent of all COVID-19 deaths by mid-July had come in care homes.[112] In a disastrous blunder, New York governor Andrew Cuomo and his health commissioner, Howard Zucker, obliged nursing homes to accept, without testing, "medically stable" patients discharged from hospitals. The result was the death of about 6 percent of all the state's nursing home residents.[113] Around the world, deaths in nursing homes as a share of total COVID-19 deaths ranged from zero percent in Hong Kong and South Korea to 72 percent in New Zealand, though absolute numbers were small there. In Europe, where absolute numbers were much higher, the shares ranged from 35 percent in France (14,341) to 38 percent in England and Wales (19,700) to 50 percent in Belgium (6,213).[114]

"The ancient Sardi of Sardinia," Henry Johnston wrote in 1889, "regarded it as a sacred . . . duty for the young to kill their old relations." The nineteenth-century Russian historian Nikolai Karamzin defined "senicide" as "the right of children to murder parents overburdened by senium [old age] and illnesses, onerous to the family and useless to fellow citizens." The explorers Knud Rasmussen and Gontran de Poncins reported that senicide was still practiced by the Netsilik of King William Island as recently as the 1930s. But who foresaw senicide in the 2020s, least of all in modern, developed democracies? The answer is the Austrian-born economist Friedrich von Hayek, who predicted, in *The Constitution of Liberty* (1960), that "concentration camps for the aged unable to maintain themselves are likely to be the fate of an old generation whose income is entirely dependent on coercing the young."[115]

The locations, from stuffy buses to senicidal old folks' homes, are only part of the story of networked contagion—the stage sets, not the actors. It also

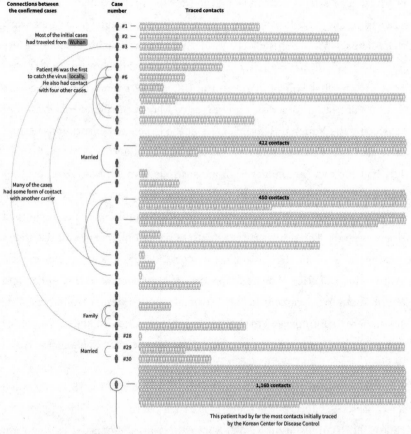

Patient 31 was a South Korean superspreader who passed COVID-19 to more than a thousand other people. In the two weeks before she tested positive, the sixty-one-year-old woman attended meetings in Seoul and Daegu. On February 6, she was involved in a minor traffic accident in Daegu and received treatment at the Saeronan Oriental Medicine Hospital. While being treated at that hospital, she attended two two-hour services at the Daegu branch of the Shincheonji Church of Jesus, on February 9 and again on February 16. Despite developing a fever, she also had lunch with a friend at the Queen Vell Hotel.

swiftly became apparent in early 2020 that, as in previous pandemics, from AIDS to SARS and MERS, a key role was being played by individual super-spreaders. The infectious disease ecologist Jamie Lloyd-Smith, who had devised the dispersion factor, k, with respect to earlier coronavirus outbreaks, was able to calculate that it was almost as low for COVID-19 as for SARS.[116] For SARS-CoV-2, k was estimated to be around 0.1, "suggesting that 80 per cent of secondary transmissions may have been caused by a small fraction of infectious individuals (~10 per cent)."[117] In Hong Kong it turned out to be nearly a perfect 20:80 Pareto ratio.[118] This meant that multiple sparks from the Wuhan bonfire were necessary—and not just one or two—to create a global pandemic. It also meant that a relatively small number of superspreaders and superspreader events were responsible for fanning the sparks into uncontrollable blazes.[119] There was the Chinese woman who flew to Munich on January 19 after a visit from her Wuhan-based parents and gave the virus to sixteen other employees of the German firm she worked for.[120] There was the Sussex businessman who caught the virus in Singapore in January and then went skiing near Mont Blanc before flying home to Gatwick in time for a pint at his local.[121] There was the gregarious patient 31 in South Korea, who unwittingly spread the virus to more than a thousand people in Daegu and Seoul, including her fellow worshippers at the Shincheonji Church of Jesus.[122] There was "Mattia," patient one in northern Italy, who went to the hospital three times when he felt ill in February but continued his social life between appointments.[123] A biotech conference at Boston Marriott Long Wharf in late February was initially believed to have led to eighty-nine COVID-19 cases.[124] A subsequent study raised that number to an estimated twenty thousand.[125] Of the sixty-one members of a choir in Skagit County, Washington, who attended a practice on March 10, fifty-three caught the virus, three were hospitalized, and two died.[126]

The critical insight of network science was that in order to prevent the spread of the new virus, existing social networks had to be to some extent broken up—especially those that promoted proximity and conversation in confined spaces—and the small world rendered somewhat larger.[127] This should have applied to the elite social links from Westchester County to Aspen to

Palm Beach.[128] It should also have applied to the tight social networks of the Latino population of Los Angeles or of the Baptist churches of the South. As we shall see, however, this insight was largely lost on policymakers and citizens in the United States. And yet it need not have been. In Taiwan, under the influence of Digital Minister Audrey Tang, a variety of online platforms were used to share information about symptoms and exposure, to ration face masks when they were scarce, and to enforce quarantines.[129] Had there been an outbreak in Taipei, officials had a plan to subdivide the city into separated neighborhoods.[130] In South Korea, the government and the private sector collaborated to ramp up testing rapidly; at the same time, a cellphone-based system of contact tracing was deployed. Under legislation passed at the time of MERS, the government had the authority to collect mobile-phone, credit-card, and other information from anyone who tested positive and use it to reconstruct their recent whereabouts. Those data, stripped of personal identifiers, were then shared on social media apps, allowing others to determine whether or not they had crossed paths with an infected person.[131] As in Taiwan, quarantines were strictly enforced. Hong Kong was somewhat different, because the initiative here passed to the pro-democracy movement, but the approach was the same: to use technology to track the contagion, and masks and quarantines to limit it.[132] Singapore's approach was similar, but it had to rely more on manual contact tracing, because its app was downloaded by too few people.[133] And it was not only Asians who adopted the right strategies. Even without such extensive (some would say intrusive) use of technology, Germany and Greece, in their different ways, showed that early detection and early action were achievable and effective.[134] If every American state had responded to early cases as effectively as Washington State did, the United States would have fared a great deal better.[135]

SOL

Who was to blame for the fact that the two biggest English-speaking countries handled the first wave of COVID-19 so much worse than their Asian and European peers? For most journalists, the answer was blindingly obvious: the two populist leaders, Boris Johnson and Donald Trump. Neither can be said to have handled the crisis ably, to put it mildly. But to turn the story of COVID-19 into a morality play—The Populists' Nemesis—is to miss the more profound systemic and societal failure that occurred, in a way that future historians will surely see as facile.

The British case is illustrative. It was not the job of the prime minister to determine whether Britain faced a deadly pandemic and, if so, what ought to be done. That responsibility lay with Chris Whitty, the government chief medical adviser; John Edmunds, of the London School of Hygiene and Tropical Medicine; and Neil Ferguson, of Imperial College London, the key epidemiological experts on the New and Emerging Respiratory Virus Threats Advisory Group (NERVTAG); and the Scientific Advisory Group for Emergencies (SAGE), which reported directly to Johnson and whichever group of ministers he chose to assemble in the Cabinet Office Briefing Rooms (COBRA). First, the experts dithered: as late as February 21, NERVTAG recommended keeping the threat level at "moderate."[136] On March 9, four days after the UK's first death, SAGE rejected the idea of a Chinese-style lockdown, as it would only lead to a "large second epidemic wave once the measures were lifted." It seems clear that the experts were thinking of the virus as a new strain of influenza. On Friday, March 13, Chief Scientific Adviser Sir Patrick Vallance told the BBC that the government was aiming to reach herd immunity, but in a managed way, so as to avoid overwhelming the National Health Service.[137] Then the experts panicked. On March 16, Ferguson published his paper, predicting that without both "mitigation" (social distancing) and "suppression" (lockdowns)—maintained until there was a vaccine—there would be "approximately 510,000 deaths in GB and 2.2 million in the US."[138] With public apprehension mounting, and with the encouragement of Dominic Cummings, the prime minister's chief strategist, herd immunity was ditched in favor of an unprecedented shutdown of British social and economic life. Having achieved this U-turn, Ferguson then hopelessly confused matters by stating that, under the new dispensation, UK deaths in 2020 would amount to "20,000 or less, two thirds of which would have died this year from other causes" anyway (i.e., a net 6,700).[139]

Events veered between farce and tragedy in the subsequent days. Ferguson himself developed COVID-19 symptoms—and both Johnson and Health Minister Matt Hancock tested positive on March 27. Johnson was hospitalized on April 5 and moved to intensive care the next day. Ferguson was caught violating the distancing rules he himself had recommended in a romantic tryst; Cummings was also spotted on an illicit cross-country trip. Private-sector computer programmers then got hold of Ferguson's model and tore it apart.[140] The crucial point, however, was not these dramas, diverting as they were to a people confined to their homes. The point was that the failure was at the level of the public health professionals as much as at the top.[141] We seem to see here some version of Feynman's *Challenger* postmortem.

From "We have it under control. It's going to be just fine" (January) to "By April, you know, in theory, when it gets a little warmer, it miraculously goes away" (February) to "I like this stuff. I really get it. People are surprised that I understand it" (March), there is an overabundance of evidence that President Trump misread the seriousness of the crisis he faced in the early months of 2020.[142] Alternatively, he understood its seriousness as early as February 7 but chose to "play it down."[143] Nothing, therefore, is easier than to lay all the blame for the U.S. handling of COVID-19 on Trump, the "single point of failure: an irrational president."[144] Journalists have not held back from writing this story, over and over again, seldom if ever asking themselves why so many current and former officials might wish to share their thoughts so frankly with *The New York Times* and its peers.[145] Nor has there been much remorse expressed about the idiotic pieces that appeared in the *Times, The Washington Post,* and *Vox* in January and February, downplaying the threat of a pandemic and denouncing Trump's Chinese travel ban as racist.*[146] This is not to defend Trump, who made the grave and ultimately irreparable error—sagely avoided by his predecessor during the opioid epidemic—of putting himself front and center of the crisis without having the faintest understanding of it ("When

---

*On January 29, *The New York Times* warned us to "beware the pandemic panic." On January 31, *The Washington Post* urged us to "get a grippe," as "the flu" was a "much bigger threat." On January 31, *Vox* tweeted (the tweet has since been deleted), "Is this going to be a deadly pandemic? No." On February 3, the *Post's* headline was "Why We Should Be Wary of an Aggressive Government Response to Coronavirus: Harsh Measures Tend to Scapegoat Already Marginalized Populations." On February 5, the *Times* dismissed the ban on Chinese citizens flying into the U.S. as an "extreme reaction" unwarranted by evidence—a "top-down decision" that could "morph into outright racism within the general population." On February 7, *Vox* made it clear that anti-Chinese xenophobia was the thing we really needed to worry about.

somebody is the president of the United States, the authority is total and that's the way it's got to be"—April 13). Trump was generally dismissive of COVID-19 throughout January and February, was eventually persuaded to take it seriously in March ("I've felt it was a pandemic long before it was called a pandemic"—March 17), and for a brief time enjoyed an improvement in his approval rating as he gave the appearance of being in charge. Trump's popularity bump in March was short-lived, however. His daily press conferences were discontinued. His insistence that increased testing was undesirable, as if tests somehow caused the cases they revealed, was manifestly idiotic. Many voters changed their minds after March: Trump's average approval rating went from 47 percent at the end of that month to 41 percent at the end of June.[147] This was all part of a circus, in which journalists and Trump made believe that it was all about him—and still insisted it was all about him even when he followed the advice of Mark Meadows, the White House chief of staff, and handed responsibility over to the state governors. (Had he not done so, he would of course have been castigated with equal indignation.) In truth, what happened was in large measure a disastrous failure of the public health bureaucracy at the Department of Health and Human Services, and particularly at the Centers for Disease Control and Prevention, a subject much less discussed in the press.

On paper, the United States was well prepared for a pandemic. In 2006, Congress passed a Pandemic and All-Hazards Preparedness Act; in 2013 a Reauthorization Act of the same name; and in June 2019 a Pandemic and All-Hazards Preparedness and Advancing Innovation Act.[148] In October 2015, the bipartisan Blue Ribbon Study Panel on Biodefense, co-chaired by Joe Lieberman and Tom Ridge, published its first report.[149] In 2019, the Study Panel was renamed the Bipartisan Commission on Biodefense "to more accurately reflect its work and the urgency of its mission."[150] Since August 2017, Robert Kadlec, a career USAF doctor, had been assistant secretary for preparedness and response at HHS. In September 2018, the Trump administration published a thirty-six-page National Biodefense Strategy.[151] Its implementation plan included, as one of its five goals, "Assess the risks posed by research, such as with potential pandemic pathogens, where biosafety lapses could have very high consequences." As Earl "Judge" Glock of the Cicero Institute has pointed out,[152] there was a profusion of pandemic plans in the years after 2006.* Yet despite all this planning—or perhaps because of it—no one appeared quite sure who was in charge when a pandemic actually struck. It was evidently not the assistant secretary for pandemic preparedness and response, who was more or less invisible throughout the first half of 2020.† According to the CDC's founding legislation, it "has an essential role in defending against and combatting public health threats domestically and abroad," which seemed to give its director, Robert R. Redfield, considerable responsibility. But the surgeon general, Jerome M. Adams, was also invested with a similar role by Congress, though he reported to the assistant secretary for health at HHS, Brett P. Giroir. As the CDC director and the assistant secretary for health both reported to the secretary of HHS, Alex M. Azar—as did the commissioner of the Food and Drug Administration and the director of the National Institutes of Health— one might have inferred that the secretary was in overall charge. However, also in charge (at least according to its own mandate) was the Federal Emergency Management Agency (administrator: Peter T. Gaynor), who reported to the acting secretary of homeland security, Chad F. Wolf—or possibly to the acting deputy secretary—not forgetting the White House's own Coronavirus Task Force, which was led by a "response coordinator," Deborah Birx, whose day job was U.S. global AIDS coordinator. Despite all this, the public health official who was most often in the public spotlight was Anthony S. Fauci, the director of the National Institute of Allergy and Infectious Diseases.

Clearly, at least some officials had suspected that there would be trouble if a pandemic struck. On October 10, 2018, Assistant Secretary Kadlec had given a lecture at the University of Texas's Strauss Center on the evolution of

---

*He lists the following: a White House Homeland Security Council National Strategy for Pandemic Influenza, a National Strategy for Pandemic Influenza Implementation Plan, a Department of Defense Implementation Plan for Pandemic Influenza, a Department of Health and Human Services Pandemic Influenza Plan (issued in 2005, 2009, and 2017), an annual Department of Homeland Security National Response Framework, a Federal Interagency Operational Plan, a National Health Security Strategy for the United States, a White House National Security Strategy, a National Security Council Playbook for Early Response to High-Consequence Infectious Disease Threats and Biological Incidents, a United States Health Security National Action Plan, and a North American Plan for Animal and Pandemic Influenza.
†Assistant Secretary Kadlec's sole newsworthy contribution was the summary firing of Dr. Rick Bright as head of the Biomedical Advanced Research and Development Authority.

biodefense policy. "If we don't build this [an insurance policy against a pandemic]," he said, "we're gonna be 'SOL' [shit out of luck] should we ever be confronted with it." He added, "We're whistling in the dark, a little bit."[153] If a further illustration was needed for the hypothesis that U.S. public institutions (and some private ones) have suffered a great degeneration in the past two or three decades, here it was.[154]

What went wrong was therefore much more than just the president's errors of judgment. Intelligence agencies appear to have done their part, warning of the seriousness of the threat posed by the initial outbreak in Wuhan, despite the lack of American CDC representatives in China following the Trump administration's winding down of the "Predict" program (set up in 2009 with funding from the U.S. Agency for International Development as part of its Emerging Pandemic Threats initiative).[155] CDC, HHS, and the National Security Council were all aware of the threat by the first week of January. Peter Navarro, one of the president's advisers on trade, repeatedly and correctly warned of the danger of a "severe pandemic" emanating from China.[156] Other influential figures who grasped the seriousness of the situation were Deputy National Security Adviser Matt Pottinger, Senator Tom Cotton, and Representative Liz Cheney.[157] "This will be the biggest national security threat you face in your presidency," Trump's national security adviser, Robert O'Brien, told him on January 28. "This is going to be the roughest thing you face."[158] The travel bans imposed on Chinese and European visitors to the United States were too late to be effective and poorly executed, but they were directionally the right things to do.[159] Those who now say a total closure of American airspace was warranted are forgetting how much even those limited measures were condemned by much of the media.[160]

The much bigger failure was the CDC's centralization and general hampering of testing. It not only declined to use WHO testing kits but also impeded other U.S. institutions from doing their own tests and then distributed a test that did not work. Matters were not helped by the need for the federal Food and Drug Administration (FDA) to approve non-CDC tests. As late as February 28, the CDC had done a grand total of 459 tests.[161] By March 7 the number was 1,895—whereas 66,650 people were tested in South Korea within a week of that country's first case of community transmission.[162] There were also serious problems with false negative results.[163] The CDC's monitoring of travelers was equally botched. This fiasco had little, if anything, to do with the White House; nor could it credibly be blamed on a lack of resources.[164] It reflected classic bureaucratic sclerosis. "It's not our culture to intervene," a former CDC official admitted. The agency was weighed down by "indescribable, burdensome hierarchy." "Here is an agency that has been waiting its entire existence for this moment," said a former FDA official. "And then they flub it. It is very sad. That is what they were set up to do."[165]

Just as happened in Britain, in mid-March there was a flip from insouciance to panic. Trump had already declared a public health emergency under the Public Health Service Act on January 31, but on March 13 he issued two national emergency declarations, under both the Stafford Act and the National Emergencies Act, as well as invoking emergency powers via executive order under the Defense Production Act five days later. The CDC suddenly warned of "between 160 million and 214 million people" being infected. "As many as 200,000 to 1.7 million people could die," *The New York Times* reported; "2.4 million to 21 million people in the United States could require hospitalization."[166] It was only at this point that the chronic shortage of masks became an issue, as did the enormous regional variation in intensive care unit capacity.[167] So much for "pandemic preparedness." Numerous articles were written, envisioning the entire United States suffering the fate of Hubei Province or northern Italy, in defiance of the obvious differences: overall, U.S. population density is much lower, and urban population density is also much lower.*[168] Italians use public transport three times more than Americans. The correct analogy was between New York City and Wuhan or Milan. Nevertheless, the majority of U.S. states had imposed travel restrictions by late March, leading to drastic declines in traffic volumes of between around 50 and 90 percent in most major cities (according to TomTom data). Cities in counties with "shelter-in-place" orders were the hardest hit, but the steep decline in mobility hap-

---

*The population density of Wuhan is 2.6 times greater than that of San Francisco. Milan's density is 1.6 times greater than New York's—and New York is by far the most densely populated of American cities.

pened almost everywhere. Planes continued to fly, but they were empty: from March 26 to May 20, passenger volumes were below 10 percent of their level over the same period in 2019.[169]

Another policy failure has gone largely unremarked. In Asia, as we have seen, the countries that dealt most successfully with COVID-19 made use of smartphone technology to operate sophisticated systems of contact tracing. Why did this not happen in the United States, the land where the internet was born, the home of the world's biggest technology companies, with the greatest quantities of data on every aspect of their users' lives? The conventional answer—"Because Americans would never endure such a violation of their civil liberties"—is unconvincing. An entire population under varying degrees of house arrest hardly has much in the way of civil liberty. Apart from one *Washington Post* story on March 17,[170] there was no evidence until April 10 of any plan to make use of the location data and social network graphs that Google, Apple, and Facebook could easily have supplied to facilitate contact tracing.[171] Finally, there was an announcement just before Easter: "Apple and Google Partner on COVID-19 Contact Tracing Technology." A more accurate headline would have been "Apple and Google Partner to Block COVID-19 Contact Tracing Technology." For it would appear that Big Tech's lawyers saw too much potential risk in enabling digital contact tracing. Silicon Valley first argued that it needed to design a global standard, then opted to punt the problem to the state governments, which clearly lacked the competence to deliver effective systems, even if state-level solutions had made sense—which they did not in the absence of border controls between states. By early September, just six states had launched apps.[172] The only thing location data were used for was to trace the spread of COVID-19 across the country—for example, from the beaches of Florida over spring break and from New York City in the first half of March, before panic was declared.[173] America had come to a near standstill by April 11, with traffic to retail and recreation destinations down 45 percent and to workplaces down 48 percent, and with most regions sheltering in place—after the virus had spread everywhere. Once again, the travel restrictions came too late to be effective.[174]

The United States is a federal system. In 2020, as in 1918, the power to impose non-pharmaceutical interventions properly lay with states and cities, not with Washington. State governors were not reluctant to seize the opportunity this presented. But their performances were mixed, and those who received the most media coverage generally performed worst. We have already seen how numerous state governments, including New York, committed senicide in eldercare homes. Their next feat was an unseemly scramble for ventilators, which turned out to be unnecessary, as these were both plentiful in the United States and not a very effective way of saving the lives of COVID patients.[175] By May, California was claiming victory for having locked down more quickly than New York.[176] This turned out to be an illusory victory, as California case numbers rose sixfold between mid-May and late July, overtaking New York. In any case, it was in large measure vanity to claim that shelter-in-place orders were crucial. In fact, Americans all across the nation seem to have adopted social distancing before the first shelter-in-place orders were issued in California, on March 16—illustrating the importance of autonomous behavioral change by citizens, which often anticipated government orders.[177] Variations in the extent of social distancing may have had more to do with the character of individual towns and neighborhoods: those with a strong sense of local community, ironically, were less willing to practice social distancing, whereas those with high individual political engagement were more willing.[178]

There is no need to idealize the federal government of the Eisenhower era any more than one should view 1950s American society through rose-tinted spectacles (see chapter 7). It is enough simply to observe that the rise of the "administrative state" has produced pathologies every bit as harmful, and perhaps in the long run more so, than the virus SARS-CoV-2.[179] The historian Philip Zelikow was not wrong, in 2019, to be "struck (and a bit depressed) that the quality of U.S. policy engineering is actually much, much worse in recent decades than it was throughout much of the 20th century."[180] In the words of Francis Fukuyama, "The overall quality of the American government has been deteriorating steadily for more than a generation," notably since the 1970s. In the United States, "the apparently irreversible increase in the scope of government has masked a large decay in its quality."[181] One may blame this on a failure of will, as the venture capitalist Marc Andreessen does, or on the triumph of "vetocracy" or "kludgeocracy,"[182] but the problem is clearly systemic, and much more profound and harder to remedy than one president's personal shortcomings, manifest as those were.

PLANDEMIC INFODEMIC

If a population is to make good choices, good information is vital. Government officials, including the president, did a poor job of this, to say the least. But their mixed (not to say downright misleading) messages—on everything from mask wearing to potential remedies for COVID-19—were not the biggest obstacle to public understanding in 2020. Unfortunately, the failure of Congress to achieve any meaningful reform of the laws and regulations governing internet network platforms, despite the problems exposed by the 2016 election and the manifest insincerity of the Big Tech companies' attempts to reform themselves,[183] ensured that not only the United States but the world as a whole was awash with fake news about the new virus within weeks of its existence being confirmed.* "No country is safe from virus tentacles," reported an Australian website (news.com.au), with an accompanying picture purporting to show "the mobile phone and flight data of 60,000 of an estimated five million Wuhan residents who fled during the critical two weeks before the outbreak city was placed under lockdown." It was nothing of the kind, as the BBC reported on February 19, but simply a ten-year-old map of all the air routes in the world.[184] The misleading description was nevertheless reproduced on countless websites and social media accounts.

Sources of fake news were plentiful, including highly respected newspapers. *The Washington Post* had to correct a story that falsely claimed the Trump administration had shut down the CDC's Global Health Security Agenda.[185] A number of Fox anchors, particularly Sean Hannity (but not

---

*I had intended to devote two chapters to this crucial part of the story of 2020: one on the problems that had been exposed in 2016's election ("The Structural Change of the Public Sphere") and the other on the failure of legislators and regulators to achieve anything more than marginal improvements by 2020 ("What Was Not Done"). However, for reasons of space these chapters had to be cut.

Tucker Carlson), encouraged viewers to regard the threat from COVID-19 as exaggerated. This had measurable effects on behavior, leading to higher case and fatality numbers among Hannity viewers.[186] On the whole, higher Fox viewership predicted lower social distancing.[187] Yet more exotic notions than these swiftly gained credibility.

One conspiracy theory in particular was actively promoted by the Chinese government. In a series of tweets, the deputy director of the Information Department at the Chinese Ministry of Foreign Affairs, Zhao Lijian, sought to suggest that the pandemic had in fact originated in the United States. "When did patient zero begin in US?" Zhao wrote on March 12, first in English and separately in Chinese. "How many people are infected? What are the names of the hospitals? It might be US army who brought the epidemic to Wuhan. Be transparent! Make public your data! US owe us an explanation!"[188] (This appeared to be a reference to the Military World Games, which were held in Wuhan in October 2019 and in which seventeen U.S. teams participated.) Zhao's tweets went viral on China's most prominent social media platform, Weibo.[189] At around the same time, fake messages began to appear in millions of Americans' direct messaging apps, warning that Trump was about to lock down the entire country. "They will announce this as soon as they have troops in place to help prevent looters and rioters," read one such message, citing an unnamed source in the Department of Homeland Security. (Other, similar messages referred to different government departments.) "He said he got the call last night and was told to pack and be prepared for the call today with his dispatch orders." American intelligence identified the Chinese government as the source of the messages.[190] An important role in amplifying conspiracy theories, as in 2016, was played by "bots." Carnegie Mellon University researchers analyzed more than two hundred million tweets discussing COVID-19 and found that roughly half the accounts—including 62 percent of the one thousand most influential retweeters—appeared to be bots. Among tweets about "reopening America," 66 percent came from accounts that were possibly humans using bot assistants, while 34 percent came directly from bots. Of the top fifty influential retweeters, 82 percent were bots. "It looks like it's a propaganda machine, and it definitely matches the Russian and Chinese playbooks," commented Kathleen Carley, the director of the Center for Computational Analysis of Social and Organizational Systems.[191] On June 3, Twitter took down 23,750 accounts that had tweeted 348,608 times, all of which the company concluded were being run by the Chinese government.[192]

Yet Chinese information warfare, like Russian infowar in 2016, was only a small, if influential, part of the fake news network, and it is clear that most of the fake Chinese accounts had few followers. The most widely circulated snake oil was neither Chinese nor Russian. The former Sheffield professor Piers Robinson, of the Bristol-based Organisation for Propaganda Studies (OPS), posed the question "Is Coronavirus the New 9/11?" His fellow OPS director, Mark Crispin Miller, of New York University, suggested that the virus was a bioweapon. Some theories claimed that 5G masts were lowering resistance to the virus (which led to attacks on masts in the UK). Other theories touted quack remedies of varying degrees of harmlessness. According to the Iraqi cleric Muqtada al-Sadr, same-sex marriage was one of the causes of the pandemic.[193] The most common conspiracy theories, however, related to vaccines. Tim Hayward, a professor of environmental political theory at the University of Edinburgh, was among those who retweeted claims that Bill Gates had ulterior motives for prioritizing the search for a COVID-19 vaccine.[194] A version of this theory inspired the widely watched conspiracy film *Plandemic*.[195] The World Health Organization belatedly grasped that, alongside the biological pandemic, there was an "infodemic" of conspiracy theories about the pandemic. Eight of the top ten sites promoting false information ran disinformation about COVID-19, with headlines such as "STUDY: 26 Chinese Herbs Have a 'High Probability' of Preventing Coronavirus Infection" and "Why Coronavirus Is a Punishment from God."[196]

As with the real pandemic, the infodemic could not be understood apart from the network structure that spread it. New conspiracy theories are grist to the mill of established networks such as the anti-vaccination ("anti-vax") movement and the QAnon cult, both of which ran multiple groups and pages on Facebook.[197] The data company Pulsar tracked the rise and fall of twelve different conspiracy themes online—5G Towers, Made in a Lab, Garlic Remedy, Aliens, Eyes of Darkness, Russian Lions, Chinese Bioweapon, Vodka Hand

Sanitizer, Cocaine Prevents Corona, Just Like Flu, Population Control, and New World Order—and related their transmission to clusters of online influencers, notably "Anti–Deep State Trump Fans" and "Republican Patriots."[198] In this context, Facebook's decisions not to change its algorithms to suggest a wider range of Facebook groups than users would ordinarily encounter and to reduce the influence of "supersharers"—the online equivalent of superspreaders—proved highly consequential.[199] In a March survey of American voters, 10 percent of respondents characterized as "probably or definitely true" the theory that the U.S. government had created the virus; 19 percent reported believing that the CDC was exaggerating the danger posed by the virus to "hurt Trump"; and 23 percent endorsed as probably or definitely true the notion that the virus had been created by the Chinese government.[200] British polling revealed a similar readiness to believe that the coronavirus came out of a lab.[201] In a U.S. poll in mid-May, half of all those who said that Fox News was their primary television news source believed the theory that Bill Gates was planning to use a COVID-19 vaccine to implant microchips in people in order to monitor their movements.[202] Pandemic disinformation was also being directed at European societies by China, Russia, Iran, and Turkey, but their aggregate impact appeared to be smaller.[203]

On June 24, at a Florida county commissioners' workshop, a young woman argued against making masks mandatory, accusing the proponents of such a measure of being in league with the devil, 5G, Bill Gates, Hillary Clinton, "the pedophiles," and the deep state.[204] A Houston doctor named Stella Immanuel, who insisted she had cured patients of COVID-19 with hydroxychloroquine, turned out also to believe that endometriosis, cysts, infertility, and impotence were caused by sexual intercourse with "nephilim" (demons in human form) and that "alien DNA" was currently being used in medical treatments.[205] The fact that President Trump retweeted a video of Dr. Immanuel's hydroxychloroquine claim—a clip that was viewed more than thirteen million times on social media—neatly encapsulated the nature of the dual plague the world confronted in 2020.

10

==

THE ECONOMIC CONSEQUENCES
OF THE PLAGUE

We have long become overgrown with calluses; we no longer hear
people being killed.

—Yevgeny Zamyatin, "X"

THE LONG AND THE SHORT

It was shortly after his recovery from what may well have been the Spanish
flu in 1919 that John Maynard Keynes wrote the inflammatory tract that made
him famous, *The Economic Consequences of the Peace*. In it, he deplored the pu-
nitive terms of the Versailles Treaty—which imposed on Germany an unspec-
ified but potentially vast war reparations debt—and predicted an inflationary
economic disaster, followed by a political backlash.[1] Keynes's concluding prophecy was ultimately validated:

> If we aim deliberately at the impoverishment of Central Europe, ven-
> geance, I dare predict, will not limp. Nothing can then delay for very long
> that final war between the forces of Reaction and the despairing convul-
> sions of Revolution, before which the horrors of the late German war will
> fade into nothing.[2]

However, his short-term prediction that the German currency would weaken proved wrong: in the spring of 1920, it unexpectedly stabilized along with other European currencies. The stabilization did not endure, but Keynes's losses on short positions in the franc, mark, and lira came close to bankrupting him.[3]

What will be the economic consequences of the pandemic? Plainly, it belongs on the list of large economic disasters. If the International Monetary Fund (IMF) is right about U.S. gross domestic product in 2020 (in June, it forecast a decline of 8 percent, though by October its projection was a less drastic minus 4.3 percent), it will be the American economy's worst year since 1946.[4] In April, the U.S. unemployment rate reached its highest point since the Depression. Elsewhere it was even worse. In May, the Bank of England forecast the worst recession since the "Great Frost" of 1709.[5] But what more could be said, aside from the fact that output would fall and unemployment would rise in most countries? In the course of 2020, a significant number of commentators inferred from the dismal public health response of the United States, the crushing impact of lockdowns on the economy, and the unprecedented expansion of government borrowing and central bank money creation, that the end of the dollar's dominance in the world economy must be drawing nigh. Yet Keynes's experience in 1920 reminds us that there are few easy predictions in the history of exchange rates. Speaking at an online forum in early August 2020, former Treasury secretary Lawrence Summers—arguably the nearest thing to Keynes that the other Cambridge has ever produced—observed, "You cannot replace something with nothing." What other currency was preferable to the dollar as a reserve and trade currency "when Europe's a museum, Japan's a nursing home, China's a jail, and Bitcoin's an experiment"?[6]

At first, when it was a Chinese epidemic, COVID-19 seemed to pose a threat mainly to global supply chains that ran through Wuhan and its environs.[7] After Beijing regained control of the virus, the question became: How fast can China come back, and how much would recovery be held back by new outbreaks of the disease?[8] On the supply side, to judge by indicators such as energy consumption, the recovery looked decidedly like a V—the contraction in the first quarter had been the deepest since the time of Mao (with GDP shrinking 6.8 percent from the last quarter of 2019), but it was swiftly reversed. On the demand side, however, to judge by traffic and transit indicators in the major cities, it was much slower going.[9] In May, the government dropped its explicit growth target in favor of a jobs target and announced the equivalent of $500 billion in new local government infrastructure bonds, as well as continued monetary easing.[10] Yet policymakers at the People's Bank of China and regulators at the China Banking and Insurance Regulatory Commission were wary of credit growth and inflation—not so much of consumer prices as of asset prices—with the attendant risk of financial crisis.[11] The rapid recovery of the Chinese stock market was not necessarily an indication of a full-fledged macroeconomic recovery. The decision to allow street vendors to operate once again in major cities was a sign of the party leadership's deep anxiety about unemployment.

As the virus spread around the world in the early months of 2020, there was a cascade of cancellations. The number of air travelers collapsed. At Changi, Singapore's usually thronged airport, traffic plunged from 5.9 million passengers in January to a mere 25,200 in April—a 99.5 percent drop.[12] A slew of airlines declared bankruptcy. Tourism slumped.[13] Automobile sales crashed. Together, the cessation of travel, combined with still buoyant supply, caused the price of oil briefly to turn negative as costs of storage exceeded market prices. Between March 8 and March 26, restaurants ceased to operate in every region covered by the app Open Table. Dining out was still dead two months later, except in Germany and a handful of American states that had not locked down as aggressively as California and New York: Arizona, Florida, Ohio, Texas.[14] Bars were closed; cafés, too.[15] Across retail, only groceries and pharmacies continued to function at anything close to a normal level. The only growth was in online electronics and retail, as housebound consumers turned to the internet to satisfy their needs. All around the world, workers were laid off or "furloughed" at rates not seen since the early 1930s. Financial market volatility leapt to heights last recorded in the worst days of the global financial crisis of 2008–9. By March 23, the main U.S. stock market index, the S&P 500, was down 34 percent. European and British investors were hit comparably hard, though East Asian markets fared somewhat better. For a moment, even the stocks of the big technology companies were marked down, with the exception of Amazon. Bitcoin sold off, falling below $4,000 on March 12. Only gold and (at first) U.S. Treasuries seemed safe. It felt as if the Great Depression were being replayed, but what had taken a year then happened this time in just a month.

The financial panic reached its climax in the wake of the emergency announcement by the Federal Reserve, on the night of Sunday, March 15, that it was cutting interest rates and buying $700 billion of bonds. Far from reassuring investors, this triggered runs on a number of money market funds and hedge funds.[16] Wall Street stared into the abyss of mass defaults in the bond market, with the energy sector especially vulnerable.[17] As in 2008–9, there was a short-term dollar squeeze as dollar debtors around the world scrambled for cash.[18] But what concerned Fed officials most were the signs of unusual stress in the market for U.S. government bonds, supposedly the safest and most liquid in the world.[19]

For the Trump administration, it might have been possible to equivocate about a pandemic; there could be no equivocation about such a large stock market crash. (This was the kind of panic Trump had been seeking to avoid by playing down the threat posed by the virus.) Unlike the public health response, the monetary and fiscal response was swift—and on a massive scale. The Federal Reserve, by its own admission, "crossed red lines" with a plethora of programs, including unprecedented pledges to buy even junk bonds. On March 23, the Fed committed to buying as many U.S. government bonds and mortgage-backed securities as needed "to support smooth market functioning."[20] In all, fourteen new facilities were announced to lend to financial firms, foreign central banks, nonfinancial businesses, and state and local governments. Between March 11 and June 3, the Fed's balance sheet grew by 53 percent, from $4.3 trillion to $7.2 trillion.[21] Although thirteen of the fourteen facilities were of doubtful legality,[22] they had the desired effect. Financial conditions eased significantly after the spasm of mid-March.

At the same time, in the small hours of March 25, congressional leaders reached an agreement on a $2 trillion fiscal package to send checks of $1,200 to all Americans below a certain income level; expand unemployment insurance and increase state-level unemployment benefits by $600 a week for four months; provide $500 billion in aid to corporations; fund $350 billion in loans to small businesses; and give healthcare providers an additional $150 billion. This came on top of earlier legislation that had allocated $8.3 billion to vaccine development and $100 billion to paid leave.[23] Goldman Sachs projected that the federal budget deficit would be roughly $3.6 trillion (18 percent of GDP) in fiscal year 2020 and $2.4 trillion (11 percent of GDP) the following year, taking the share of the federal debt held by the public above 100 percent of GDP and the gross debt to 117 percent.[24] (In fact, nearly all the newly issued bonds in the first quarter of 2020 were bought by the Fed.)

If their sole objective was to avert a financial crisis, these measures were an immense success. Stocks rallied and by early August were back in positive territory for the year. As made intuitive sense, the stocks of the big information technology companies accounted for much of the rally: the pandemic had clearly served to accelerate multiple trends from the physical world to the virtual world. With market conditions distorted by monetary policies previously seen only in times of world war, these "growth stocks" seemed likely to retain their high multiples. On the other hand, the policy implications of what had just been done were startling. It was almost as if the pandemic had rendered two hitherto radical ideas—modern monetary theory and universal basic income—mainstream in mere months. Just how long ordinary people could be expected to endure being shut up in their homes, even if they were receiving more generous unemployment benefits than usual, was not much discussed.

President Trump's strong instinct was to return American life to normal as rapidly as possible, preferably by Easter. By the last week of March, public approval for his administration's handling of the crisis was at 94 percent with Republicans, 60 percent with independents, and even 27 percent with Democrats.[25] But Trump understood that this support would swiftly evaporate if the lockdowns persisted for too long—especially in those states not yet much affected by COVID-19, where the logic of suspending economic life seemed less than obvious. Beginning in April, sentiment began to shift away from

Trump and toward the more prominent governors and public health officials, notably Anthony Fauci.[26] The mood of mid-April was one of public anxiety: in one poll, two thirds of those surveyed said they were more worried that state governments would lift restrictions on public activity too soon, rather than too late. Nearly three quarters feared the worst was yet to come.[27] A stark partisan divide emerged: Democrats continued to worry about COVID-19; between mid-April and mid-May, Republicans stopped doing so.[28] In reality, the worst of the American epidemic's first wave was over in terms of excess mortality by the beginning of June, as we shall see. But the economic consequences of the pandemic had barely begun to make themselves felt.

SCHRÖDINGER'S VIRUS

It was at around this time that a wit coined the phrase "Schrödinger's virus," a play on the physicist Erwin Schrödinger's famous cat that (to illustrate a problem in quantum mechanics) was simultaneously alive and dead:

> We all have Schrödinger's virus now.
>
> Because we cannot get tested, we can't know if we have the virus or not.
>
> We have to act as if we have the virus so that we don't spread it to others.
>
> We have to act as if we've never had the virus because if we didn't have it, we're not immune.
>
> Therefore, we both have and don't have the virus.[29]

This was a predicament that could be endured if the alternative of uncontrolled contagion was sufficiently terrifying. Recall that in mid-March, the epidemiologists at Imperial College London had warned of up to 2.2 million dead Americans without social distancing and lockdowns. In one paper, they claimed that "in the absence of interventions, COVID-19 would have resulted in 7.0 billion infections and 40 million deaths globally this year."[30] Such counterfactuals were widely cited in the press, legitimizing the hardship of shel-

week, total mortality was 10 percent above the five-year average. In the subsequent three weeks (ending April 17), excess mortality soared tenfold to 113 percent, with nearly twelve thousand excess deaths, of which three quarters were attributed to COVID-19.[47] The rate then declined more gradually than it had risen, reaching just 7 percent in the week ending June 5, seven weeks after the peak.[48] Because of lags in data collection, the actual peak of excess mortality was likely around April 8.[49] That was also the week when the number of patients who died in hospitals in England and tested positive for COVID-19 at the time of death peaked at 5,486. By the week ending June 19, the figure was 334.[50] There is no question, then, that Britain had its worst excess mortality in five years in April and May 2020. Though London had the highest excess mortality rate of any region, the whole of the UK was affected. Around a dozen Spanish and Italian cities (e.g., Bergamo) had even higher rates than London.[51] Compared with other countries, however, the UK had the highest excess morality relative to population.[52] Yet in a longer-term perspective, going back to 1970, Britain's worst week for excess death in 2020—week 16—finishes in twenty-first place. The winters of 1969–70, 1989–90, and 1975–76 were all worse than the spring of 2020. The excess mortality rate in the first week of 1970 was a third higher than in mid-April 2020.[53]

The United States had an experience that was similar to Britain's but less severe—or perhaps it would be more accurate to say that the northeastern states had a similar experience, because the rest of America initially followed a different path. In mid-July, cumulative U.S. excess mortality was estimated at 149,200, or 23 percent above the average level in recent years. That was more or less the same as the Swedish rate.[54] Relative to population, U.S. excess mortality was between the Swiss and Austrian figures.[55] Relative to the previous four years, April–May 2020 stood out for the share of deaths attributed to pneumonia, influenza, and COVID-19.[56] Media comparisons to seasonal flu were wildly off: the number of COVID-19 deaths for the week ending April 21 was between ten and forty-four times larger than the number of influenza deaths in the peak week of the previous seven influenza seasons.[57] At its height, COVID-19 was the number-one cause of death in America.[58] Yet not all states experienced excess mortality. And not all excess mortality was attributable to COVID-19.[59] As in Europe, the global pandemic was, on closer inspection, heavily concentrated in a few regions. In Italy, it was Bergamo and its environs.[60] In Spain, excess mortality was recorded in Aragón, Castilla y León, Castilla–La Mancha, Cataluña, Extremadura, Madrid, País Vasco, Navarra, La Rioja, and Valencia, but not in Andalucía, Asturias, the Balearic Islands, the Canaries, Cantabria, Ceuta, Galicia, or Murcia.[61] In France it was Île-de-France and the far northeast that suffered most. In the United States, a third of COVID-19 deaths occurred in New York and New Jersey.[62] Excess mortality in New York City was exceptionally high. From March 11 to April 13, 2020, there were roughly 3.6 times the number of deaths that would have been expected based on the averages for the same dates between 2013 and 2017. Just under 17 percent of all excess mortality up to mid-July came in New York City, a share similar to London's in the UK total (15 percent).[63] There was similar concentration in California: 45 percent of cases and 56 percent of deaths were in Los Angeles.[64]

The U.S. COVID-19 pandemic began in the week ending March 28, peaked in the week ending April 11, when excess mortality was 36 to 41 percent above normal, and seemed close to over by the week ending June 25 (5 to 9 percent above normal). Unlike in the UK and Europe, however, excess mortality did not revert entirely to normal. From a low of 7 to 11 percent above normal in mid-June, it rose back to 20 to 25 percent above normal in late July, declining thereafter but not returning to its expected level.[65]

The impatience of many Americans, especially Republican voters in predominantly "red" states with few COVID-19 cases, was understandable. Even if their sources of information had been the best possible, uncertainty would have reigned. How many people had the virus? Early estimates ranged widely. Eleven studies suggested, variously, that asymptomatic carriers could be between 18 and 86 percent of all infected people. On the basis of serological tests, which of course varied in their accuracy, estimates of the total percentages infected ranged from 0.33 percent in Austria to 5 percent in Spain to 36 percent in a Boston homeless shelter to 73 percent in an Ohio jail.[66] In New York, 26 percent of people tested positive in early July; in the Corona neighborhood of Queens it was 68 percent.[67] Estimates of the all-important infection fatality rate were similarly dispersed. A California study suggested 0.12 to 2.0 percent.[68] European figures ranged from 0.05 percent (Iceland) to 1.18 percent (Spain), with almost everything in between.[69] A UK study published in August suggested 0.3 percent or 0.49 percent.[70] Surveys arrived at unhelpfully wide ranges, such as 0.02 to 0.78 percent.[71] By mid-2020, some kind of consensus had formed around 0.53 to 0.82 percent.[72] But it was clear that the variance in IFRs between age groups was huge, with those over sixty-five ten times more at risk than the average, and workers in healthcare also much more vulnerable (because severity of sickness correlates with the scale of viral load, which is generally a function of exposure).[73] Even if Americans had not been under a bombardment of fake news about the COVID-19 "plandemic," they could have been forgiven for thinking the lockdowns were overkill and that by July 4, if not Memorial Day (May 25), it was time to get back to normal life.

THE DUMB REOPENING

Were the lockdowns a mistake? In April, a number of people tried to show that the timing of lockdowns had been crucial to limiting the extent of contagion.[74] This correlation evaporated on closer scrutiny.[75] Researchers at Oxford University's Blavatnik School of Government showed that there was in fact no relationship whatever between the stringency of government measures and the extent to which the disease was contained.[76] "While Germany had milder restrictions than Italy," as one commentator noted in May, "it has been much more successful in containing the virus." Taiwan had the lowest stringency and the least contagion. The statistically significant relationship was between stringency and the extent of economic collapse.[77] A growing body of research offered an alternative interpretation. Containment of the contagion was a function of social distancing in all its forms.[78] This did not need to be mandated, though it generally was more effective when it was. If social distancing was done effectively, lockdowns were more or less superfluous. School closures and bans on public meetings sufficed. This seemed to be the lesson learned in Singapore[79] and even in China.[80] The most comprehensive study to date of government measures suggested that mandated social distancing* was a far more effective policy than closing businesses and making everyone work from home, including all those who patently could not.[81] Other measures that should have been more widely adopted would have focused on isolating the elderly and otherwise vulnerable populations.[82] The most effective measures, however, were those that quarantined superspreaders and banned superspreader events. A lockdown was far too indiscriminate a response to a virus with as low a dispersion factor as that of SARS-CoV-2.[83]

Beginning in mid- to late April, countries such as Austria, Denmark, Germany, Norway, and Switzerland began phased, partial reopenings of stores and schools, followed later by cafés and restaurants.[84] By mid-June, mobility data suggested that traffic was back to normal in Berlin, Geneva, Milan, Paris, and Stockholm (which had never locked down).[85] By the summer, Germany was running largely as usual.[86] There were significant jumps in case numbers in Spain, as well as in a number of East European countries, but on the whole European reopening was going reasonably well as the summer holidays drew to a close. Case numbers reflected positive tests, not illnesses, and there was no sign of excess mortality. In Britain, by contrast, the end of excess mortality was not followed by a return to normal. Mobility remained exceptionally depressed: around 25 percent below its pre-pandemic level at the end of July. Neither government nor people seemed to have the confidence to return

---

*The study in question covers a multitude of measures under the umbrella "other social distancing": "[1] *Isolate certain populations:* recommend or mandate the isolation of populations such as the elderly, immunocompromised or those who have recently returned from a cruise. [2] *If outside the home, [people] must abide by social distancing standards:* require a six foot minimum distance from others outside the home, maintain distance when riding public transportation, ask that businesses restrict the number of people within storefront at a time, as well as restricting certain types of activities that involve physical interaction with customers (e.g., bagging groceries, taking cash payment). [3] *Mandate mask wearing:* require people to wear a mask outside the home. [4] *Close public facilities:* close libraries, museums, flea markets, historic sites, memorials, and polling locations. [5] *Close outdoor facilities:* close beaches, state parks, public parks, public toilets, lakes, and campgrounds. [6] *Social distance restriction of visitation to certain facilities:* restrict visitation to prisons, long term care facilities, child care facilities, and homeless shelters, stop elective medical and veterinary procedures, and bar short term rental accommodations. [7] *Suspend non-critical state operations/government services:* close government buildings, stop in person meetings of people working for the state, suspend court operations, waive or extend licensing, and permit certain types of work to be carried out remotely, [which] normally could not (e.g., notaries, police work, licensing)." Some of these restrictions were themselves superfluous. Closures of beaches and parks ceased to make sense as it became clear that nearly all transmission of the virus occurred indoors.

to anything resembling business as usual.[87] New restrictions on social gatherings had to be imposed in September.

In the United States, it was a different story. There, even in April, a rising share of voters were ready to get back to work "right now"—especially Republicans and especially people aged forty-five to sixty-three. (Younger people, less at risk, were paradoxically more reluctant to return to normal.)[88] This was also the president's strong inclination, as we have seen. However, whereas Europeans undertook a qualified reopening during the summer, maintaining social distancing norms and in some places increasing mask wearing, the American approach was to race back recklessly to the old normal. Social distancing had largely stopped in most of America by mid-June. Mobility picked up as Americans—especially Republicans—took to the roads again.[89] But the country returned to normality on a state-by-state basis, with governors and mayors relaxing restrictions as they saw fit. All this was done without the advisable prerequisites of more widespread and rapid testing[90] and an effective system of contact tracing (except perhaps in Massachusetts).[91] As the tech executive Tomas Pueyo pointed out in a vivid phrase, the rational strategy for governments against COVID-19 could be characterized as "the Hammer and the Dance."[92] What the United States was attempting was whack-a-mole with a blindfold on. Nothing was easier to predict than that this would lead to second waves in many states that had seen improvement, and ongoing first waves in most of the rest. That was what happened in June and July, especially in the South (notably Georgia, Florida, and Texas) and the West (Arizona), where summer temperatures meant that dining, shopping, and socializing took place indoors with air-conditioning.[93] The economist John Cochrane's prediction of a "dumb reopening" was fulfilled.[94] Cochrane was also right that when the numbers of cases, hospitalizations, and deaths jumped upward, people's behavior would adapt again. Research bore his hypothesis out. It was adaptive behavior, not government orders, that determined the trajectory of the American contagion.[95] This meant that by early August the numbers of new cases and hospitalizations flattened out and then fell again. But it also meant that a return to complete economic normality grew less and less likely.

It was frequently asserted by economists in the first half of 2020 that natural disasters tend to cause relatively short, if sharp, economic crises. The argument was therefore made that economies should experience rapid V-shaped recoveries after the COVID-19 pandemic was over—like a seaside town that shuts for the winter and then reopens at the end of May.[96] That might have been true of those countries where, by the summer of 2020, new-case numbers had dropped to very low levels. But it did not apply to a country such as the United States, where the pandemic was still ongoing and a dumb reopening had been partially aborted. The IMF, the Organization for Economic Cooperation and Development, and the World Bank were all more circumspect, recognizing the risks of a second wave.[97] Some academic economists were even more pessimistic, predicting a long, deep recession driven by uncertainty—a "Frankenstein recession," combining the size of the Great Depression, the speed of Hurricane Katrina, and the labor reallocation costs of World War II.[98] As the economists debated, with increasing absurdity, whether the recovery would be V-shaped, W-shaped, K-shaped, "Nike swoosh"–shaped, or inverse-square-root-shaped, my suggestion in early April was that it would be shaped more like a giant tortoise: as output came down off the shell, it plummeted to the base of the tortoise's neck, then climbed upward, leveling off on its head, some distance below its starting point atop the shell. Wall Street had been bailed out (again), but Fed policies were doing little to help small businesses—which were working at half to three-quarters capacity by the second week of May—and even the Paycheck Protection Program (forgivable loans for small businesses to stop them from laying off workers) seemed to have helped rather a lot of quite large firms.[99]

The best-known economists struggled to make sense of it all. For the arch-liberal Paul Krugman, the lockdown was "the economic equivalent of a medically induced coma," but the Keynesian remedy of government borrowing would provide the necessary relief and stimulus. "There may be a slight hangover from this borrowing," he wrote on April 1, "but it shouldn't pose any major problems."[100] By contrast, Kenneth Rogoff—no Keynesian on fiscal questions—wrote of an "economic catastrophe . . . likely to rival or exceed that of any recession in the last 150 years," with lingering effects, potentially leading to a "global depression." The pandemic, Rogoff argued, was akin to an "alien invasion."[101] The grisly metaphor favored by Lawrence Summers was that "physical isolation is chemotherapy and the goal is remission. The problem is that chemo is . . . increasingly toxic over time." He foresaw an "accordion-like dynamic" until a vaccine was generally available.[102] John Cochrane, the sharpest commentator of the Chicago School, saw a "big *shift* in demand . . . from the carefree economy to the permanently social distanced economy" and "a negative permanent technology shock."[103]

All of these speculations would have benefited from some economic history. A pandemic is not like a hurricane (or, for that matter, winter on Cape Cod), because its duration is highly uncertain. COVID-19 could fizzle out, like SARS and MERS, if humanity modifies its behavior intelligently, or it could be with us for years, like AIDS, killing many more people than we currently can imagine. The key economic point was that a relatively rapid supply-side recovery might be possible—China had already made that clear—but getting consumer demand to revive in the face of a continued but nebulous public health risk would be much harder.[104] The marginal propensity to consume (the key concept in Keynes's *General Theory,* a book more cited than read) had been hit hard by the pandemic and its associated surge in uncertainty and insecurity. In 1957–58, in the face of a comparably dangerous pandemic, Americans had taken excess mortality on the chin as a cost of doing business. That was not what happened in 2020. True, unemployment did not hit the Depression-era rate nearly every economist had predicted but pulled back to 13 percent in May, 11 percent in June, 10 percent in July, and 8 percent in August. But the personal savings rate soared during the lockdown, when people could not spend, and it remained elevated in June, at 19 percent, three times its average over the previous nineteen years and more than double its average since 1959.[105] Many people certainly wanted to rush back to normality in June.[106] But the second wave of cases in the Sun Belt, along with "reclosing" or "pausing" measures in more than twenty states,[107] choked off the consumer recovery. Based on the mid-April-to-mid-June trend in Google mobility data, it had seemed in June as if retail and recreation trips would return to their baseline by July 10. By the end of July, that steep path back to the good old days had flattened into a plateau between 10 and 20 percent below the baseline. Transportation Security Administration checkpoint passenger numbers were stuck at a quarter of their normal level.[108] Foot traffic was still 25 to 50 percent below normal in Washington, D.C., Miami, Seattle, Los Angeles, Boston, New York, and San Francisco.[109] Even driving was still down 10 to 16 percent in San Francisco.[110] As of August 3, small business revenue was slipping back to 17 percent below its January level; consumer spending was flatlining at 6 percent below its January level, with wealthy households retrenching the most.[111] Having briefly returned to normal, electricity consumption fell back to 4 percent below its pre-pandemic level.[112]

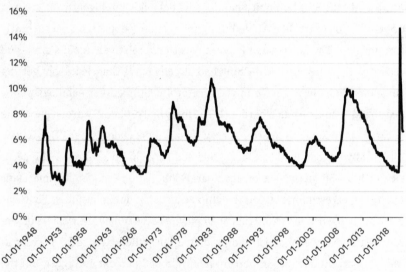

The U.S. unemployment rate (seasonally adjusted) since 1948.

Meanwhile, the most counterintuitive stock market rally of modern times continued, seemingly oblivious to the ongoing pandemic and the failure of the dumb reopening, effacing all the losses sustained during March's panic attack. How to account for this? The obvious explanation was that swift and expansive fiscal and monetary relief measures had successfully mitigated the worst economic effects of the lockdowns, supporting U.S. firms and households with tens of millions of checks. Yet as this strange summer wore on, unease began to grow. If COVID-19 declined to go away simply because many Americans were tired of it, how long could government money prop up the economy, when around a third of the job losses resulted from small businesses closing down?[113] Would the bitter partisan enmities of Congress stand in the way of the fiscal bailouts many states and municipalities needed to avoid mass layoffs of government workers?[114] How should the Treasury manage its much enlarged debt: with short-term borrowing or nineteenth-century-style perpetual bonds?[115] Had the Federal Reserve implicitly lost its independence, returning to a pre-1951 state of debt servitude?[116] Was it secular stagnation we had to fear or a return of inflation?[117] True, in the short run the pandemic was deflationary.[118] But explosively rapid monetary growth—one measure of the U.S. monetary aggregate M3 was growing at 23 percent a year in June—must at some future date have consequences.[119] World trade was down 12 percent, foreign direct investment down even further.[120] If all restraint on monetary and fiscal policy had been cast aside under a Republican administration, what was to prevent a weakening of the dollar[121] similar to that which had begun in the late 1960s, when Keynesian policies on a far more modest scale ran out of control in the face of twin crises—the slide to defeat in Vietnam and the crisis in urban America that the "Great Society" welfare programs failed to resolve? Was the stock market in a delusional bubble inflated by neophyte day traders like Dave Portnoy?*[122]

THE GREAT EXPIATION

As with almost everything in U.S. politics, except perhaps China, COVID-19 became a partisan issue. Among Democrats, concern about "a coronavirus outbreak in your local area" remained high (80 percent more people concerned than unconcerned, according to the online polling company Civiqs). Among Republicans, it had vanished by August (net 31 percent unconcerned). Independents were in the middle (net 25 percent concerned).[123] On balance, by

---

*Portnoy had two rules for making money in stock markets. Rule one was that "stocks only go up," as he frequently reminded his 1.5 million Twitter followers. Rule two: "When in doubt whether to buy or sell see Rule One."

July, Americans other than die-hard pro-Trump Republicans had changed their minds: far from handling the pandemic well, as they had believed in April, Trump had screwed it up. Polls, as well as prediction markets, clearly pointed to a Joe Biden victory on November 3.[124] Both the impact of the pandemic and the impact of the recession made it seem increasingly hard for Trump to win in the crucial "big three" states that had delivered the White House to him in 2016: Michigan, Pennsylvania, and Wisconsin. Other states that seemed to be in play included Arizona, Florida, Georgia, Iowa, North Carolina, Ohio, and Texas. It seemed likely that, if Biden won the White House, the Democrats would also win control of the Senate. Given the prospect of a Democratic sweep and the growing influence of the progressive left over the party, it also seemed reasonable to anticipate higher corporate tax rates in 2021. Moreover, as we have seen, the COVID-19 crisis had led to the unwitting normalization by Republicans of more radical policies such as universal basic income and modern monetary theory. A "blue wave" would therefore mean further fiscal stimulus for the economy.

However, an important lesson of 2016 had been to be wary of polls as a basis for predictions about U.S. presidential elections. It remained to be seen whether or not Trump's campaign team could damage Biden's credibility as a potential president—the classic strategy for winning a second term since Bill Clinton beat Bob Dole in 1996—by deploying the social-media dark arts that had been unknown in those days. What was beyond doubt was that Trump was far ahead of his rival in spending on Facebook advertising.[125] It was also significant that, unlike Jack Dorsey at Twitter, Mark Zuckerberg continued to resist the pressure to intervene editorially in political ads, despite intense pressure from inside and outside Facebook (including a frontal attack from the Biden campaign).[126] And no matter how invisible his campaign kept Biden in the summer of 2020, voters' concerns about his age and mental fitness persisted.[127]

The key problem for the Trump campaign was simple: a pandemic—especially if it is exacerbated by economic lockdowns that trigger a recession—hurts a great many people in a host of ways. Some of those affected would never even consider voting Republican, but 2020's experiences might make them more likely to turn out to vote Democratic. This could be especially true of black voters, whose lower turnout had been one of the biggest differences between 2012 and 2016. Conversely, some of the voters hit hardest by the pandemic and the recession were lifelong conservatives, but 2020's experiences might make them less likely to turn out to vote Republican—especially if they were seniors confronted with a new COVID-19 wave around election time.

Disaster can bring people together, increasing altruistic behavior, and there is some evidence that this happened in 2020.[128] But the American pandemic had struck a highly unequal society; its effect, as it became commonplace to observe, was to exacerbate the inequality.[129] Early in the crisis, when it seemed that only the rich could get COVID-19 tests, Trump was asked to comment. He expressed disapproval but added, "Perhaps that's been the story of life."[130] The lockdown was like a pressure cooker. Crime went down—as did road accidents—but domestic violence went up.[131] Excess mortality was due not just to COVID-19 but to above-normal deaths from diabetes and heart disease, probably because people were avoiding hospitals and surgeries.[132] As in China, mental health problems and substance abuse habits got worse.[133] Suspected drug overdoses jumped by 18 percent in March, 29 percent in April, and 42 percent in May.[134] As in England, mortality rates in poor areas (such as the Bronx) were roughly double what they were in rich ones (such as Manhattan).[135] Economic policy was most successful at reflating financial asset prices, disproportionately owned by the wealthy. It did little to help those with no savings.[136] It was not just that black Americans were disproportionately vulnerable to COVID-19. They were also harder hit economically: the prepandemic convergence of the black and white unemployment rates abruptly reversed itself.[137] Young people were also harder hit economically than older ones.[138] Women were more likely to lose their jobs than men.[139]

Something had to give. At 8:00 p.m. on Monday, May 25, a black man named George Floyd entered Cup Foods in Minneapolis, Minnesota. A store clerk alleged that he had paid for cigarettes with a counterfeit $20 bill and called the police. Derek Chauvin, a white police officer who may have known Floyd from security work at a local club, knelt down on Floyd's neck behind a police vehicle outside the store. For eight minutes and forty-six seconds,

Chauvin pressed his knee into Floyd's neck in silence as his captive gasped repeatedly that he could not breathe. Bystanders pleaded for Chauvin to desist, but—as cellphone video showed—he continued to kneel on Floyd for another two minutes and fifty-three seconds after he had ceased to struggle. Floyd was pronounced dead at 9:25 p.m. Four nights of mayhem in Minneapolis ensued.[140] Chauvin's killing of Floyd appeared the perfect illustration of the claim by the Black Lives Matter movement that American police disproportionately used lethal violence against black people because of systemic racism. What followed was a new contagion, of a sort that should now be familiar to the reader. From May 26 to June 28, between fifteen and twenty-six million people participated in demonstrations in support of Black Lives Matter. The protests peaked on June 6, when half a million people turned out in nearly 550 locations across the country. Of the 315 largest U.S. cities, only thirty-four did not see a protest. Two fifths of all counties saw at least some form of demonstration. The scale of the protests at their peak was less than the three to five million who had turned out for the January 21, 2017, Women's March, but the 2020 protests were much more prolonged; indeed, they were said to exceed in size every public demonstration since the birth of the republic.[141] Unlike the Women's March, however, these protests were hastily organized and often unruly. In around half of the cities where protesters marched, violence was reported.[142] Another study insisted that just 7 percent of the protests were violent, though in Oregon (principally Portland) the proportion rose from 17 to 42 percent after federal forces were deployed.[143]

Attorney General Bill Barr blamed much of the trouble on "anarchic and . . . far-left extremist groups, using Antifa-like tactics."[144] There was some evidence to support this, but on the whole the protests resembled similar mass movements around the world the year before—from Hong Kong to Beirut to Santiago—that were essentially acephalous. "If you were to ask anyone who is leading these marches, I'd be surprised if anyone could tell you," said Eric Adams, the Brooklyn borough president and a former police captain.[145] The other key feature of the protests was that in a number of cities there were abject collapses of authority. On the night of May 28, Minneapolis mayor Jacob Frey ordered the city's Third Police Precinct evacuated. The building was promptly set ablaze. On May 29, Minnesota governor Tim Walz explained that he was not mobilizing the National Guard, to avoid appearing "oppressive." New York mayor Bill de Blasio called on police to use a "light touch" in response to violence and vandalism by protesters.[146] Pledges by mayors such as Eric Garcetti, of Los Angeles, to reduce police budgets (a response to the protesters' call to "defund the police") did nothing to bolster the morale of beleaguered officers.[147] Parts of Portland descended into anarchy.

Whoever enforces the law of unintended consequences is mischievous. Many feared that to hold mass rallies amid a pandemic would spread the virus further. It did not, because overall social distancing went up during the protests as most people shut themselves up indoors, especially where violence was reported.[148] What did spread was crime. In Minneapolis, 111 people were shot in the four weeks after the death of George Floyd. New York City recorded 125 shootings in the first three weeks of June, double the number in the same period in 2019. In Chicago, more than 100 people were shot in a single weekend, the worst since 2012.[149] There was some reason to believe that the protests and the crime wave might help Trump politically, as violent protest had helped Richard Nixon in 1968,[150] by moving the national topic of conversation from pandemic unpreparedness to Trump's preferred political terrain: the culture war. Only 38 percent of people in a June 2–3 poll said they disapproved of the protests, but three quarters said they disapproved of the property destruction.[151] To be sure, support for Black Lives Matter surged in 2020, especially among young people.[152] Yet there was reason to be skeptical about such polling. Public criticism of BLM (the organization, not the proposition) was a career-endangering activity as "cancel culture" spread out from academia to corporate America. When Tucker Carlson inveighed against BLM, some companies withdrew advertising from his show. But his ratings soared.[153]

The protests of June 2020 produced some strange scenes, reminiscent in some ways of the religious acts of expiation that occurred in Europe in the heyday of the bubonic plague. In a ritual in Cary, North Carolina, on June 8, several white police officers washed the feet of pastors Faith and Soboma Wokoma, of the Legacy Center Church, after a "unity walk" from the city center to the police station—a "multiracial, multiethnic, multicultural response" to the death of Floyd.[154] A young white man with an English accent knelt and intoned through a megaphone, "On behalf of all white people . . . all of our white race . . . We stand here, Lord, confessing repentance. . . . Lord, I ask for your forgiveness for putting in our hearts such hatred that we would perpetrate slavery, Lord, that we would perpetrate injustice, that we would perpetrate prejudice, even to this very day, even in our legal system, can I ask for your forgiveness?" In Bethesda, protesters knelt on the pavement with upraised arms, chanting their renunciation of white privilege and all its works.[155] On a similar occasion, white protesters knelt down before black people and prayed for forgiveness (a gesture that was reciprocated).[156] On another, BLM activists denounced white protesters for engaging in self-flagellation (or at least painting whip stripes on their backs).[157] In a surreal encounter in Washington, D.C., a young white female protester got into an argument with a group of white and black cops, to whom she set out to explain the meaning of systemic racism. "America has a sin problem," responded one of the black officers. "The world has a sin problem, ma'am. Okay? Jesus said, 'I am the way, the truth, and the light. No one comes to the Father except through me.' America and the world have a sin problem. That's where racism, injustice, and hate and anger and violence come from. It's not about racism. Read the Bible. Read the Bible. Read the Bible, that's real."[158] The Great Awokening had met its match.

In addition to these religious manifestations, there was a wave of iconoclasm. Like the Protestants in the sixteenth century, like the Taiping in the nineteenth, like the Bolsheviks and the Maoists in the twentieth, the protesters tore down or vandalized statues. Most were of slaveholders and Confederate generals: John Breckenridge Castleman, in Louisville, Kentucky; Robert E. Lee, in Montgomery, Alabama; Raphael Semmes, in Mobile, Alabama; and Edward Carmack in Nashville, Tennessee. But that was not enough. Christopher Columbus must also be removed from sight, and Juan de Oñate in Albuquerque, New Mexico, and George Washington in Portland, Oregon. Ulysses Grant was not spared, nor Theodore Roosevelt in New York, nor even the Emancipation Memorial of Lincoln, in Washington's Lincoln Park.[159] There were similar imitative bouts of iconoclasm in England, unconsciously echoing a radical tradition going back to the sixteenth century.[160] And as in past revolutions, children took to denouncing their parents. As Pavlik Morozov informed on his father in Soviet Gerasimovka, so American teenagers took to social media to accuse their parents of racism.[161] Even adults descended to this level. One economist unleashed the Twitter mob against another for daring to express skepticism about Black Lives Matter.[162] The lesson of history is that biological and political contagions often coincide. As we have seen, the Russian Civil War ran more or less in tandem with the Spanish flu of 1918–19, not to mention rampant typhus. A similar phenomenon of twin contagions threatened to arise in early July 2020.

For many ordinary Americans, all this was odious. In a Rasmussen poll, 56 percent of all voters said the government should criminally prosecute those who had damaged or destroyed historical monuments. And 73 percent agreed that "together we are part of one of the greatest stories ever told—the story of America . . . the epic tale of a great nation whose people have risked everything for what they know is right"—words from a Trump speech.[163] Revealed preferences in one area, at least, told a very different story from the headline polls on the presidential race. Background-check statistics pointed to a surge of gun purchases in 2020. Small Arms Analytics and Forecasting put total firearms sales in June 2020 at 2.4 million units, 145 percent higher than in June 2019. Most were handguns.[164] Gun ownership had been a very accurate predictor of Trump votes in 2016.[165] Not surprisingly, all this new weaponry was also associated with higher gun violence and gun accidents.[166]

Finally, a nagging anxiety in early August 2020 was that the ultimate result of the election three months hence might end up being similar to that of 2000—too close to call on election night, but this time with the results in multiple states being called into question—or 1876, when the Senate and the House could not agree on which candidate had won, a scenario not necessarily ruled out by the Electoral Count Act of 1887.[167] Republicans, led by the president, were already casting aspersions on votes cast by mail, an issue on which public opinion was divided—along, of course, partisan lines.[168] Democrats countered with allegations of deliberate voter suppression in red states. The ingredients seemed to be in place for a result that lacked legitimacy, which, if there was still a problem of urban disorder—to say nothing of a new wave of COVID-19, perhaps coinciding with seasonal influenza[169]—was a less than cheering prospect, if not quite the prelude to Civil War II feared by some.

GUESS NOT

Swayed by epidemiological models, and against President Trump's initial instincts, the United States belatedly went down the European (though not the Swedish) road of suppression of COVID-19 through not just social distancing but also economic lockdowns. These measures certainly limited the percentage of the population that became infected and perhaps prevented some American hospitals from being overwhelmed, as Lombardy's had been. However, the economic shock of sustained lockdowns was enormous. A more rational strategy would have been to keep that share of the working population employed that could not work from home while mandating social distancing, enforcing mask wearing, and isolating older and vulnerable people. Returning to work without any of those precautions—and with a system of testing, contact tracing, and isolating that was wholly ineffective—made an ongoing first wave or a significant second wave inevitable. By early August, however, those second waves seemed to be cresting. By the end of the month, the period of excess mortality appeared to be coming to an end. If there was no further wave in the fall, if one or more vaccines came through their Phase III trials, if the economy caught up with the stock market, then Trump would claim the credit for having averted the disaster feared by the epidemiologists at a tolerable cost. The question was whether he would be believed—or simply blamed for the economic hardships and the chaos of the protests. As Henry Kissinger long ago pointed out, leaders are rarely rewarded for avoided disasters, and more often blamed for the painful prophylactic remedies they recommended. Trump's political future seemed clear in August: defeat in November. In September and October, events did not go his way: a third wave of COVID-19 cases swept the country, the Midwest especially; no vaccine could be approved before the election; and the stock market briefly sagged despite very strong third-quarter growth. Yet conventional political analysis, wedded to the methodologies of a bygone era, still tended to understate the ongoing role of online disinformation, domestic and foreign—and that may help explain why the 2020 election result proved to be much closer than polls had predicted. Even after the election, it was still unclear what would become of the escalating cold war between the United States and China—a confrontation that Trump had persuaded a significant proportion of Americans was necessary. As we shall see in the next and final chapter, this superpower conflict was another reason why some commentators in 2020 foresaw a decline and fall of the U.S. dollar. However, they were forgetting the hard lessons the foreign exchange market once taught John Maynard Keynes.

He may have been the most influential economist of the twentieth century, but Keynes was a remarkably mediocre forex trader. Not only did he nearly bankrupt himself in 1920; he made a similar miscalculation twelve years later. Having shorted the dollar more or less unprofitably between October 1932 and February 1933, he closed his position on March 2, 1933—just eight days before the suspension of the U.S. dollar's gold convertibility. By the year-end, the dollar had depreciated 50 percent relative to the pound. Keynes ruefully concluded, "Exchange rates are now dominated by guesses."[170] And what the fourth quarter of 2020 would bring—medically, economically, and politically—was indeed anybody's guess.

11

THE THREE-BODY PROBLEM

To derive a basic picture of cosmic sociology . . . you need two other important concepts: chains of suspicion and the technological explosion.

—Liu Cixin, *The Dark Forest*

THE FOOTHILLS OF A COLD WAR

In Liu Cixin's extraordinary science fiction novel *The Three-Body Problem,* China recklessly creates, then ingeniously solves, an existential threat to humanity. During the chaos of Mao's Cultural Revolution, Ye Wenjie, an astrophysicist, discovers the possibility of amplifying radio waves by bouncing them off the sun and in this way beams a message to the universe. When, years later, she receives a response from the highly unstable and authoritarian planet Trisolaris, it takes the form of a stark warning not to send further messages. Deeply disillusioned with humanity, she does so anyway, betraying the location of Earth to the Trisolarans, who are seeking a new planet because their own is subject to the chaotic gravitational forces exerted by three suns (hence the book's title). So misanthropic that she welcomes an alien invasion, Ye cofounds the Earth-Trisolaris Organization as a kind of fifth column, in partnership with a radical American environmentalist. Yet their conspiracy to help the Trisolarans conquer Earth and eradicate mankind is ingeniously foiled by the dynamic duo of Wang Miao, a nanotechnology professor, and Shi Qiang, a coarse but canny Beijing cop.[1]

The nonfictional threat to humanity we confronted in 2020 was not, of course, an alien invasion. The coronavirus SARS-CoV-2 did not come from outer space, though it shared with the Trisolarans an impulse to colonize us. The fact, however, is that the first case of COVID-19—the disease the virus causes—was in China, just as the first messages to Trisolaris were sent from China. Rather as in *The Three-Body Problem*, China caused this disaster—first by covering up how dangerous the new virus SARS-CoV-2 was, then by delaying the measures that might have prevented its worldwide spread. But then— again as in Liu Cixin's novel—China sought to claim the credit for saving the world from the disaster it had started by liberally exporting testing kits, face masks, and ventilators to afflicted countries, and promising to do the same with any successful vaccine. Not only that, but the deputy director of the Chinese Foreign Affairs Ministry's Information Department went so far as to endorse a conspiracy theory that the coronavirus had originated in the United States (see chapter 9).

It was already obvious in early 2019 that a new cold war—between the United States and China—had begun.[2] What had started out in early 2018 as a trade war—a tit for tat over tariffs while the two sides argued about the American trade deficit and Chinese intellectual property piracy—by the end of that year had metamorphosed into a technology war over the global dominance of the Chinese company Huawei in 5G network telecommunications; an ideological confrontation in response to the Chinese Communist Party's (CCP's) treatment of the Uighur minority in the Xinjiang region and the pro-democracy protesters in Hong Kong; and an escalation of old frictions over Taiwan and the South China Sea. In November 2019, Henry Kissinger himself—the master builder of Sino-American "coevolution" since 1971— acknowledged the new reality when I interviewed him at the Bloomberg New Economy Forum in Beijing. "We are," he said, "in the foothills of a cold war."[3]

The COVID-19 pandemic merely intensified Cold War II, at the same time revealing its existence to those who previously doubted it was happening. Chinese scholars such as Yao Yang, a professor at the China Center for Economic

Research and dean of the National School of Development at Peking University, now openly discussed it.[4] Proponents of the era of U.S.-China "engagement" after 1971 now wrote engagement's obituary, ruefully conceding (in Orville Schell's words) that it had foundered "because of the CCP's deep ambivalence about the way engaging in a truly meaningful way might lead to demands for more reform and change and its ultimate demise."[5] A growing number of Western observers of China now accepted the Australian John Garnaut's argument that Xi Jinping was in fact the doctrinaire Marxist-Leninist heir of Stalin and Mao.[6] Critics of engagement were eager to dance on its grave, urging that the People's Republic be economically "quarantined," its role in global supply chains drastically reduced. To quote Daniel Blumenthal and Nick Eberstadt, "The maglev from 'Cultural Revolution' to 'Chinese Dream' does not make stops at Locke Junction or Tocqueville Town, and it has no connections to Planet Davos."[7] Moves in the direction of economic quarantine began in the spring of 2020. The European Union Chamber of Commerce in China said that more than half its member companies were considering moving supply chains out of China. Japan earmarked ¥240 billion ($2.3 billion) to help manufacturers leave China. "People are worried about our supply chains," Prime Minister Shinzo Abe said in April. "We should try to relocate high added value items to Japan. And for everything else, we should diversify to countries like those in ASEAN," the Association of Southeast Asian Nations.[8] In the words of Republican senator Josh Hawley of Missouri, "The international order as we have known it for thirty years is breaking. Now imperialist China seeks to remake the world in its own image, and to bend the global economy to its own will. . . . We must recognize that the economic system designed by Western policymakers at the end of the Cold War does not serve our purposes in this new era."[9] In early May, his state's attorney general filed a lawsuit in a federal court that sought to hold Beijing responsible for the coronavirus outbreak.[10]

To be sure, many voices were raised to argue against a second cold war. Yao Yang urged China to take a more conciliatory line toward Washington, acknowledging what had gone wrong in Wuhan in December and January and eschewing nationalistic "wolf warrior" diplomacy. A similar argument for reconciliation to avoid the "Thucydides Trap" (of war between a rising and an incumbent power) was made by the economists Yu Yongding and Kevin Gallagher.[11] Eminent architects of the strategy of engagement, notably Henry Paulson and Robert Zoellick, argued eloquently for its resurrection.[12] Wall Street remained as addicted as ever to the financial symbiosis that Moritz Schularick and I had christened "Chimerica" in 2007,[13] and Beijing's efforts to attract big U.S. financial firms such as American Express, Mastercard, J.P. Morgan, Goldman Sachs, and BlackRock into the Chinese market proceeded apace.[14] Nevertheless, the political trend by mid-2020 was quite clearly in the other direction. In the United States, public sentiment toward China had become markedly more hawkish since 2017, especially among older voters.[15] By 2020 there were few subjects about which there was a genuine bipartisan consensus in the United States. China was about the only one. On the eve of Cold War II, 51 percent of Republicans and 47 percent of Democrats had an unfavorable view of China. By July 2020, those shares had risen to, respectively, 83 and 68 percent.[16]

It was therefore to state the obvious that this new cold war would be the biggest challenge to world order, whoever was sworn in as president of the United

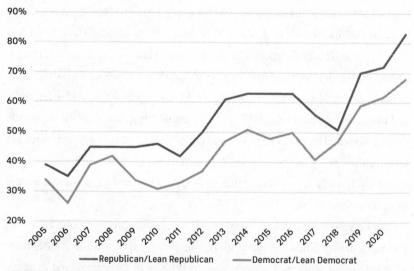

The one bipartisan issue. Percentages of Republicans and Democrats who say they have an "unfavorable" opinion of China. Most recent poll conducted June 16–July 14, 2020.

States in January 2021, for most of that person's term in office. Armed with John Bolton's new memoir—which revealed President Donald Trump to be privately a good deal more conciliatory toward his Chinese counterpart, Xi Jinping, than he had been in public—Joe Biden's campaign could claim that their man would be tougher on China than Trump.[17] According to the Beijing-controlled *Global Times,* Chinese netizens had taken to mocking the American president as Chuan Jianguo, or "Build-up-the-country Trump"—a kind of parody Manchurian Candidate.[18] By contrast, the language of some potential cabinet-level appointees in a Biden administration was so tough in 2020 as to be indistinguishable in places from that of the increasingly belligerent secretary of state Mike Pompeo. A *Foreign Affairs* article by Michèle Flournoy featured fighting words that might equally well have been spoken by the late senator John McCain.[19] Indeed, they echoed the arguments made by McCain's former aide, Christian Brose, in his book *The Kill Chain*.[20]

Commentators (and there are many) who doubted the capacity of the United States to reinvigorate and reassert itself implied, or stated explicitly, that this was a cold war the Communist power could win. "Superpowers expect others to follow them," the former Singaporean diplomat Kishore Mahbubani told *Der Spiegel* in April 2020. "The United States has that expectation, and China will too, as it continues to get stronger."[21] In an interview with *The Economist,* he went further: "History has turned a corner. The era of Western domination is ending."[22] This view had long had its supporters among left-leaning or Sinophile Western intellectuals, such as Martin Jacques[23] and Daniel Bell.[24] The COVID-19 crisis made it more mainstream. Yes, the argument ran, the fatal virus might have originated in Wuhan; nevertheless, after an initially disastrous sequence of events, the Chinese government had brought its own epidemic under control with remarkable speed, illustrating the strengths of the "China model."[25]

By contrast, the U.S. had badly bungled its pandemic response. "America is first in the world in deaths, first in the world in infections and we stand out as an emblem of global incompetence," the distinguished diplomat William Burns told the *Financial Times* in May 2020. "The damage to America's influence and reputation will be very hard to undo."[26] The editor in chief at

Bloomberg, John Micklethwait, and his coauthor, Adrian Wooldridge, wrote in a similar vein in April.[27] "If the 21st century turns out to be an Asian century as the 20th was an American one," argued Lawrence Summers in May, "the pandemic may well be remembered as the turning point."[28] Nathalie Tocci, an adviser to the European Union's high representative (foreign minister), likened the 2020 coronavirus crisis to the 1956 Suez crisis.[29] The American journalist and historian Anne Applebaum lamented, "There is no American leadership in the world. . . . The outline of a very different, post-American, post-coronavirus world is already taking shape. . . . A vacuum has opened up, and the Chinese regime is leading the race to fill it."[30] The Princeton historian Harold James went so far as to draw an analogy between Trump's America and the twilight of the Soviet Union.[31] The Canadian anthropologist Wade Davis wrote of the "unraveling" of "a failed state, ruled by a dysfunctional and incompetent government." "The hinge of history," he concluded, "opened to the Asian century."[32] Those who took the other side of this argument—notably the columnist Gideon Rachman and the political scientist Joseph Nye—were in a distinct minority.[33] Even Richard Haass, who insisted that "the

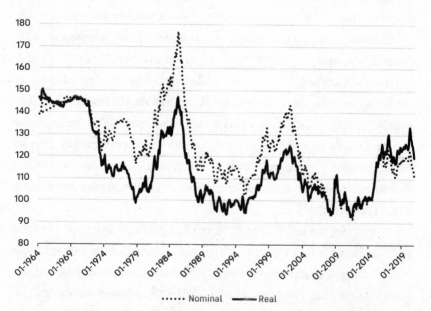

U.S. dollar, nominal and real trade-weighted effective exchange rate since 1964.

world following the pandemic is unlikely to be radically different from the one that preceded it," foresaw a dispiriting future of "waning American leadership, faltering global cooperation, great-power discord."[34] Meanwhile, those who believed in historical cycles, such as the investor turned financial historian Ray Dalio, were already sounding the death knell of a dollar-dominated world economy.[35] Peter Turchin had made a similar argument on the basis of "structural demographic theory," predicting in 2012 that the year 2020 would be "the next instability peak [of violence] in the United States."[36] Who, under the circumstances of 2020, could blame the playwright David Mamet for being haunted by Cassandra's prophecies?[37] Yet again, it seemed, we were doomed.

As Kissinger argued in an April essay, the pandemic would "forever alter the world order. . . . The world will never be the same after the coronavirus." But how exactly would the international system change? One possible answer was that COVID-19 had reminded many countries of the benefits of self-reliance. In Kissinger's words:

> Nations cohere and flourish on the belief that their institutions can foresee calamity, arrest its impact and restore stability. When the Covid-19 pandemic is over, many countries' institutions will be perceived as having failed. Whether this judgment is objectively fair is irrelevant.[38]

Not everyone shared Daniel Bell's ecstatic assessment of the performance of the Chinese Communist Party. True, COVID-19 was not likely to be Xi Jinping's Chernobyl. Unlike its Soviet counterpart in 1986, the Chinese Communist Party had the ability to weather the storm of a disaster and to restart the industrial core of its economy. Yet by mid-2020 there was no plausible way that Xi could meet his cherished goal of a 2020 gross domestic product in China that would be double that of 2010: the pandemic necessitated the abandonment of the growth target that was necessary to achieve that. Nor did Xi look politically unassailable. A second major disaster—the collapse of the Three Gorges Dam when the summer floods were at their height, for example— would have posed a major threat to his and perhaps even CCP's position: it would have seemed as if the Mandate of Heaven had been withdrawn. It was a naive assumption that China would be the principal geopolitical beneficiary of the pandemic.

However, the United States hardly seemed likely to emerge from the pandemic with its global primacy intact. It was not just that Trump had bungled his response to the crisis, though he certainly had. Much more troubling was the realization that the parts of the federal government that were primarily responsible for handling such a crisis had also bungled it. As we have seen, this was not for lack of legislation or pandemic preparedness plans. As a consequence, the United States had fallen back on the 1918–19 playbook of pandemic pluralism—states did their own thing; in some states a lot of people died—but combined with the 2009–10 playbook of financial crisis management. The dumb reopening ensued, followed by an equally predictable slowing of the economic recovery. As this debacle played out, I sometimes felt I was watching all my earlier visions of the endgame of American empire—in the trilogy *Colossus* (2004), *Civilization* (2011), and *The Great Degeneration* (2012)—but speeded up.

A CATALOG OF CATASTROPHES

To each administration comes the disaster it is least prepared for, and most deserves. That, in any event, is one way of thinking about American history since the end of the Cold War.

Bill Clinton was elected in 1992 precisely because the forty-year contest with the Soviet Union had ended the year before. With every expectation of a "peace dividend," the public no longer had need of George H. W. Bush's exceptional experience in war, diplomacy, and intelligence. Bush had fought in World War II as a Navy pilot, narrowly avoiding death when his Grumman Avenger was shot down over Chichijima, north of Iwo Jima.[39] By contrast, Clinton had done his utmost to avoid being drafted during the Vietnam War. He had participated in protests against the war while a Rhodes Scholar at Oxford. Back in the United States, he had unsuccessfully sought to join the National Guard or the Air Force and had applied to join the Reserve Officers' Training Corps (ROTC) program at the University of Arkansas purely to avoid being sent to Vietnam. A philanderer, a saxophonist, a voracious consumer of chicken enchiladas, Clinton seemed ideally qualified to lead the baby boomers into an eight-year-long party. History handed him the breakup of Yugoslavia and the Rwandan genocide.

Clinton's administration intervened to end the war in Bosnia and Herzegovina only after years of procrastination and did nothing whatever to prevent mass slaughter in Rwanda.[40] When the issue of Bosnia was raised during the 1992 presidential campaign, Clinton argued that American troops should not be sent "into a quagmire that is essentially a civil war"—shorthand for "another Vietnam." His defense secretary, William Cohen, unwittingly gave a green light to Serbian attacks on Goražde when he declared that the United States would not enter the war to avert its fall.[41] Only with the greatest difficulty did Tony Lake, Richard Holbrooke, and increasingly negative press convince Clinton that the United States could stop the war with a modest military effort.[42] By that time, nearly 100,000 people had been killed and 2.2 million displaced.[43] In the case of Rwanda, the Clinton administration's attitude was determined, once again, by the fear of American casualties. The decision to send a risibly small force of two hundred U.S. troops to the Kigali airport in 1994 was based on the repulsive calculation that (as an American military officer told the head of the UN peacekeeping mission) "one American casualty is worth about 85,000 Rwandan dead."[44] Between half a million and a million people died in Rwanda between April and July 1994, most of them ethnic Tutsis murdered by their Hutu countrymen.

George W. Bush had campaigned in 2000 to reduce American commitments overseas. Then, in the first year of a presidency he had won only by a hair's breadth, came 9/11—an event prophesied by Richard Clarke, among others. In 1992, Clarke had been appointed by Bush's father to chair the Counterterrorism Security Group and sit on the National Security Council. Bill Clinton had kept Clarke and even promoted him to national coordinator for security, infrastructure protection, and counterterrorism. Despite repeated efforts, however, Clarke could not persuade the senior members of Bush's national security team to prioritize the threat posed by Osama bin Laden and al-Qaeda. "Al Qaeda plans major acts of terrorism against the U.S.," he told a meeting of deputy secretaries in April 2001. "It plans to overthrow Islamic governments and set up a radical multination Caliphate." Paul Wolfowitz was dismissive. Clarke would later argue that Wolfowitz and his boss, Defense Secretary Donald Rumsfeld, had already made up their minds to intervene in Iraq, and 9/11 merely furnished the pretext.[45] In the immediate aftermath of the attacks on New York and Washington, the Bush administration embarked on an ambitious strategy not merely to penalize the Afghan government for sheltering bin Laden—action that Al Gore might also have taken, had he been elected president—but also to reshape the "Greater Middle East" by overthrowing Saddam Hussein, the Iraqi dictator. Typical of the new mindset was a briefing given in November 2001 by CIA director George Tenet, Vice President Dick Cheney, and National Security Adviser Condoleezza Rice on the subject of al-Qaeda's potential access to Pakistani nuclear weapons expertise. Cheney observed that the United States had to confront a new type of threat, a "low-probability, high-impact event," and therefore, if there was "a 1% chance that Pakistani scientists are helping al-Qaeda build or develop a nuclear weapon, we have to treat it as a certainty in terms of our response. It's not about our analysis. . . . It's about our response."[46] Allied to this "one percent doctrine" was a neocolonial hubris on the part of some administration officials. As the journalist Ron Suskind reported, an unnamed Bush adviser told him that

> guys like me were "in what we call the reality-based community," which he defined as people who "believe that solutions emerge from your judicious study of discernible reality." I nodded and murmured something about enlightenment principles and empiricism. He cut me off. "That's not the way the world really works anymore," he continued. "We're an empire now, and when we act, we create our own reality. And while you're studying that reality—judiciously, as you will—we'll act again, creating other new realities, which you can study too, and that's how things will sort out. We're history's actors . . . and you, all of you, will be left to just study what we do."[47]

This was not the way most ordinary Americans thought, much as they thirsted to see bin Laden and his confederates brought to justice. "I think we're trying to run the business of the world too much," a Kansas farmer told the British author Timothy Garton Ash in 2003, "like the Romans used to."[48] To assuage such feelings of unease, President Bush declared on April 13, 2004, "We're not an imperial power. . . . We're a liberating power."[49] Secretary of Defense Rumsfeld echoed this. "We don't take our forces and go around the world and try to take other people's real estate or other people's resources, their oil," he told Al Jazeera. "That's just not what the United States does. We never have, and we never will. That's not how democracies behave."[50] Very few people outside the United States believed a word of such assurances.

The costs to Americans of the "global war on terror" were low by the standards of their country's Cold War conflicts. In "Operation Iraqi Freedom" (2003–10), 3,490 U.S. service personnel were killed in action and 31,994 wounded. A further 59 were killed in the Middle East in the subsequent operations "New Dawn" and "Inherent Resolve." In Afghanistan, the casualties were 1,847 killed in action and 20,149 wounded, plus another 66 killed and 571 wounded since the end of 2014, when "Operation Enduring Freedom" formally ended and "Operation Freedom's Sentinel" began.[51] (These figures should be compared with those for the Korean and Vietnam wars, which together left 81,110 U.S. personnel dead from combat and 245,437 wounded.) It is not easy to argue today that these interventions were hugely successful, however, even if the counterfactuals of nonintervention are hard to imagine, much less compute. Certainly, if the goal was to remake Iraq and Afghanistan as prosperous democracies, aligned diplomatically with the United States, the outcomes fell far short. The human costs for those on the receiving end of these policies, by contrast, were much higher than were foreseen. According to Iraq Body Count, the total number of violent deaths since the U.S. invasion was 288,000, of whom between 185,000 and 208,000 were civilians.[52] The Afghan death toll has been estimated at 157,000, including 43,000 civilians.[53] The total financial cost of these wars to the United States has been estimated at around $6.4 trillion.[54] Yet the "one percent doctrine" turned out to apply only to external threats. The Bush administration was caught flat-footed by Hurricane Katrina in August 2005 and entirely failed to anticipate the financial crisis that was already detectable in late 2006 but erupted into a full-blown run on the banking system with the bankruptcy of Lehman Brothers in September 2008. Strategic and financial risk management appeared to exist in two completely separate domains.[55]

At a press briefing on February 12, 2002, Rumsfeld was asked a question about the administration's central and almost certainly erroneous allegation that there were ties between Saddam Hussein and al-Qaeda. The exchange was revealing:

JOURNALIST: In regard to Iraq weapons of mass destruction and terrorists, is there any evidence to indicate that Iraq has attempted to or is willing to supply terrorists with weapons of mass destruction? Because there are reports that there is no evidence of a direct link between Baghdad and some of these terrorist organizations.

RUMSFELD: Reports that say that something hasn't happened are always interesting to me, because as we know, there are known knowns; there are things we know we know. We also know there are known unknowns; that is to say we know there are some things we do not know. But there are also unknown unknowns—the ones we don't know we don't know. And if one looks throughout the history of our country and other free countries, it is the latter category that tend to be the difficult ones.[56]

The idea of unknown unknowns can be traced back to a 1955 paper by the psychologists Joseph Luft and Harrington Ingham.[57] Rumsfeld himself attributed it to NASA administrator William Graham, with whom he had worked in the 1990s on the congressional Commission to Assess the Ballistic Missile Threat to the United States.[58] As we saw in chapter 8, NASA managers had good reason to be concerned about unknown unknowns. But they, like Rumsfeld, might have devoted more attention to the "unknown knowns"—perfectly obvious dangers (such as the risk of an O-ring failing or an insurgency in post-Saddam Iraq) that decision makers unconsciously ignore because they do not accord with their preconceptions. Just over a year later, with Saddam gone and Iraq already descending into anarchy, Rumsfeld faced the press again. Looting in Baghdad, Rumsfeld explained, was a result of "pent-up feelings" that would soon subside. "Freedom's untidy, and free people are free to make mistakes and commit crimes and do bad things," Rumsfeld said. "Stuff happens."[59]

With Bush's approval down to 25 percent by October 2008, the freshman senator Barack Obama—who had opposed the Iraq invasion—comfortably defeated a Republican nominee best known for his belligerent temperament. (John McCain did not help himself when he told an antiwar activist at a New Hampshire town hall meeting that the U.S. military could stay in Iraq for "maybe a hundred years" and that "would be fine with me."[60]) Yet it was easier said than done to extricate America from the Middle East. In August 2011, as revolution swept the Arab world, Obama told the Syrian dictator Bashar al-Assad to "step aside." However, the president declined to will the means by arming the Free Syrian Army. The most he would do, in 2012, was to approve CIA training of ten thousand rebel fighters, who proved ineffectual at best. Between July 2012 and August 2013, the White House said that if Assad used chemical weapons he would be deemed to have "crossed a red line." Chemical weapons were used anyway, but on August 30, 2013—after consulting only Denis McDonough, his chief of staff—Obama decided to call off the planned air strikes, to the dismay of his national security team. He then allowed the Russian government to broker a deal under which Assad handed over (some of) his chemical weapons. In an address to the nation on September 10, 2013, Obama announced that the United States was no longer the "world's policeman."[61] Less than a year later, the terrorist group Islamic State (ISIS)—which had emerged from the ashes of al-Qaeda in Iraq after Obama withdrew U.S. forces—decapitated James Foley and other Western hostages, leading Obama to authorize joint air strikes with the Gulf states against ISIS in Syria. In September 2015, after a Russian proposal for joint action was rejected by Obama, President Vladimir Putin sent not only three dozen aircraft but also fifteen hundred troops to Latakia and warships to the Caspian Sea.

It was at around this time that the White House came up with the crude slogan "Don't do stupid shit." (According to Ben Rhodes, Obama's deputy national security adviser for strategic communication, "The questions we were asking in the White House were 'Who exactly is in the stupid-shit caucus? Who is pro–stupid shit?'") Letting Putin into the Syrian conflict was referred to by Rhodes and others as the "Tom Sawyer approach"—meaning that "if Putin wanted to expend his regime's resources by painting the fence in Syria, the U.S. should let him."[62] The consequences, as the Syrian Civil War dragged on, were a death toll of more than 500,000, nearly half of them civilians;[63] around 13.4 million forcibly displaced people, 6.6 million of them now outside Syria;[64] and a flood of two to three million refugees and migrants—not only Syrians but people from all over the Muslim world who seized the moment—pouring into Europe. The escalation of the conflict also had grave strategic consequences, not the least of which was the return of Russia to the region as a major player for the first time since the early 1970s. In short, the consequences of American nonintervention in Syria were, in many ways, as bad as the consequences of American intervention in Iraq, though far fewer American lives and dollars were expended.[65]

There was rich irony here. In one of their preelection debates in 2012, Obama had taunted the Republican candidate Mitt Romney: "The 1980s are now calling to ask for their foreign policy back because the Cold War's been over for twenty years." The allusion was to Romney's description of Russia as "our number one geopolitical foe."[66] A year after his second inaugural, in January 2014, Obama complacently told the editor of *The New Yorker,* "I don't really even need George Kennan right now,"[67] an allusion to the architect of the Cold War strategy of "containing" Soviet expansion. Before the following month was over, Russian troops had occupied Crimea, the annexation of which followed on March 18. Fighting over Donetsk and Luhansk, where Russian-backed separatists seized control of a significant amount of Ukrainian territory, continues to this day.

Yet the biggest disaster of the Obama presidency was not foreign but domestic. Though regarded by conservatives as a left-leaning Democrat at the time of his election, Obama presided over a profound socioeconomic crisis that stemmed partly from the financial mess he had inherited and partly from longer-term trends. Measures intended to stimulate economic recovery, notably the Federal Reserve's program of "quantitative easing," indirectly benefited owners of financial assets. The share of total net worth held by the top 1 percent of Americans rose from 26 percent in the first quarter of 2009 to 32 percent in the last quarter of 2016.[68] Meanwhile, middle- and lower-class white Americans experienced not only economic stagnation but an epidemic of what the Princeton economists Anne Case and Angus Deaton called "deaths of despair," principally drug overdoses, alcohol poisonings, and suicides, as well as marked increases in disability, pain, and insecurity. According to Case and Deaton, had the white mortality rate "continued to fall at its previous (1979–1998) rate of decline of 1.8% per year, 488,500 deaths would have been avoided in the period 1999–2013."[69] Three waves of opioid overdoses (first of prescription opioids, then of heroin, and then of synthetic opioids such as fentanyl) produced a surge of deaths during the Obama presidency, more than doubling the opioid-related death rate from 6.4 per 100,000 in 2008 to 13.3 in 2016.[70] More than 365,000 Americans died of drug overdoses between 2009 and 2016. Each year saw more deaths than the year before. The most affected age groups were those between twenty-five and fifty-four, for whom the overdose rates in 2016 were between 34 and 35 per 100,000, which meant that the total of life years lost approached that of the 1918–19 influenza pandemic.[71] It was rarely pointed out that a major source of synthetic opioids and fentanyl precursors was China.[72]

Though the media assigned almost no blame to Obama for his administration's failure to deal with the opioid epidemic, such social trends did much to explain Donald J. Trump's success as a populist outsider in 2016, first in winning the Republican nomination, then in defeating Hillary Clinton to win the presidency itself. His argument that Middle America had experienced "carnage" resonated with many voters, especially key voters in midwestern swing states such as Michigan and Wisconsin; his skill was to use old populist tropes to channel popular resentment not against bankers—the preferred target of the populists of the left—but against China (globalization), Mexico (immigration), and Clinton herself, the personification of a wealthy liberal elite, disconnected from the concerns of "real people," sneeringly dismissing half of Trump's supporters as a "basket of deplorables . . . racist, sexist, homophobic, xenophobic, Islamaphobic—you name it."[73] Obama's many admirers in the bureaucratic, academic, and corporate elites were appalled by Trump's election. The most obvious manifestations of elite horror were protests such as the 2017 Women's March, in which—according to one sample—more than half the participants had a graduate as well as a bachelor's degree.[74]

More subtle was the steady stream of briefings against Trump by Obama appointees. John MacWilliams, a former investment banker turned Department of Energy risk officer under Obama, warned Michael Lewis of five risks: a "broken arrow" (a lost or damaged nuclear missile or bomb), North Korean and Iranian nuclear aggression, an attack on the electrical power grid, and a "fifth risk": a decay of government program management. The fifth risk, Lewis explained, was "the risk a society runs when it falls into the habit of responding to long-term risks with short-term solutions. . . . 'Program management' is the existential threat that you never really even imagine as a risk. . . . It is the innovation that never occurs and the knowledge that is never created, because you have ceased to lay the groundwork for it. It is what you never learned that might have saved you."[75] It was, in short, Rumsfeld's unknown unknown. But does this really explain what went wrong in 2020, when COVID-19 struck? Only if one has a somewhat ingenuous view of the way government works. For if any administration should have been ready for a threat made in China that could best be met by tight border controls, it was the anti-China, pro-borders Trump administration. The "Wuhan flu" should have been the ideal disaster for a populist president.

Commentators for whom life is wonderfully simple have, without hesitation, blamed Trump for the excess mortality in 2020 due to COVID-19. No doubt the buck of responsibility stopped with him, as with every president. Without question, Trump made matters worse. He downplayed the risk. He touted quack remedies. He made bad appointments. He disparaged masks. He tweeted downright lies. He campaigned with a callous disregard for the health of those around him. These sins of omission and commission far outweighed the things his administration got right, notably "Operation Warp

Speed." Yet arguing that Trump could have *averted* the public health disaster is rather like saying that Bill Clinton could have prevented the dismemberment of Bosnia or the Rwandan genocide. It is like claiming that Bush could have saved New Orleans from Hurricane Katrina or avoided the 2008 financial crisis, or that Obama had the power to avert or end quickly the Syrian Civil War—or the capacity to save hundreds of thousands of Americans from opioid overdoses. All these arguments are versions of Tolstoy's Napoleonic fallacy that do a violence to the complexity of political disaster by imagining the U.S. president as an omnipotent executive, rather than an individual perched atop a bureaucratic hierarchy that would appear to have become steadily worse at managing disasters over a period of several decades.

THE RETURN OF NONALIGNMENT

The truth is that the pandemic exposed the weaknesses of all the big players on the world stage: not only the United States but also China and, for that matter, the European Union.[76] This should not have surprised us. As we have seen, plagues are generally bad for big empires, especially those with porous frontiers (witness the reigns of the Roman emperors Marcus Aurelius and Justinian). City-states and small nation-states are better positioned to limit contagion. The key point is that there are diseconomies of scale when a new pathogen is on the loose. Yet Taiwan, South Korea, Singapore, New Zealand, and (initially) Israel—among the smaller states to handle the pandemic competently—could never be more than the modern equivalent of city-states; great-power status was beyond their grasp. The question remained: Who would gain from this demonstration that, in a real crisis, small is beautiful? China's increasingly omniscient surveillance state might seem to have proved its superiority over decreasingly competent American democracy when it came to pandemic containment. On the other hand, the fate of Hong Kong was hardly an alluring advertisement for integration into the Chinese imperial panopticon. Moreover, the centrifugal forces unleashed by the pandemic posed, at least in theory, a more profound threat to a monolithic one-party state than to a federal system that was already in need of some decentralization.

As Kissinger observed, "No country . . . can in a purely national effort overcome the virus. . . . The pandemic has prompted an anachronism, a revival of the walled city in an age when prosperity depends on global trade and movement of people." Ultimately, Taiwan could not prosper in isolation; no more could South Korea. "Addressing the necessities of the moment," Kissinger wrote, "must ultimately be coupled with a global collaborative vision and program. . . . Drawing lessons from the development of the Marshall Plan and the Manhattan Project, the U.S. is obliged to undertake a major effort . . . [to] safeguard the principles of the liberal world order."[77] This seemed to many like wishful thinking. The reputation of the Trump administration had sunk to rock bottom in the eyes of most scholars of international relations long before COVID-19. The president was seen as a wrecking ball, taking wild swings at the very institutions on which global stability supposedly depended, notably the World Trade Organization and, most recently, the World Health Organization, to say nothing of the Joint Comprehensive Plan of Action on Iran's nuclear program and the Paris Agreement on climate change. Yet reasonable questions could be asked about the efficacy of all of these institutions and agreements with respect to the Trump administration's core strategy of engaging in "strategic competition" with China.[78] If the administration was judged by its actions in relation to its objectives, rather than by presidential tweets in relation to some largely mythical liberal international order, a rather different picture emerged.[79] In four distinct areas, the Trump administration had achieved, or stood a chance of achieving, at least some success in its competition with China.

The first was financial. For many years, China had toyed with the idea of making its currency convertible. This had proved to be impossible because of the pent-up demand of China's wealth owners for assets outside China. More recently, Beijing had sought to increase its financial influence through large-scale lending to developing countries, some of it (though not all) through its One Belt One Road initiative. The crisis unleashed by the COVID-19 pandemic presented the United States with an opportunity to reassert its financial leadership of the world. In response to the severe global liquidity crisis in March, the Federal Reserve opened two channels—swap lines and a new repo facility for foreign and international monetary authorities (FIMA)—through which other central banks could access dollars. The first already applied to Europe, the UK, Canada, Japan, and Switzerland and was extended to nine more countries, including Brazil, Mexico, and South Korea. At its peak, the amount of swaps outstanding was $449 billion.[80] In addition, the new repo facility made dollars available on a short-term basis to 170 foreign central banks. At the same time, the International Monetary Fund—an international institution the Trump administration showed no inclination to undermine—dealt with a spate of requests for assistance from about a hundred countries, canceling six months of debt payments due from twenty-five low-income countries such as Afghanistan, Haiti, Rwanda, and Yemen, while the G20 countries agreed to freeze the bilateral debts of seventy-six poorer developing countries.[81] As international creditors braced themselves for a succession of defaults, reschedulings, or restructurings by countries such as Argentina, Ecuador, Lebanon, Rwanda, and Zambia, the United States was in a much stronger position than China. Since 2013, total announced lending by Chinese financial institutions to One Belt One Road projects amounted to $461 billion, making China the single biggest creditor to emerging markets.[82] The lack of transparency that characterized these loans—the failure to publish their terms and conditions—had for some time aroused the suspicions of Western scholars, notably Carmen Reinhart, now chief economist at the World Bank.[83]

It was one thing to lament the dominance of the dollar in the international payments system; it was another to devise a way to reduce it.[84] Unlike in the 1940s, when the U.S. dollar stood ready to supplant the British pound as the international reserve currency, the Chinese renminbi in 2020 remained far from being a convertible currency, as Henry Paulson and others pointed out.[85] Chinese and European experiments with central bank digital currencies posed no obvious threat to dollar dominance. As for Facebook's grand design for a digital currency, Libra, as one wit observed, it had "about as much chance of displacing the dollar as Esperanto has of replacing English."[86] The most that could be said in mid-2020 was that the United States was lagging behind Asia, Europe, and even Latin America when it came to adopting new financial technology. But it was hard to see how the most ambitious alternative to the dollar—a projected East Asian digital currency consisting of the renminbi, the Japanese yen, the South Korean won, and the Hong Kong dollar—would even come to fruition, in view of the profound suspicions many in Tokyo and Seoul felt toward the financial ambitions of Beijing.[87]

The second area where U.S. dominance seemed likely (though not certain) to be reasserted was in the race to find a vaccine against the SARS-CoV-2 virus.[88] According to the Milken Institute, there were more than two hundred vaccine research projects under way at the time of writing, five of which were already in Phase III human trials. Eight candidates—including those of Oxford/Vaccitech and Moderna—were being given U.S. government funding as part of the Trump administration's "Operation Warp Speed."[89] True, three of the vaccines in Phase III trials were Chinese, but they were inactivated whole virus vaccines, an earlier generation of medical science than Moderna's mRNA-1273.[90] As an April survey in *Nature* noted, "Most COVID-19 vaccine development activity is in North America, with 36 (46%) developers of the confirmed active vaccine candidates compared with 14 (18%) in China, 14 (18%) in Asia (excluding China) and Australia, and 14 (18%) in Europe."[91] It was possible one of the Chinese contenders might beat the odds and produce a vaccine. It was nevertheless worth remembering the recurrent problems the People's Republic had experienced with vaccine safety and regulation, most recently in January 2019, when children in Jiangsu Province had received out-of-date polio shots,[92] and before that in July 2018, when 250,000 doses of vaccine for diphtheria, tetanus, and whooping cough had been found to be defective.[93] It was only fourteen years ago that Zheng Xiaoyu, the former head of the Chinese State Food and Drug Administration, was sentenced to death for taking bribes from eight domestic drug companies.[94] Both Chinese and Russian vaccine projects seemed to be using 1950s methods of development and testing, with all the attendant risks.

Third, in 2020 the United States was pulling ahead of China in the "tech war." The Trump administration's pressure on allied countries not to use 5G hardware produced by Huawei began yielding results. In Germany, Norbert Röttgen, a prominent member of Chancellor Angela Merkel's Christian Democratic Union, helped draft a bill that would bar any "untrustworthy" company from "both the core and peripheral networks."[95] In Britain, Conservative MP Neil O'Brien, cofounder of the China Research Group, and a group of thirty-eight rebel Tory backbenchers succeeded in changing Prime Minister Boris Johnson's mind about Huawei, much to the fury of the editors of *China Daily*.[96] More significant were the U.S. Commerce Department rules announced on May 15, and further tightened on August 17, that, from mid-September, cut Huawei off from advanced semiconductors produced anywhere in the world using U.S. technology or intellectual property. This included the chips produced in Taiwan by Taiwan Semiconductor Manufacturing Company (TSMC), the world's most advanced manufacturer. The new U.S. rules posed a potentially mortal threat to Huawei's semiconductor affiliate HiSilicon.[97]

Finally, the United States' lead in artificial intelligence research, as well as in quantum computing, began to look commanding, though the decision by President Trump to restrict H-1B visas for computer programmers and other skilled workers threatened ultimately to reduce that lead.[98] One 2020 study showed that while "China is the largest source of top-tier AI researchers . . . a majority of these Chinese researchers leave China to study, work, and live in the United States."[99] An Oxford survey of the tech war concluded, "If we look at the 100 most cited patents since 2003, not a single one comes from China. . . . A surveillance state with a censored internet, together with a social credit system that promotes conformity and obedience, seems unlikely to foster creativity."[100] If Yan Xuetong, dean of the Institute of International Relations at Tsinghua University, was correct that Cold War II would be a purely technological competition, without the nuclear brinkmanship and proxy wars that had made Cold War I so risky and so costly, then the United States must be the favorite to win it.[101]

It could hardly be claimed that the Trump administration was "safeguard[ing] the principles of the liberal world order." That was never its raison d'être. It would nevertheless be fair to say that, in practice, the administration was quite effective in at least some of the steps it took to achieve its stated goal of competing strategically with China. There was, however, a potential flaw in the strategy. The great achievement of the various strategies of containment pursued by the United States during the First Cold War was to limit and ultimately reverse the expansion of Soviet power without precipitating a third world war. Might strategic competition prove less successful in that regard? It was possible. First, there was a clear and present danger that information warfare and cyberwarfare operations, honed by the Russian government and now adopted by China, could cause severe disruption to the U.S. political and economic system.[102] Second, the United States could find itself at a disadvantage in the event of a conventional war in the South China Sea or the Taiwan Strait, because U.S. aircraft carrier groups, with their F-35 fighters, were now highly vulnerable to new Chinese weapons such as the DF-21D ("the carrier killer"), the world's first operational anti-ship ballistic missile.[103] One could imagine without too much difficulty an American naval defeat and diplomatic humiliation.[104] This would be disaster on a different scale from COVID-19, regardless of the death toll.

Third, the United States already found it difficult to back up words with actions. In the summer of 2020, China imposed new national security laws on Hong Kong, dealing a blow to the territory's autonomy and surely violating the terms of the 1984 Sino-British Joint Declaration, which guaranteed the "one country, two systems" model until 2047. Adding various Chinese agencies and institutions to the Commerce Department's entity list did not deter Beijing from going ahead. Nor did the broader economic sanctions threatened by indignant senators. Secretary of State Pompeo went out of his way to show friendliness toward the Taiwanese government in 2020, publicly congratulating President Tsai Ing-wen on her reelection in January. Even Richard Haass, a pre-Trump Republican and the personification of East Coast establishment strategy, argued for an end to the "ambiguity" of the U.S. commitment to defend Taiwan. "Waiting for China to make a move on Taiwan before deciding whether to intervene," wrote Haass in September, "is a recipe for disaster."[105] Yet how effectively could the United States counterattack if Beijing decided to launch a surprise amphibious invasion of the island? Such a step was openly proposed by nationalist writers on Chinese social media as the solution to the threat that Huawei will be cut off from TSMC. One lengthy post on this subject was headlined: "Reunification of the Two Sides, Take TSMC!"[106]

The reunification of Taiwan and the mainland was and remained Xi Jinping's most cherished ambition, as well as being one of the justifications for his removal of term limits. Xi may well have wondered if there would ever again be a more propitious time to force the issue than in late 2020, with the United States emerging from a lockdown-induced recession and with a deeply divisive election unlikely to reduce the country's internal frictions. While the Pentagon remained skeptical of China's ability to execute a successful invasion of Taiwan, the People's Liberation Army had been rapidly increasing its amphibious capabilities.[107] With good reason, Harvard's Graham Allison warned that the administration's ambition to "kill Huawei" could play a similar role to the sanctions imposed on Japan between 1939 and 1941, which culminated in the August 1941 oil embargo.[108] It was this and other economic pressure that ultimately drove the imperial government in Tokyo to gamble on the war that began with the surprise attack on Pearl Harbor.[109] If it were the United States that suddenly found itself cut off from TSMC, the boot would be on the other foot, as the Taiwanese company's new foundry in Arizona would take years to complete and, in terms of size, would be no substitute for the much larger facilities it had in Taiwan.[110]

Cold wars can deescalate in the process we remember as détente. But they can also escalate: a recurrent feature of the period from the late 1950s until the early 1980s was fear that brinkmanship might lead to Armageddon. At times, as John Bolton made clear, President Trump inclined to a very crude form of détente. There were important members of his administration who leaned in that direction, too. In mid-2020 there was occasionally melodious mood music about the Phase One trade deal announced late in 2019, despite abundant evidence that Beijing was far from fulfilling its commitments to purchase U.S. goods.[111] Yet the language of the American secretary of state grew increasingly combative. To be sure, his meeting with Yang Jiechi, the director of the CCP Office of Foreign Affairs, in Hawaii on June 17 was notable for the uncompromising harshness of the language used in the official Chinese communiqué released afterward.[112] But that might have been exactly what Secretary Pompeo wanted on the eve of his speech to the Copenhagen Democracy Summit, which was clearly intended to raise his European audience's awareness of the Chinese threat.[113]

How likely was it that the Atlantic Alliance could be resuscitated for the purpose of containing China? In some quarters not at all. The Italian foreign minister, Luigi Di Maio, was one of a number of Italian politicians all too ready to swallow Beijing's aid and propaganda in March, when the COVID-19 crisis in northern Italy was especially bad. "Those who scoffed at our participation in the Belt and Road Initiative now have to admit that investing in that friendship allowed us to save lives in Italy," Di Maio declared in an interview.[114] The Hungarian prime minister, Viktor Orbán, was equally enthused. "In the West, there is a shortage of basically everything," he said in an interview with Chinese state television. "The help we are able to get is from the East."[115] "China is the only friend who can help us," gushed Serbian president Aleksandar Vučić, who kissed a Chinese flag when a team of doctors flew from Beijing to Belgrade.[116] However, mainstream European sentiment, especially in Germany and France, reacted very differently. "Over these months China has lost Europe," Reinhard Bütikofer, a German Green Party member of the European Parliament, declared in an interview in April.[117] "The atmosphere in Europe is rather toxic when it comes to China," said Jörg Wuttke, president of the EU Chamber of Commerce in China. On April 17, the editor in chief of Germany's biggest tabloid, *Bild,* published an open letter to General Secretary Xi Jinping, entitled "You Are Endangering the World."[118] In France, too, "wolf warrior diplomacy" backfired on the wolves. A late summer tour of European capitals by Chinese foreign minister Wang Yi was notably autumnal in its atmosphere.[119] Survey data published in early October showed that it was not just in the United States but in all advanced economies, including the major EU countries, that anti-Chinese feeling had surged in 2020.[120]

One reason for China's failure to increase its influence in Europe was that, after an initial breakdown in early March, when *sauve qui peut* was the order of the day, European institutions rose to the challenge posed by COVID-19.[121] In a remarkable interview published on April 16, the French president declared that the EU faced a "moment of truth" in deciding whether it was more than just a single economic market. "You cannot have a single market where some are sacrificed," Emmanuel Macron told the *Financial Times.* "It is no longer possible . . . to have financing that is not mutualized for the spending we are undertaking in the battle against Covid-19 and that we will have for the economic recovery. . . . If we can't do this today, I tell you the populists will win—today, tomorrow, the day after, in Italy, in Spain, perhaps in France and elsewhere."[122] His German counterpart agreed. Europe, declared Angela Merkel, was a "community of fate" (*Schicksalsgemeinschaft*). To the surprise of skeptical commentators, the result was very different from the cheeseparing that had characterized the German response to the global financial crisis. The "Next Generation EU" plan, presented by the European Commission on May 27, proposed €750 billion of additional grants and loans, to be financed through bonds issued by the EU and to be allocated to the regions hit hardest by the pandemic.[123] Perhaps even more significantly, the German federal government adopted a supplementary budget of €156 billion (4.9 percent of GDP), followed by a second fiscal stimulus package worth €130 billion (or 3.8 percent of GDP), which—along with large-scale guarantees from a new economic stabilization fund—was intended to ignite recovery with a "ka-boom," in the words of finance minister Olaf Scholz.[124] Such fiscal measures, combined with large-scale asset purchases by the European Central Bank, hardly constituted a "Hamilton moment" analogous to the first U.S. Treasury secretary's consolidation of the states' debts in 1790. The European Recovery Fund did almost nothing to resolve the looming Italian debt crisis. It was not obvious that it could be repeated, if necessary, in the event of a second wave of COVID-19 (which the autumn duly brought as students returned to universities). However, the ERF did help to dampen support for the populist right in most EU member states.

This successful reassertion of the European solidarity—made easier by the departure of the United Kingdom from the EU—had an unexpected consequence from the vantage point of Washington. Europeans—especially young Europeans and especially Germans—had never, since 1945, been more disenchanted with the transatlantic relationship. This was true almost from the moment of Trump's election. In one pan-European survey conducted in mid-March, 53 percent of young respondents said they had more confidence in authoritarian states than democracies when it came to addressing the climate crisis.[125] In a poll published by the Körber Foundation in May, 73 percent of Germans said that the pandemic had worsened their opinion of the United

States—more than double the number of respondents who felt that way toward China. Just 10 percent of Germans considered the United States to be their country's closest partner in foreign policy, as compared with 19 percent in September 2019. And the proportion of Germans who prioritized close relations with Washington over close relations with Beijing had decreased significantly, from 50 percent in September 2019 to 37 percent, roughly the same share as those who preferred China to the United States (36 percent).[126] Increased anti-Chinese sentiment, in other words, was offset by increased anti-American sentiment.

In Cold War I, it is sometimes forgotten, there was a Non-Aligned Movement, which had its origins in the 1955 Bandung Conference, hosted by Indonesian president Sukarno and attended by Indian prime minister Jawaharlal Nehru, Egyptian president Gamal Abdel Nasser, his Yugoslav counterpart, Josip Broz Tito, and the president of Ghana, Kwame Nkrumah, as well as North Vietnam president Ho Chi Minh, Chinese premier Zhou Enlai, and Cambodian prime minister Norodom Sihanouk. Formally constituted in 1956 by Tito, Nehru, and Nasser, the NAM's goal was (in the words of one Arab leader who joined the movement) to enable the newly free countries of the Third World "to safeguard their independence and remain a vocal force in a world where the rules are made by the superpowers."[127] For most Western Europeans and many East and Southeast Asians, however, nonalignment was not an attractive option. That was partly because the choice between Washington and Moscow was a fairly easy one—unless the Red Army tanks were rolling into a country's capital city. It was also because the NAM's geopolitical nonalignment was not matched by a comparable ideological nonalignment, a feature that became more prominent with the ascendancy of the Cuban dictator Fidel Castro in the 1970s, finally leading to a near breakup of the movement over the Soviet invasion of Afghanistan. The Arab leader quoted above was Saddam Hussein, who had intended to host the 1981 NAM conference in Baghdad, a plan stymied by his country's war with equally nonaligned Iran.

In 2020, by contrast, the choice between Washington and Beijing looked to many Europeans like a choice between the frying pan and the fire or, at best, the kettle and the pot. As the Körber poll mentioned above suggested,

"The [German] public [was] leaning toward a position of equidistance between Washington and Beijing." Even the government of Singapore made it clear that it "fervently hope[d] not to be forced to choose between the United States and China." "Asian countries see the United States as a resident power that has vital interests in the region," the Singaporean prime minister, Lee Hsien Loong, wrote in *Foreign Affairs*. "At the same time, China is a reality on the doorstep. Asian countries do not want to be forced to choose between the two. And if either attempts to force such a choice—if Washington tries to contain China's rise or Beijing seeks to build an exclusive sphere of influence in Asia—they will begin a course of confrontation that will last decades and put the long-heralded Asian century in jeopardy. . . . Any confrontation between these two great powers is unlikely to end as the Cold War did, in one country's peaceful collapse."[128]

Lee was right in at least one respect. The fact that both world wars had the same outcome—the defeat of Germany and its allies by Britain and its allies—did not mean that Cold War II would end the same way as Cold War I, with the victory of the United States and its allies. Cold wars are usually regarded as bipolar; in truth, they are always three-body problems, with two superpower alliances and a third, nonaligned network in between. This may indeed be a general truth about war itself: that it is seldom simply a Clausewitzian contest between two opposing forces, each bent on the other's subjugation, but more often a three-body problem, in which winning the sympathies of the neutral third parties can be as important as inflicting defeat on the enemy.[129]

The biggest problem facing the president of the United States today, and for years to come, is that many erstwhile American allies are seriously contemplating nonalignment in Cold War II. And without a sufficiency of allies, to say nothing of sympathetic neutrals, Washington may find this Second Cold War to be unwinnable.

THE DARK FOREST

The crux of the matter, in August 2020, is how fearful of China the rest of the world is—or can be persuaded to be. As long as Europeans believe that

Donald Trump started Cold War II, the urge to be nonaligned will persist. Yet that view attaches too much importance to the change in U.S. foreign policy since 2016, and not enough to the change in Chinese foreign policy that came four years earlier, when Xi Jinping became general secretary of the Chinese Communist Party. Future historians will discern that the decline and fall of Chimerica began in the wake of the global financial crisis, as a new Chinese leader drew the conclusion that there was no longer any need to hide the light of China's ambition under the bushel that Deng Xiaoping had famously recommended. When Middle America voted for Trump in 2016, it was partly a backlash against the asymmetric payoffs of engagement and its economic corollary, globalization. Not only had the economic benefits of Chimerica gone disproportionately to China, not only had its costs been borne disproportionately by working-class Americans, many of whose manufacturing jobs had gone there, but now those same Americans also saw that their elected leaders in Washington had acted as midwives at the birth of a new strategic superpower—a challenger for global predominance even more formidable, because economically stronger, than the Soviet Union.

I have argued that this new cold war is both inevitable and desirable, not least because it has jolted the United States out of complacency and into an earnest effort not to be surpassed by China in artificial intelligence, quantum computing, and other strategically crucial technologies. Yet there remains, in academia especially, significant resistance to the view that we should stop worrying and learn to love Cold War II. At a July conference on "The World Order After Covid-19," organized by the Kissinger Center for Global Affairs at Johns Hopkins University, a clear majority of speakers warned of the perils of a new cold war. Eric Schmidt, the former chairman of Google, argued instead for a "rivalry-partnership" model of "coopetition," in which the two nations would at once compete and cooperate, rather as Samsung and Apple have done for years. Graham Allison agreed, giving as another example the eleventh-century "frenmity" between the Song emperor of China and the Liao kingdom on China's northern border. The pandemic, Allison argued, had made "incandescent the impossibility of identifying China clearly as either foe or friend. Rivalry-partnership may sound complicated, but life is complicated." "The establishment of a productive and predictable US/China relationship," wrote John Lipsky, formerly of the International Monetary Fund, "is a sine qua non for strengthening the institutions of global governance." The last cold war had cast a "shadow of a global holocaust for decades," observed James Steinberg, a former deputy secretary of state. "What can be done to create a context to limit the rivalry and create space for cooperation?" The Hoover Institution's Elizabeth Economy had an answer: "The United States and China could . . . partner to address a global challenge," namely climate change. Tom Wright, of the Brookings Institution, took a similar line: "Focusing only on great-power competition while ignoring the need for cooperation actually will not give the United States an enduring strategic advantage over China."[130]

All this talk of "coopetition" may seem eminently reasonable, if linguistically jarring, apart from one thing. The Chinese Communist Party is not Samsung, much less the Liao kingdom. Rather—as was true in Cold War I, when (especially after 1968) academics tended to be doves rather than hawks—today's proponents of "rivalry-partnership" are overlooking the possibility that the Chinese are not interested in being "frenemies." They know full well that this is a cold war, because they started it. When, in 2019, I first began talking publicly about Cold War II at conferences, I was surprised that no Chinese delegates contradicted me. In September of that year, I asked one of them—the Chinese head of a major international institution—why that was. "Because I agree with you!" he replied with a smile. As a visiting professor at Tsinghua University, in Beijing, I have seen for myself the ideological turning of the tide under Xi. Academics who study taboo subjects such as the Cultural Revolution find themselves subject to investigations or worse. Those who hope to revive engagement with Beijing underestimate the influence of Wang Huning, a member since 2017 of the Standing Committee of the Politburo, the most powerful body in China, and Xi's most influential adviser. In August 1988, Wang spent six months in the United States as a visiting scholar, traveling to more than thirty cities and nearly twenty universities. His account of that trip, *America Against America* (published in 1991), is a critique—in places scathing—of American democracy, capitalism, and culture. Racial division features prominently in the third chapter.

For Ben Thompson, the author of the widely read *Stratechery* newsletter, the events of 2019 and 2020 were revelatory. Having previously played down the political and ideological motivations of the Chinese government, he came out in 2019 as a new cold warrior. China's vision of the role of technology, he argued, was fundamentally different from the West's, and it fully intended to export its antiliberal vision to the rest of the world.[131] When Trump proposed a ban on the inane Chinese-owned video-and-music app TikTok in August 2020, Thompson was inclined to agree. "If China is on the offensive against liberalism not only within its borders but within ours," he wrote in July 2020, "it is in liberalism's interest to cut off a vector that has taken root precisely because it is so brilliantly engineered to give humans exactly what they want."[132] To appreciate the danger of allowing half of American teenagers to provide their personal data to a Chinese app, consider how the Communist Party is using AI to build a surveillance state that makes Orwell's Big Brother seem primeval. (As we shall see, Xi's panopticon is actually more akin to the dystopia imagined in Yevgeny Zamyatin's 1920s novel *We*.) In the words of the journalist Ross Andersen, "In the near future, every person who enters a public space [in China] could be identified, instantly, by AI matching them to an ocean of personal data, including their every text communication, and their body's one-of-a-kind protein-construction schema. In time, algorithms will be able to string together data points from a broad range of sources—travel records, friends and associates, reading habits, purchases—to predict political resistance before it happens."[133] Many of China's prominent AI startups are the Communist Party's "willing commercial partners" in this, which is bad enough. But the greater concern, as Andersen says, is that all this technology is for export. Among the countries buying it are Bolivia, Ecuador, Ethiopia, Kenya, Malaysia, Mauritius, Mongolia, Serbia, Sri Lanka, Uganda, Venezuela, Zambia, and Zimbabwe.

The Chinese response to the American attack on TikTok gave the game away. On Twitter, Hu Xijin, the editor in chief of the government-controlled *Global Times,* called the move "open robbery," accused Trump of "turning the once great America into a rogue country," and warned that "when similar things happen time and again, the U.S. will take steps closer to its decline."

In a revealing essay published last April, the Chinese political theorist Jiang Shigong, a professor at Peking University Law School, spelled out the corollary of American decline. "The history of humanity is surely the history of competition for imperial hegemony," Jiang wrote, "which has gradually propelled the form of empires from their original local nature toward the current tendency toward global empires, and finally toward a single world empire." The globalization of our time, according to Jiang, is the "'single world empire' 1.0, the model of world empire established by England and the United States." But that Anglo-American empire is "unravelling" internally, because of "three great unsolvable problems: the ever-increasing inequality created by the liberal economy . . . ineffective governance caused by political liberalism, and decadence and nihilism created by cultural liberalism." Moreover, the Western Empire is under external attack from "Russian resistance and Chinese competition." This is not a bid to create an alternative Eurasian empire, but "a struggle to become the heart of the world empire."[134]

If you doubt that China is seeking to take over empire 1.0 and turn it into empire 2.0, based on China's illiberal civilization, then you are not paying attention to all the ways this strategy is being executed. China has successfully become the workshop of the world, as the West used to be. It now has its version of Wilhelmine Germany's weltpolitik, in the form of One Belt One Road, a vast infrastructure project that looks a lot like European imperialism as described by J. A. Hobson in 1902.[135] China uses the prize of access to its market to exert pressure on U.S. companies to toe Beijing's line. It conducts "influence operations" throughout the West, including in the United States.[136]

One of the many ways America sought to undermine the Soviet Union in Cold War I was by waging a "cultural cold war."[137] This was partly about being seen to beat the Soviets at their own games—chess (Fischer vs. Spassky); ballet (Rudolf Nureyev's defection); ice hockey (the "Miracle on Ice" of 1980). But it was mainly about seducing the Soviet people with the irresistible temptations of American popular culture. In 1986, Régis Debray, the French leftist philosopher and comrade in arms of Che Guevara, lamented, "There is more power in rock music, videos, blue jeans, fast food, news networks and TV satellites than in the entire Red Army."[138] The French left sneered at "Coca-

Colonization." But Parisians, too, drank Coke. Now, however, the tables have been turned. In a debate I hosted at Stanford in 2018, the tech billionaire Peter Thiel used a memorable aphorism: "AI is Communist, crypto is libertarian."[139] TikTok validates the first half of that. In the late 1960s, during the Cultural Revolution, Chinese children denounced their parents for rightist deviance.[140] In 2020, when American teenagers posted videos of themselves berating their parents for racism, they did it on TikTok.

The work of Jiang Shigong and others make it clear that China today understands itself to be in a cold war that, like the last one, is a struggle between two forms of empire. Yet the book that provides the deepest insight into how China views America and the world today is not a political text, but a work of science fiction. *The Dark Forest* was Liu Cixin's 2008 sequel to *The Three-Body Problem*. It would be hard to overstate Liu's influence in contemporary China: he is revered by the tech companies of Shenzhen and Hangzhou and was officially endorsed as one of the faces of twenty-first-century Chinese creativity by none other than Wang Huning.[141] *The Dark Forest,* which continues the story of the invasion of Earth by the ruthless and technologically superior Trisolarans, introduces Liu's three axioms of "cosmic sociology." First, "Survival is the primary need of civilization." Second, "Civilization continuously grows and expands, but the total matter in the universe remains constant." Third, "chains of suspicion" and the risk of a "technological explosion" in another civilization mean that in space there can only be the law of the jungle. In the words of the book's hero, the "Wallfacer" Luo Ji:

> The universe is a dark forest. Every civilization is an armed hunter stalking through the trees like a ghost . . . trying to tread without sound. . . . The hunter has to be careful, because everywhere in the forest are stealthy hunters like him. If he finds other life—another hunter, an angel or a demon, a delicate infant or a tottering old man, a fairy or a demigod—there's only one thing he can do: open fire and eliminate them. In this forest, hell is other people. . . . Any life that exposes its own existence will be swiftly wiped out.[142]

Henry Kissinger is often thought of—in my view, wrongly—as the supreme American exponent of realpolitik. But this is something much harsher than realism. This is intergalactic Darwinism. It is not up to us whether or not we have a cold war with China, if China has already declared cold war on us. Not only are we already in the foothills of that new cold war; those foothills are also impenetrably covered in a dark forest of China's devising. The question that lingers—and the best argument in favor of Cold War—is whether or not we can avoid stumbling into a hot war in that darkness. If we do stumble into such a war, the outcome could be a disaster far greater in its impact than even the worst-case scenario for COVID-19.

Conclusion

―――――

FUTURE SHOCKS

"In fact," said Mustapha Mond, "you're claiming the right to be unhappy."

"All right, then," said the Savage defiantly. "I'm claiming the right to be unhappy."

—Aldous Huxley, *Brave New World*

WHAT DOESN'T KILL ME

"Can it be true . . . that whole countries are laid waste, whole nations annihilated, by these disorders in nature? The vast cities of America, the fertile plains of Hindostan, the crowded abodes of the Chinese, are menaced with utter ruin. Where late the busy multitudes assembled for pleasure or profit, now only the sound of wailing and misery is heard. The air is empoisoned, and each human being inhales death, even while in youth and health, their hopes are in the flower. . . . Plague had become Queen of the World."

Toward the end of Mary Shelley's *The Last Man* (1826), the hero stands alone on the shore, the sole survivor of a catastrophic pandemic. Set in the late twenty-first century, the book describes how a new Black Death, originating in Istanbul and accompanied by extreme weather events, civil strife, and waves of religious fanaticism, has annihilated mankind. For close to two hundred years—from Shelley's pioneering work of dystopian fantasy to Margaret

Atwood's MaddAddam trilogy—writers have imagined the human race ending in some such fashion. We once read such books as works of science fiction,
not prophecies. Amid a real pandemic, they exerted a ghoulish appeal, as did
movies with the same theme. I cannot have been the only reader in 2020 who
belatedly bought Emily St. John Mandel's novel *Station Eleven,* a contribution
to the plague genre I had hitherto overlooked. Nor, as I prepared to leave town
for a rural retreat, was I alone in thinking uneasily of Edgar Allan Poe's
"Masque of the Red Death."

But COVID-19 turned out not to be the Red Death or the Black Death or
even the Spanish influenza. At least that was how it seemed in August 2020.
It was more like the influenza of 1957–58, a major crisis of global public health
at the time, but fifty years later largely forgotten. It appeared that, with a regime of mass testing, contact tracing, social distancing, and targeted quarantining, a country could contain the spread of SARS-CoV-2, as the virus relied
heavily on superspreaders for its transmission and disproportionately sickened or killed people past retirement age. The chances were that a vaccine
would be widely available by the time this book was published, if not sooner.
Unlike World War I, this pandemic might even be over, if not by Christmas,
then by Easter. Similarly, there was a chance that the world economy would
snap back to life once this became clear. True, there was a worse scenario, in
which we would spend years playing whack-a-mole with an endemic, evolving
SARS-CoV-2, with no vaccine that really worked and no immunity that really
lasted. By the standards of past pandemics, this one might still be at an early
stage—perhaps not even at the end of the first quarter. Further waves could
not be ruled out, if the great pandemics of the past were any guide.[1] And perhaps COVID-19 would turn out to do more lasting harm to those who caught
it—even when they were young and fit—than we yet realized. In the first week
of August 2020, COVID-19 case numbers were rising in sixty-four countries.
Still, it was hard to believe that it would ever join the elite of pandemics—the
twenty or so in recorded history that killed upwards of 0.05 percent of humanity.[2] For some countries there had been no disaster worth talking about.
Only a minority had experienced excess mortality higher than 25 percent
above normal, and only for a few weeks. Only a handful of those nations that

fought World War II had lost more people per day to COVID than they had lost to the Axis powers. The United States was one of those countries.[3] This illustrated the central point of this book—that all disasters are at some level manmade political disasters, even if they originate with new pathogens. Politics explained why World War II killed twenty-five times as many Germans as Americans. Politics explains why COVID-19 has thus far killed eighteen times as many Americans as Germans.

This plague began as a gray rhino, predicted by many. It struck as a black swan, somehow completely unforeseen. Could it become a dragon king? As we have seen, disasters of any kind become truly epoch-making events only if their economic, social, and political ramifications amount to more than the excess mortality they cause. Could this medium-size disaster nevertheless alter our lives permanently and profoundly? Let me now hazard three guesses.

First, COVID-19 will be to social life what AIDS was to sexual life: it will change our behavior, though by no means enough to avert a significant number of premature deaths. I myself welcome a new age of social distancing, but then I am a natural misanthrope who hates crowds and will not greatly miss hugs and handshakes. Most people, however, will be unable to resist the temptations of post-lockdown gregariousness. There will be unsafe socializing just as there still is unsafe sex, even after more than three decades and thirty million deaths from HIV.

Second, and for that reason, most big cities are not "over." Do we all now head from Gotham or the Great Wen to the villages, there to cultivate our vegetable gardens in splendid, rustic isolation? Do nearly half of us continue to work from home, as we did during the pandemic—more than three times more than before?[4] Probably not. It takes a lot to kill a city. True, just over a century after Thomas Mann wrote *Death in Venice* (1912), Venice is pretty much dead. But it was not cholera that killed it—it was the shifting pattern of international trade. Likewise, COVID-19 will not kill London or New York; it will just make them cheaper, grungier, and younger. Some billionaires will not return. Some firms and many families will move to the suburbs or even farther afield. Tax revenues will drop. Crime rates will jump. As Gerald Ford supposedly did in 1975, when the city asked for a federal bailout, another president may tell New York to "drop dead." San Francisco will lose talent to Austin. But inertia is a powerful thing. Americans these days relocate less than they used to. Only a third of jobs can really be done at home; everyone else will still need to work in offices, shops, and factories. Workplaces will just be different—more spacious and campus-like, as they already are in Silicon Valley. Commuting will no longer involve being packed like sardines on a subway.[5] No more unwelcome intimacies on elevators. Masks over most faces. No more tut-tutting at the hijab and the niqab. Perforce, we are all modest now.

What of the pandemic's impact on the generational imbalances that had grown so intolerable in many societies by 2020? Was COVID-19 sent by Freya, the goddess of youth, to emancipate millennials and Generation Z from bearing the fiscal burden of an excessive number of elderly people? It is tempting to marvel at this ageist virus. No previous pandemic was so discriminating against the elderly and in favor of the young. But in truth, the impact of COVID-19 in terms of excess mortality will probably not be great enough to balance the intergenerational accounts. In the short run, the majority of old people will remain retired; relatively few will die prematurely—hardly any in the most elderly of countries, Japan. The young, meanwhile, will be the ones struggling to find jobs (other than with Amazon) and struggling almost as much to have fun. An economy without crowds is not a "new normal." It may be more like the new anomie, to borrow Émile Durkheim's term for the sense of disconnectedness he associated with modernity. For most young people, the word "fun" is almost synonymous with "crowd." The era of distancing will be a time of depression in the psychological as well as the economic sense. The gloom will be especially deep for Generation Z, whose university social lives—half the point of college, if not more—have been wrecked. They will spend yet more time on electronic devices—perhaps an hour a day more than before the pandemic. It will not make them happier.

As I write, we cannot know for sure what the political and geopolitical consequences of the pandemic will be. Will the populist right benefit because the vital importance of national borders is no longer in doubt? Or will the left now be able to make the case for even bigger government, despite big (but in-competent) government's conspicuous failure in the United States and the United Kingdom? Is Bruno Maçães right that, in the wake of "the great pause," we shall henceforth think of the economy more as a giant computer to be pro-grammed than as a natural organism?[6] Will we get to relive the Roaring Twenties? Or are we destined for a reprise of the 1970s, with the promise of modern monetary theory leading to the disappointment of stagflation lite?[7] What will people prefer to the dollar: the euro, gold, or bitcoin? What will be the consequences—if any—of the wave of protest and flagellation that followed the killing of George Floyd in Minneapolis? Will the quality of American po-licing improve or deteriorate? Does Cold War II between China and the United States intensify? Does it even turn into a hot war over Taiwan? Following the outbreak of COVID-19, Russia and Turkey carved out zones of influence in Libya, Chinese and Indian soldiers skirmished hand to hand on their border, and Lebanon metaphorically (and the port of Beirut literally) blew up. Is peace at hand? Probably not. Did the Black Death stop the Hundred Years' War? Did the Spanish flu prevent the Russian Civil War?

Pandemics, like world wars and global financial crises, are history's great interruptions. Whether we consider them man-made or naturally occurring, whether they are prophesied or strike like bolts from the blue, they are also moments of revelation. A catastrophe divides us all up into three groups: the prematurely dead, the lucky survivors, and the permanently wounded or trau-matized. A catastrophe also separates the fragile from the resilient and the antifragile—Nassim Taleb's wonderful word to describe something that gains strength under stress. (Remember Nietzsche: "What doesn't kill me makes me stronger.") Some cities, corporations, states, and empires collapse under the force of the shock. Others survive, though weakened. But a third, Nietzschean category emerges stronger. I suspect that, despite appearances, the United States is in category two, not one, while the People's Republic of China may ultimately prove to be in category one, not two, much less three. The Repub-lic of China, Taiwan, is in category three—unless Beijing annexes it.

Plagues do not halt progress if progress is happening. The same London that suffered the last great bubonic plague outbreak of 1665 (and the Great Fire the following year) was about to become the central hub of an extraordinary commercial empire, a humming hive of scientific and financial innovation, the pivotal city of the world for roughly two centuries. No pathogen could stop that. Our plague is likely to have the biggest disruptive impacts on places where progress had already ceased and stagnation had set in. First in line for disruption should be the bureaucracies that in some countries, including Britain and America, so badly failed to deal with this crisis. Next should be those universities that were more interested in propagating "woke" ideology than in teaching all that can profitably be learned from science and the human past. I would hope, too, that the second contagion—of lies and nonsense about the first one—will at last prompt a challenge to the current combination of monopoly and anarchy that characterizes the American (and hence much of the global) public sphere. The East India Companies of the internet have plundered enough data; they have caused enough famines of truth and plagues of the mind. Finally, the pandemic ought to force some changes on those media organizations that insisted on covering it, childishly, as if it were all the fault of a few wicked presidents and prime ministers. If stagnating institutions are shaken up by this disaster, there is just a chance that we shall see a return to progress in places where, up until 2020, the most striking trend had been degeneration. By killing those parts of our system that failed this test, COVID-19 might just make us stronger.

RUSSIAN ROULETTE

What disaster will come to test us next? Surely not another pandemic—that would be too obvious to be plausible history. It is nevertheless possible. A new strain of swine flu is never far away,[8] nor some new Asian respiratory disease.[9] Antibiotic-resistant microbes such as *Staphylococcus aureus* already exist;[10] we await with trepidation an antibiotic-resistant strain of the plague.[11] If not one of these—alongside which COVID-19 may one day seem a mild distemper— then which global catastrophic risk will it be? There are many to choose from.[12] Already, as one disaster so often begets another, COVID-19—with the help of swarms of locusts—is causing a potential crisis of nutrition in Africa and parts of South Asia. The World Food Programme has warned that the number of people suffering acute hunger could double from 135 million in 2019 to 265 million by the end of 2020.[13] Matters are being made worse by the disruption of established vaccination programs. Diphtheria is spreading in Pakistan, Bangladesh, and Nepal; cholera in South Sudan, Cameroon, Mozambique, Yemen, and Bangladesh; measles in the Democratic Republic of the Congo. Polio might even be reviving in Pakistan and Afghanistan. COVID-19 is also disrupting the treatment of HIV/AIDS, tuberculosis, and malaria.[14]

Then there is the continuing danger that steadily rising global temperatures could lead to disastrous climate change, as James Hansen and many others have warned.[15] Since 2013–14, when the Intergovernmental Panel on Climate Change published its Fifth Assessment Report, the worst of its "representative concentration pathways," RCP8.5, has grown more, not less probable, implying accelerating rises over this century in greenhouse gas emissions, temperatures, precipitation, and sea levels.[16] The argument has been made that this is a slow-moving problem that can be addressed with affordable mitigation measures, and that some of the drastic remedies touted by youthful millenarians could do much more harm than good.[17] Still, the uncertainties surrounding the future behavior of the complex system that is the world's climate argue strongly against the current combination of procrastination and virtue signaling. In the late summer of 2020, large tracts of California were ablaze, though as much because of chronic forest mismanagement as because of abnormally high temperatures.[18] An unusually rainy summer in China posed a meaningful threat to the integrity of the Three Gorges Dam.[19] A small earthquake could have delivered the coup de grâce. Then again, a huge earthquake in California and Oregon could make wildfires seem a small problem, and would have nothing to do with CO_2 emissions. The eruption of the Yellowstone supervolcano,[20] the caldera of which is less than one hundred miles from where I sit, would render discussion of man-made climate change superfluous in the brief period before mass extinction ensued.

There could be other, even bigger surprises. Alien invasion—a favorite of conspiracy theorists as well as sci-fi writers—is the least likely of these. The distances involved simply seem too vast.[21] More likely are the extraterrestrial threats posed by fluctuations in solar or stellar activity, such as a coronal mass ejection or a gamma ray burst from a supernova or "hypernova."[22] Also conceivable is another large, climate-altering asteroid strike.[23] Tiny black holes could swallow up the planet. Negatively charged stable "strangelets"— hypothetical particles of subatomic quarks—could catalyze the conversion of all the ordinary matter on Earth into "strange matter." A phase transition of a vacuum could cause the universe to expand exponentially.[24]

In addition to these exogenous threats are the various technologies we as a species have devised or are devising that have the potential to destroy us. The world was always vulnerable; we have made it more so.[25] Since the late 1950s, we have had the capacity for suicide—or at least catastrophic self-harm—by means of nuclear weapons. A nuclear war between two major powers or a major act of nuclear terrorism could kill in a matter of hours more people than COVID-19 has in eight months, and without regard for youth. The nuclear winter that would follow a nuclear war would render large parts of the planet uninhabitable.[26] Biological weapons of the sort the Soviet Union contemplated could have comparably catastrophic consequences, were they to be deployed or accidentally released.[27] Genetic engineering is a more recent innovation that, like nuclear energy, could be used for malign as well as benign purposes. It was a revolutionary discovery that genes could be "edited" using the Cas9 protein and the "clustered regularly interspaced short palindromic repeats" (CRISPR) that characterize DNA.[28] Gene editing's great flaw is that, unlike nuclear fission, it is cheap to do. A "genetic engineering home lab kit" was available in 2020 for just $1,845.[29] The danger here is not that someone will synthesize the master race, but that some kind of readily reproducible but undesirable modification could be created by mistake.[30]

In the realm of computer technology, new dangers have also arisen or could shortly arise. The existing "Internet of Things" has created multiple vulnerabilities in the event of unfettered cyberwarfare, in the sense that a country's critical power, command, control, and communications infrastructure could be wholly or partly disabled.[31] Artificial intelligence systems can already teach themselves how to beat human champions at games such as chess and go.

However, artificial general intelligence—a computer as intelligent as a human—
is still probably around half a century away. Eliezer Yudkowsky, who leads the
Machine Intelligence Research Institute at Berkeley, argues that we may unwittingly create an unfriendly or amoral AI that turns against us—for example,
because we tell it to halt climate change and it concludes that annihilating
Homo sapiens is the optimal solution. Yudkowsky warns of a modified Moore's
law: every eighteen months, the minimum IQ necessary to destroy the world
drops by one point.[32] A final nightmare scenario is that nanotechnology—
molecular manufacturing—leads to some self-perpetuating and unstoppable
process that drowns us in gloop.[33] One brave attempt to attach a probability
to "human extinction or the unrecoverable collapse of civilization" happening
in the next hundred years puts it at 1 in 6.[34] Life itself turns out to be Russian
roulette, but with many different fingers randomly pulling on the trigger.

A number of authors have proposed ways in which humanity might protect itself against destruction and self-destruction, acknowledging that, as
presently constituted, few if any national governments are incentivized to
take out meaningful insurance against catastrophic threats of uncertain probability and timing.[35] One suggestion is that there should be official Cassandras within governments, international bodies, universities, and corporations,
and a "National Warnings Office" tasked with identifying worst-case scenarios, measuring the risks, and devising hedging, prevention, or mitigation
strategies.[36] Another proposal is to "slow the rate of advancement towards
risk-increasing technologies relative to the rate of advancement in protective
technologies," ensuring that the people involved in the development of a new
technology are in agreement about using it for good, not evil, ends, and to
"develop the intra-state governance capacity needed to prevent, with extremely high reliability, any individual or small group . . . from carrying out
any action that is highly illegal."[37]

Yet when one considers what all this implies, it turns out to be an existential threat in its own right: the creation of a "High-tech Panopticon," complete with "ubiquitous-surveillance-powered preventive policing . . . effective
global governance [and] some kind of surveillance and enforcement mechanism that would make it possible to interdict attempts to carry out a destructive

act."[38] This is the road to totalitarianism—at a time when the technologies that would make possible a global surveillance state already exist. In the economist Bryan Caplan's words, "One particularly scary scenario for the future is that overblown doomsday worries become the rationale for world government, paving the way for an unanticipated global catastrophe: totalitarianism. Those who call for the countries of the world to unite against threats to humanity should consider the possibility that unification itself is the greater threat."[39] According to the Israeli historian Yuval Noah Harari, "once we begin to count on AI to decide what to study, where to work, and whom to date or even marry, human life will cease to be a drama of decision making. . . . We are now creating tame humans who produce enormous amounts of data and function as efficient chips in a huge data-processing mechanism." The advance of artificial intelligence, he argues, dooms mankind to a new totalitarianism, rendering liberal democracy and free-market economics "obsolete." We shall soon be to data what cows are to milk.[40] Even that bleak prospect might be too optimistic. The track record of totalitarian regimes is that they kill as well as milk their helots.

DYSTOPIAN WORLDS

To all of these potential disasters it is impossible to attach more than made-up probabilities. So how should we envision them? The best answer would seem to be that we must strive to imagine them. For the past two centuries, since Mary Shelley, this has been the role of science fiction writers. A lethal plague is only one of many forms that mankind's doom has taken in their imaginations.

Dystopian fiction reads as a history of the future—surely a contradiction in terms. In reality, whether their authors' purpose was to satirize, to provoke, to sound a warning, or merely to entertain, imagined dystopias have echoed present fears—to be precise, the anxieties of the literary elite. To study science fiction is therefore to gain an understanding of past worries, some of which have themselves played consequential roles in history. Ray Bradbury once said, "I am a preventor of futures not a predictor of them."[41] But how many policy decisions have been influenced by dystopian visions? And how often did those decisions turn out to be wise ones? The policy of appeasement, for example, was based partly on an exaggerated fear that the Luftwaffe could match Wells's Martians when it came to the destruction of London. More often, nightmare visions have failed to persuade policymakers to act preemptively. Yet science fiction has been a source of inspiration, too. When the pioneers of Silicon Valley were thinking through the potential applications of the internet, they often turned to writers such as William Gibson and Neal Stephenson for ideas. Today, no discussion of the implications of artificial intelligence is complete without at least one reference to *2001: A Space Odyssey* or the *Terminator* movies, just as nearly all conversations about robotics include a mention of Philip K. Dick's *Do Androids Dream of Electric Sheep?* or the movie it inspired, *Blade Runner.*

Now that the long-feared pandemic has arrived—along with rising sea levels, virtual reality, and at least prototypes of flying cars, not to mention levels of state surveillance undreamt of even by George Orwell—we can turn back to science fiction and ask: Who got the future most right? For the truth is that dystopia is (at least in some respects) now, not at some future date. The history of the future deserves our attention, partly because it may help us to think more rigorously about the shape of the next things to come. Historical data remain the foundation for all kinds of forecasting. Models based on theory may work, but without past statistics we cannot verify them. Yet future technological changes are not easy to infer from the past. Science fiction provides us with a large sample of imagined discontinuities that might not occur to us if we looked only backward.

In Mary Shelley's *Frankenstein* (1818), the eponymous scientist creates a synthetic man, the first of many such experiments in literature to go disastrously wrong. Like Prometheus, who stole the technology of fire, Frankenstein is punished for his presumption. Shelley followed this with *The Last Man* (1826), in which, as we have seen, a plague wipes out all but one specimen of humanity. With its vision of mass extinction and a depopulated world, *The Last Man* deserves to be regarded as the first true dystopian novel. It was not a commercial success. By the 1890s, however, H. G. Wells had established the popularity of the genre. In *The Time Machine* (1895), Wells envisioned a nightmare future Earth—the year is 802,701—where the Eloi, an incurious vegetarian people, are preyed upon by the subterranean Morlocks. Speciation has occurred, in other words, dividing humanity into two degenerate halves: airhead cattle and rapacious troglodytes. Traveling ever further forward in time, Wells's protagonist witnesses the last gasp of life on an inert planet. In *The War of the Worlds* (1898), invading Martians annihilate Londoners with weaponry eerily reminiscent of the intra-terrestrial world wars that lay ahead. Humanity in this case is saved by a pathogen against which the invaders have no immunity.

In our time, anxieties about man-made climate change have promoted environmental disaster as a subject for dystopian fiction. Margaret Atwood's *Oryx and Crake* (2003) reprises Shelley's *Last Man* but with the addled "Snowman" as one of just a handful of survivors of a world ravaged by global warming, reckless genetic engineering, and a disastrous attempt at population reduction that resulted in a global plague. In Cormac McCarthy's *The Road* (2006), cannibals roam a blasted wasteland. Paolo Bacigalupi's *The Windup Girl* (2009) ingeniously combines rising sea levels with rampant contagion caused by genetic engineering gone wrong. These works, too, have their precursors. During the Cold War, visions of climatic disaster were key drivers of both the antinuclear and environmental movements. In *On the Beach* (1957), by Nevil Shute, regular people are entirely helpless in the face of the slowly spreading fallout from nuclear war. In J. G. Ballard's *The Drowned World* (1962), rising temperatures (owing to solar activity, not pollution) have submerged most cities underwater.

Finally, there are the dystopias inspired by mass migration. For example, in Michel Houellebecq's 2015 novel *Submission,* the French left sides with an Islamic fundamentalist party rather than help the right-wing Front National take power. The new government purges non-Muslims from state and academic positions, legalizes polygamy, and distributes attractive wives. The novel ends as the protagonist submits to the new order. Although Houellebecq was widely accused of Islamophobia at the time of its publication, the book is actually a satire of France's fragile institutions and of the urban intellectuals' failure to defend them.

As the example of *Submission* suggests, science fiction is as much concerned with political catastrophe as with the natural or technological variety. A recurrent dystopia since the 1930s has been that of a fascist America. This fear has persisted from Sinclair Lewis's *It Can't Happen Here* (1935) to Suzanne Collins's *The Hunger Games* (2008), by way of Stephen King's *The Running Man* (1982), Margaret Atwood's *The Handmaid's Tale* (1985), and Philip Roth's *The Plot Against America* (2004). The alternative political nightmare was of a Stalin-like totalitarianism. In Ayn Rand's *Anthem* (1937), the hero ("Equality 7-2521") revolts against an egalitarian tyranny by rejecting his fate as a street sweeper and striving for freedom. Evelyn Waugh's *Love Among the Ruins* (1953) depicts an absurd England of mass incarceration and state-run euthanasia centers. Ray Bradbury's *Fahrenheit 451* (published in 1953 but set in 1999) describes an illiberal America where the government has banned all books and the job of firemen is to burn prohibited literature. (Though the novel is sometimes interpreted as a critique of McCarthyism, Bradbury's real message was that the preference of ordinary people for the vacuous entertainment of television and the willingness of religious minorities to demand censorship together posed a creeping threat to the book as a form for serious content.) Of all these dystopian visions of totalitarianism, however, none has surpassed George Orwell's *Nineteen Eighty-Four* (1949) in its readership and influence.

In a remarkable letter written in October 1949, Aldous Huxley—who had been the young Eric Blair's French teacher at Eton—warned Orwell that he was capturing his own present rather than the likely future. "The philosophy of the ruling minority in Nineteen Eighty-Four," Huxley wrote, "is a sadism which has been carried to its logical conclusion. . . . Whether in actual fact the policy of the boot-on-the-face can go on indefinitely seems doubtful. My own belief is that the ruling oligarchy will find less arduous and wasteful ways of governing and of satisfying its lust for power, and these ways will resemble those which I described in Brave New World."[42] In Huxley's 1932 novel, we arrive at a very different dystopia (in AD 2540): one based on Fordism plus eugenics, not Stalinism. Citizens submit to a caste system of rigid structural inequalities because they are conditioned to be content with the satisfaction of their shallow physical desires. Self-medication ("soma"), constant entertainment (the "feelies"), regular holidays, and ubiquitous sexual titillation are the basis for mass compliance. Censorship and propaganda play a part, too, as in *Nineteen Eighty-Four,* but overt coercion is rarely visible. The West today thus seems much more Huxley than Orwell: there is a good deal more corporate distraction than state brutality.

Yet there are other and better fits than Huxley or Orwell when we seek to make sense of today's dystopias. China under Xi Jinping increasingly calls to mind Yevgeny Zamyatin's extraordinary *We* (written in 1921 but suppressed by the Bolshevik regime). Set in a future "One State" led by "the Benefactor," *We* depicts a surveillance state more chillingly effective than Orwell's (which it partly inspired, as it also inspired Ayn Rand's *Anthem*). All "ciphers"—who have numbers, not names, and wear standardized "unifs"—are under round-the-clock surveillance, and all apartments are made of glass, with curtains that can be drawn only when one is having state-licensed sex. Faced with insurrection, the all-powerful Benefactor orders mass lobotomization of all ciphers, because the only way to preserve universal happiness is to abolish the imagination. "What have people—from the very cradle—prayed for, dreamed about, and agonized over?" the Benefactor asks. "They have wanted someone, anyone, to tell them once and for all what happiness is—and then to attach them to this happiness with a chain."[43]

Yet, on further reflection, none of these authors truly foresaw all the peculiarities of our networked world, which has puzzlingly combined a rising speed and penetration of consumer information technology with a slackening of progress in other areas, such as nuclear energy, and a woeful degeneration of governance. The real prophets turn out, on closer inspection, to be less familiar figures—for example, John Brunner, whose *Stand on Zanzibar* (1968) is set in 2010, at a time when population pressure has led to widening social divisions and political extremism. Despite the threat of terrorism, U.S. corporations like General Technics are booming, thanks to a supercomputer named Shalmaneser. China is America's new rival. Europe has united. Brunner also foresees affirmative action, genetic engineering, Viagra, Detroit's collapse, satellite TV, in-flight video, gay marriage, laser printing, electric cars, the de-

criminalization of marijuana, and the decline of tobacco. There is even a progressive president (albeit of Beninia, not America) named "Obomi."

With comparable prescience, William Gibson's *Neuromancer* (1984) an-
ticipates the internet and artificial intelligence. Opening in the dystopian
underworld of Chiba City, Japan, the novel has as its central characters a
drug-addled hacker, a feline street samurai, and a damaged special-ops officer. But Gibson's real imaginative breakthrough is the global computer network in cyberspace called the "matrix," as well as the central plot device of
the twin artificial intelligences Wintermute and Neuromancer. An especially
popular book among Facebook employees in the company's early years, Neal
Stephenson's *Snow Crash* (1992) foresees corporate overreach and virtual reality in an almost anarchic America. The state has withered away in California;
everything has been privatized, including highways; the federal government
is vestigial. Most people spend about half their time in a virtual-reality world,
where their avatars have a lot more fun than they do in the real world. Meanwhile, vast flotillas of refugees and migrants approach the United States via
the Pacific. These cyberpunk Americas seem much closer to the United States
in 2020 than the authoritarian dystopias of Lewis, Atwood, or Roth.

If the United States is less Gilead than Chiba City, then to what extent is
modern China really a version of Zamyatin's *We*? In Chan Koonchung's *The
Fat Years* (2009)—which is banned on the mainland—tap water laced with
drugs renders people docile, but at a cost. The month of February 2011 has
somehow been removed from public records and popular memory. It turns out
that this was the month when a series of drastic emergency measures had to
be introduced to stabilize the Chinese economy, but also to assert China's primacy in East Asia. Chan is one of a number of recent Chinese authors who
have tried to envision the decline of the United States, the corollary of China's rise. *The Fat Years* is set in an imagined 2013, after a second Western financial crisis has made China the world's number-one economy. In Han Song's
2066: Red Star over America (2000), a terrorist attack destroys the World
Trade Center and the rising ocean sweeps over Manhattan. And in Liu Cixin's
The Three-Body Problem (2006), as we have seen, it is a Chinese nanotechnology expert and a Beijing cop who lead the global defense against an alien

invasion that is itself the fault of a misanthropic Chinese physicist. The Americans in the *Remembrance of Earth's Past* trilogy are either malicious or incompetent.

Yet even mainland-based Chinese authors are conscious of the People's Republic's deeply illiberal nature, as well as the recurrent instability of Chinese political history. The "problem" of *The Three-Body Problem* is introduced to the reader as a virtual-reality game, set in a strange, distant world with three suns rather than the familiar one. The mutually perturbing gravitational attractions of the three suns prevent this planet from settling into a predictable orbit with regular days, nights, and seasons. It has occasional "stable eras," during which civilization can advance, but with minimal warning these give way to "chaotic eras" of intense heat or cold that render the planet uninhabitable. The central conceit of Liu's novel is that China's history has the same pattern as the three-body problem: periods of stability always end with periods of chaos (*dong luan*).

Acute readers may also wonder if the ideology of the Earth-Trisolaris Movement (ETM)—the radically misanthropic organization dedicated to helping the Trisolarans conquer Earth—is a subtle parody of Maoism. The members of ETM "had abandoned all hope in human civilization, hated and were willing to betray their own species, and even cherished as their highest ideal the elimination of the entire human race, including themselves and their children." "Start a global rebellion!" they shout. "Long live the spirit of Trisolaris! We shall persevere like the stubborn grass that resprouts after every wildfire! . . . Eliminate human tyranny!" Little do these would-be collaborators know that the Trisolarans are even worse than humans. As one of the aliens points out, because of their world's utter unpredictability, "everything is devoted to survival. To permit the survival of the civilization as a whole, there is almost no respect for the individual. Someone who can no longer work is put to death. Trisolaran society exists under a state of extreme authoritarianism." Life for the individual consists of "monotony and desiccation." That sounds a lot like Mao's China.

True, the hero of the story is the foulmouthed, chain-smoking Beijing cop Shi Qiang. Chinese readers doubtless relish the scene in which he lectures a pompous American general about how best to save the world. But the deeper meaning of the book is surely that Trisolaris is China. The three bodies in contention are not suns but classes: rulers, intellectuals, masses. The Trisolarans, like good totalitarians, are omniscient. Their invisible "sophons" provide them with complete surveillance of humanity, enabling them effectively to prevent further scientific progress on Earth. But the inexorably approaching invaders turn out to have a weakness. Their culture of complete transparency—communication via unfiltered thought—precludes cheating or lying, so (as is revealed in *The Dark Forest*) they cannot "pursue complicated strategic thinking." With four hundred years before their estimated arrival, humanity has time to prepare its defenses and to exploit this one advantage.

Is it too much to see here an allegory of China's changing place in the world—perhaps even of the new cold war between the United States and the People's Republic? If not, it is an unnerving allegory—an enthralling intimation of a future geopolitical disaster.

"YET I ALIVE"

If, as Paul Samuelson joked, declines in U.S. stock prices have correctly predicted nine of the last five American recessions, science fiction has correctly predicted nine of the last five technological breakthroughs. Flying cars remain at the prototype stage, and time machines are nowhere to be seen. The aliens have yet to reveal themselves in the dark forest. And, of course, science fiction has predicted many more than nine of the last zero ends of the world. Nevertheless, science fiction can play an important role in helping us to think clearly about the future.

Much that lies ahead will follow the ancient, perennial rules of human history. An incumbent power will feel menaced by a rising power. Another demagogue will feel frustrated by the constraints of a constitution. Power will corrupt, and absolute power will corrupt absolutely. This much we know from history and from great literature. But in other respects, because of changes in science, medicine, and technology, the future will be different, and historians are not well qualified to foresee that kind of discontinuity, except to affirm that it happens. In *Foundation* (1951), Isaac Asimov imagined "psychohistory" as a fictional discipline that combined history, sociology, and mathematical statistics to make general predictions about the future. Though the late Israeli president Shimon Peres once assured me that Israeli scholars had succeeded in establishing a version of Asimov's "Prime Radiant," I am skeptical that such a discipline will ever exist. If the ultimate contribution of cliodynamics is just another cyclical theory of history, it will have betrayed its early promise.

History tells us to expect the great punctuation marks of disaster in no predictable order. The four horsemen of the Book of Revelation—Conquest, War, Famine, and the pale rider Death—gallop out at seemingly random intervals to remind us that no amount of technological innovation can make mankind invulnerable. Indeed, some innovations—like those fleets of jet airplanes that transported so many infected people from Wuhan to the rest of the world in January 2020—give the horsemen the opportunity to ride in their slipstream. Yet somehow the riders' arrival always takes us by surprise. For a moment, we contemplate the scenario of total extinction. We shelter in place, watching *Contagion* or reading Atwood. Perhaps the black swan becomes a dragon king and turns life upside down. But very rarely. Mostly, for the lucky many, life after the disaster goes on, changed in a few ways but on the whole remarkably, reassuringly, boringly the same. With astonishing speed, we put our brush with mortality behind us and blithely carry on, forgetful of those who were not so lucky, regardless of the next disaster that lies in wait. Think, if you doubt the truth of this, of Daniel Defoe's concluding doggerel from his *Journal of the Plague Year*:

> *A dreadful Plague in* London *was,*
> *In the Year Sixty Five,*
> *Which swept an Hundred Thousand Souls*
> *Away; yet I alive!*[44]

Acknowledgments

The writing of a book such as this is the responsibility of a single author, but he incurs numerous debts of gratitude as he writes. I am especially grateful to my friends Nicholas Christakis and John Cochrane, who painstakingly read the galleys and suggested many corrections and improvements. All errors that remain are, of course, my own fault. Research assistance was very ably and speedily provided by Sarah Wallington and Kyle Kinnie.

I am grateful to many colleagues at the Hoover Institution for ideas and inspiration, not only John Cochrane but also Victor Davis Hanson, H. R. Mc-Master, Condoleezza Rice, Manny Rincon-Cruz, and John Taylor.

At Greenmantle I am privileged to work with a remarkably talented brain trust. All of the following contributed to this book through our twice-weekly meetings to discuss the unfolding events of 2020: Pierpaolo Barbieri, Alice Han, Nicholas Kumleben, Phumlani Majozi, Jay Mens, Chris Miller, Stephanie Petrella, Emile Simpson, John Sununu, Dimitris Valatsas, and Joseph de Weck. In particular, Justin Stebbing was an indispensable guide to the relevant medical science; Gil Highet was of considerable assistance with chapter 7; and Daniel Lansberg-Rodríguez and Eyck Freymann contributed a good deal to the conclusion. Special thanks are due to those who read early drafts of the book. In addition to Pierpaolo, Alice, Jay, Chris, Dimitris, Emile, and Eyck, thanks go to Joe Lonsdale, Norman Naimark, Dan Seligson, and Tim Simms. I would also like to thank Piotr Brzezinski, Sahil Mahtani, Glen O'Hara, Ryan Orley, Jason Rockett, and Sean Xu for their insights. Though the youngest person to be named here, Thomas Ferguson also helped a good deal with chapter 8. Jim Dickson was an eagle-eyed proofreader.

Also helpful have been the many members of the applied history network at Stanford, Harvard, and elsewhere with whom I had the opportunity to discuss parts of the book, notably Graham Allison, Hal Brands, Francis Gavin, Charles Maier, and Calder Walton. Amartya Sen kindly read chapter 6.

To my editors, Scott Moyers and Simon Winder, as well as to my literary agent, Andrew Wylie, I am also deeply grateful.

On the home front, the Jones siblings—Collin, Kelsey, and Kyle—cheerfully and creatively enabled me to cope with a new life in the mountains, as did Nazha Schultz. Last, but by no means least, my wife, Ayaan, and all my children—Felix, Freya, Lachlan, Thomas, and Campbell—deserve the most heartfelt thanks for putting up with the monomaniacal mood that was necessary for this book to get written, as well as for inspiring me in countless ways. To them, and to my mother, Molly, who endured the plague year mostly alone in Oxfordshire, I dedicate this book.

Notes

Introduction

1. "Davos Man Is Cooling on Stockholm Girl Greta Thunberg," *Sunday Times,* January 26, 2020, https://www.thetimes.co.uk/edition/comment/davos-man-is-cooling-on-stockholm-girl-greta-thunberg-z2sqcx872.
2. "The Deadliest Virus We Face Is Complacency," *Sunday Times,* February 2, 2020, https://www.thetimes.co.uk/edition/comment/the-deadliest-virus-we-face-is-complacency-wsp7xdr7s.
3. "Trump May Shrug Off Coronavirus. America May Not," *Sunday Times,* March 1, 2020, https://www.thetimes.co.uk/edition/comment/trump-may-shrug-off-coronavirus-america-may-not-bmvw9rqzd.
4. "'Network Effects' Multiply a Viral Threat," *Wall Street Journal,* March 8, 2020, https://www.wsj.com/articles/network-effects-multiply-a-viral-threat-11583684394.
5. Data from Worldometer, https://www.worldometers.info/coronavirus/country/us.
6. "The First Coronavirus Error Was Keeping Calm," *Sunday Times,* March 15, 2020, https://www.thetimes.co.uk/edition/comment/the-first-coronavirus-error-was-keeping-calm-zvj28s0rp.
7. Richard J. Evans, *Death in Hamburg: Society and Politics in the Cholera Years, 1830–1910* (Oxford: Oxford University Press, 1987).
8. Niall Ferguson, *The Pity of War: Explaining World War I* (New York: Basic Books, 1999), pp. 342f.
9. Niall Ferguson, *The War of the World: Twentieth-Century Conflict and the Descent of the West* (New York: Penguin Press, 2006), pp. 144f.
10. Niall Ferguson, *Empire: The Rise and Fall of the British World Order and the Lessons for Global Power* (New York: Penguin Press, 2006), p. 65.
11. Niall Ferguson, *Civilization: The West and the Rest* (New York: Penguin Press, 2011), p. 175.
12. Niall Ferguson, *The Great Degeneration: How Institutions Decay and Economies Die* (New York: Penguin Press, 2012), p. 144.
13. Niall Ferguson, *The Square and the Tower: Networks and Power from the Freemasons to Facebook* (New York: Penguin Press, 2018), p. 203.
14. SeroTracker, Public Health Agency of Canada, https://serotracker.com/Dashboard.
15. For the precise terms of the bet, see Bet 9, Long Bets Project, http://longbets.org/9/. Rees was principally concerned with the danger of bioterrorism but included "bioerror" to mean "something which has the same effect as a terror attack, but rises from inadvertance rather than evil intent." There is some ambiguity as to whether or not "casualties" meant fatalities only: "Casualties should ideally include 'victims requiring hospitalization' and not include indirect deaths caused by the pathogen."
16. Patrick G. T. Walker et al., "The Global Impact of COVID-19 and Strategies for Mitigation and Suppression," Imperial College COVID-19 Response Team Report 12 (March 26, 2020), https://doi.org/10.25561/77735.
17. For an introduction, Ferguson, *Square and the Tower.*
18. Nassim Nicholas Taleb, *Antifragile: Things That Gain from Disorder* (New York: Random House, 2012).
19. "South Africa's 'Doom Pastor' Found Guilty of Assault," BBC News, February 9, 2018, https://www.bbc.co.uk/news/world-africa-43002701.
20. Nicole Sperling, "'Contagion,' Steven Soderbergh's 2011 Thriller, Is Climbing up the Charts," *New York Times,* March 4, 2020, https://www.nytimes.com/2020/03/04/business/media/coronavirus-contagion-movie.html.
21. Louis-Ferdinand Céline, *Journey to the End of the Night,* trans. Ralph Manheim (New York: New Directions, 1983 [1934]), p. 14.
22. Marc Bloch, *L'étrange défaite: Témoignage écrit en 1940* (Paris: Gallimard, 1997 [1946]).
23. Max H. Bazerman and Michael D. Watkins, *Predictable Surprises: The Disasters You Should Have Seen Coming, and How to Prevent Them,* 2nd ed. (Cambridge, MA: Harvard Business School Publishing,

2008); Michele Wucker, *The Gray Rhino: How to Recognize and Act on the Obvious Dangers We Ignore* (New York: Macmillan, 2016).

24. Nassim Nicholas Taleb, *The Black Swan: The Impact of the Highly Improbable* (London: Penguin/Allen Lane, 2007).

25. Didier Sornette, "Dragon Kings, Black Swans and the Prediction of Crises," Swiss Finance Institute Research Paper Series No. 09-36 (2009), available at SSRN, http://ssrn.com/abstract=1470006.

26. Keith Thomas, *Religion and the Decline of Magic: Studies in Popular Beliefs in Sixteenth and Seventeenth Century England* (London: Weidenfeld & Nicolson, 1971).

27. Norman Dixon, *On the Psychology of Military Incompetence* (London: Pimlico, 1994).

28. Christina Boswell, *The Political Uses of Expert Knowledge: Immigration Policy and Social Research* (Cambridge: Cambridge University Press, 2009).

29. Henry A. Kissinger, "Decision Making in a Nuclear World" (1963), Henry A. Kissinger papers, Part II, Series I, Yale University Library, mssa.ms.1981/ref25093.

30. Richard Feynman, *"What Do You Care What Other People Think?," Further Adventures of a Curious Character* (New York: W. W. Norton, 1988), pp. 179–84.

31. "House Approves Creation of Committee to Investigate Katrina Response," Voice of America, October 31, 2009, https://www.voanews.com/archive/house-approves-creation-committee-investigate-katrina-response.

32. J. R. Hampton, "The End of Medical History?," *Journal of the Royal College of Physicians of London* 32, no. 4 (1998), pp. 366–75.

33. Larry Brilliant, "My Wish: Help Me Stop Pandemics," February 2006, TED video, 25:38, https://www.ted.com/talks/larry_brilliant_my_wish_help_me_stop_pandemics.

34. See, in general, Nick Bostrom and Milan M. Ćirković, eds., *Global Catastrophic Risks* (Oxford: Oxford University Press, 2008).

35. Ricki Harris, "Elon Musk: Humanity Is a Kind of 'Biological Boot Loader' for AI," *Wired,* September 1, 2019, https://www.wired.com/story/elon-musk-humanity-biological-boot-loader-ai/.

Chapter 1: The Meaning of Death

1. Retirement & Survivors Benefits: Life Expectancy Calculator, Social Security Administration, https://www.ssa.gov/cgi-bin/longevity.cgi; Life Expectancy Calculator, Office for National Statistics (UK), https://www.ons.gov.uk/peoplepopulationandcommunity/healthandsocialcare/healthandlifeexpectancies/articles/lifeexpectancycalculator/2019-06-07; Living to 100 Life Expectancy Calculator, https://www.livingto100.com/calculator/age.

2. Max Roser, Esteban Ortiz-Ospina, and Hannah Ritchie, "Life Expectancy," Our World in Data (2013), last revised October 2019, https://ourworldindata.org/life-expectancy.

3. "Mortality Rate, Under-5 (per 1,000 Live Births)," World Bank Group, https://data.worldbank.org/indicator/SH.DYN.MORT; "Mortality Rate Age 5–14," UN Inter-agency Group for Child Mortality Estimation, https://childmortality.org/data/Somalia.

4. Salvator Rosa, *L'umana fragilità* ("Human Frailty"), c. 1656, Fitzwilliam Museum, Cambridge, https://www.fitzmuseum.cam.ac.uk/pharos/collection_pages/italy_pages/PD_53_1958/TXT_SE-PD_53_1958.html.

5. Philippe Ariès, *The Hour of Our Death,* trans. Helen Weaver (New York: Alfred A. Knopf, 1981).

6. Adam Leith Gollner, "The Immortality Financiers: The Billionaires Who Want to Live Forever," *Daily Beast,* August 20, 2013, https://www.thedailybeast.com/the-immortality-financiers-the-billionaires-who-want-to-live-forever.

7. Jon Stewart, "Borges on Immortality," *Philosophy and Literature* 17, no. 2 (October 1993), pp. 295–301.

8. Murray Gell-Mann, "Regularities in Human Affairs," *Cliodynamics: The Journal of Theoretical and Mathematical History* 2 (2011), pp. 53f.

9. Cynthia Stokes Brown, *Big History: From the Big Bang to the Present* (New York: New Press, 2007), pp. 53f. See also Fred Spier, *Big History and the Future of Humanity* (Chichester, UK: Blackwell, 2011), p. 68.

10. Nick Bostrom and Milan M. Ćirković, "Introduction," in *Global Catastrophic Risks,* ed. Nick Bostrom and Milan M. Ćirković (Oxford: Oxford University Press, 2008), p. 9.

11. Bostrom and Ćirković, "Introduction," p. 8.

12. See, in general, Tom Holland, *Dominion: How the Christian Revolution Remade the World* (New York: Basic Books, 2019).

13. Richard Landes, *Heaven on Earth: The Varieties of Millennial Experience* (New York and Oxford: Oxford University Press, 2011), pp. 426f. See also Paul Casanova, *Mohammed et la fin du monde: Étude critique sur l'Islam primitif* (Paris: P. Geuthner, 1911), pp. 17f.

14. Norman Cohn, *The Pursuit of the Millennium* (Oxford: Oxford University Press, 1961 [1957]), pp. 106f.

15. Holland, *Dominion,* p. 300.

16. James J. Hughes, "Millennial Tendencies in Responses to Apocalyptic Threats," in *Global Catastrophic Risks,* ed. Nick Bostrom and Milan M. Ćirković (Oxford: Oxford University Press, 2008), pp. 9, 78, 83.

17. Holland, *Dominion,* p. 451.

18. Robert Service, *Lenin: A Biography* (London: Pan Macmillan, 2011), pp. 538, 539, 594. See also Robert C. Williams, "The Russian Revolution and the End of Time: 1900–1940," *Jahrbücher für Geschichte Osteuropas,* Neue Folge, 43, no. 3 (1995), pp. 364–401.

19. "Lenin Opposed as Antichrist by Peasants in Old Russia," *New York Times,* June 21, 1919, https://www.nytimes.com/1919/06/21/archives/lenin-opposed-as-antichrist-by-peasants-in-old-russia.html.

20. Eric Voegelin, *The New Science of Politics: An Introduction,* 4th ed. (Chicago: University of Chicago Press, 1962), pp. 120f.

21. Voegelin, *The New Science,* p. 124.

22. Voegelin, *The New Science,* pp. 122, 129, 131f.

23. Landes, *Heaven on Earth,* p. 470.

24. James A. Hijiya, "The Gita of J. Robert Oppenheimer," *Proceedings of the American Philosophical Society* 144, no. 2 (June 2000).

25. Doomsday Clock, *Bulletin of the Atomic Scientists,* https://thebulletin.org/doomsday-clock/.

26. Sewell Chan, "Doomsday Clock Is Set at 2 Minutes to Midnight, Closest Since 1950s," *New York Times,* January 25, 2018, https://www.nytimes.com/2018/01/25/world/americas/doomsday-clock-nuclear-scientists.html.

27. Bulletin of the Atomic Scientists Science and Security Board, "Closer Than Ever: It Is 100 Seconds to Midnight," ed. John Mecklin, *Bulletin of the Atomic Scientists,* January 23, 2020, https://thebulletin.org/doomsday-clock/current-time/.

28. Matthew Connelly, "How Did the 'Population Control' Movement Go So Terribly Wrong?," *Wilson Quarterly* (Summer 2008), https://www.wilsonquarterly.com/quarterly/summer-2008-saving-the-world/how-did-population-control-movement-go-so-terribly-wrong/. See also Matthew Connelly, *Fatal Misconception: The Struggle to Control World Population* (Cambridge, MA: Harvard University Press, 2008).

29. Greta Thunberg, *No One Is Too Small to Make a Difference* (London: Penguin, 2019), p. 46.

30. William Cummings, "'The World Is Going to End in 12 Years If We Don't Address Climate Change,' Ocasio-Cortez Says," *USA Today,* January 22, 2019, https://www.usatoday.com/story/news/politics/onpolitics/2019/01/22/ocasio-cortez-climate-change-alarm/2642481002/.

31. "Greta Thunberg's Remarks at the Davos Economic Forum," *New York Times,* January 21, 2020, https://www.nytimes.com/2020/01/21/climate/greta-thunberg-davos-transcript.html.

32. Leonard Lyons, "Loose-Leaf Notebook," *Washington Post,* January 20, 1947.

33. "Der Krieg? Ich kann das nicht so schrecklich finden! Der Tod eines Menschen: das ist eine Katastrophe. Hunderttausend Tote: das ist eine Statistik!" Kurt Tucholsky, "Französische Witze (I)" and "Noch einmal französische Witze (II)," *Vossische Zeitung,* August 23, 1925, and September 10, 1925. The columns were reprinted in Tucholsky's book *Lerne lachen ohne zu weinen* (Berlin: Ernst Rowohlt, 1932), pp. 147–56.

34. Eliezer Yudkowsky, "Cognitive Biases Potentially Affecting Judgement of Global Risks," in *Global Catastrophic Risks,* ed. Nick Bostrom and Milan M. Ćirković (Oxford: Oxford University Press, 2008), p. 114.

35. Pasquale Cirillo and Nassim Nicholas Taleb, "Tail Risk of Contagious Diseases" (working paper, 2020); Lee Mordechai, Merle Eisenberg, Timothy P. Newfield, Adam Izdebski, Janet E. Kay, and Hendrik Poinar, "The Justinianic Plague: An Inconsequential Pandemic?," *Proceedings of the National Academy of Sciences of the United States of America* (henceforth *PNAS*) 116, no. 51 (2019), pp. 25546–54, https://doi.org/10.1073/pnas.1903797116.

36. For a good discussion of Richardson's contribution, see Brian Hayes, "Statistics of Deadly Quarrels," *American Scientist* 90 (January–February 2002), pp. 10–15.

37. The standard works are Lewis F. Richardson, *Statistics of Deadly Quarrels,* ed. Quincy Wright and C. C. Lienau (Pittsburgh: Boxwood Press, 1960), and Jack S. Levy, *War in the Modern Great Power System, 1495–1975* (Lexington: University of Kentucky Press, 1983). More recent publications of importance include Pasquale Cirillo and Nassim Nicholas Taleb, "On the Statistical Properties and Tail Risk of Violent Conflicts," Tail Risk Working Papers (2015), arXiv:1505.04722v2; Cirillo and Taleb, "The Decline of Violent Conflicts: What Do the Data Really Say?," in *The Causes of Peace: What We Know Now,* ed. Asle Toje and Bård Nikolas Vik Steen (Austin: Lioncrest, 2020), pp. 51–77; Bear F. Braumoeller, *Only the Dead: The Persistence of War in the Modern Age* (Oxford: Oxford University Press, 2019); Aaron Clauset, "On the Frequency and Severity of Interstate Wars," in *Lewis Fry Richardson: His Intellectual Legacy and Influence in the Social Sciences* (Pioneers in Arts, Humanities, Science, Engineering, Practice, vol. 27), ed. Nils Gleditsch (Berlin: Springer, 2020), pp. 113–27.

38. Cirillo and Taleb, "Statistical Properties."

39. Alfred W. Crosby, *Ecological Imperialism: The Biological Expansion of Europe, 900–1900* (New York: Cambridge University Press, 1993). For a critique of Crosby's view of the "Columbian Exchange," which stresses the effects of exploitation and enslavement on indigenous mortality, see David S. Jones, "Virgin Soils Revisited," *William and Mary Quarterly* 60, no. 4 (2003), pp. 703–42. See also Noble David Cook, *Born to Die: Disease and New World Conquest, 1492–1650* (New York: Cambridge University Press, 1998).

40. For a comprehensive discussion, see Niall Ferguson, *The War of the World: History's Age of Hatred* (London: Penguin Press, 2006), appendix, pp. 647–54.
41. Hayes, "Statistics of Deadly Quarrels," p. 12.
42. Robert J. Barro, "Rare Disasters and Asset Markets in the Twentieth Century," *Quarterly Journal of Economics* 121, no. 3 (2006), pp. 823–66, table 1.
43. John A. Eddy, "The Maunder Minimum," *Science* 192, no. 4245 (June 18, 1976), pp. 1189–1202. See also Stephanie Pain, "1709: The Year That Europe Froze," *New Scientist*, February 4, 2009, https://www.newscientist.com/article/mg20126942-100-1709-the-year-that-europe-froze/.
44. Nicholas Dimsdale, Sally Hills, and Ryland Thomas, "The UK Recession in Context—What Do Three Centuries of Data Tell Us?," *Bank of England Quarterly Bulletin* (Q4 2010), pp. 277–91. See also David Milliken and Andy Bruce, "Bank of England Sees Worst Slump in 300 Years as Coronavirus Bites," Reuters, May 6, 2020, https://www.reuters.com/article/us-health-coronavirus-britain-boe/bank-of-england-sees-worst-slump-in-300-years-as-coronavirus-bites-idUSKBN22I3BV.
45. Gita Gopinath, "Reopening from the Great Lockdown: Uneven and Uncertain Recovery," *IMFBlog*, June 24, 2020, https://blogs.imf.org/2020/06/24/reopening-from-the-great-lockdown-uneven-and-uncertain-recovery/.
46. See also Leandro Prados de la Escosura, "Output per Head in Pre-Independence Africa: Quantitative Conjectures," Universidad Carlos III de Madrid Working Papers in Economic History (November 2012).
47. "Global Data," Fragile States Index, Fund for Peace, https://fragilestatesindex.org/data/.
48. Leandro Prados de la Escosura, "World Human Development: 1870–2007," EHES Working Paper No. 34 (January 2013).
49. Allison McCann, Jin Wu, and Josh Katz, "How the Coronavirus Compares with 100 Years of Deadly Events," *New York Times*, June 10, 2020, https://www.nytimes.com/interactive/2020/06/10/world/coronavirus-history.html. See also Jeremy Samuel Faust, Zhenqiu Lin, and Carlos del Rio, "Comparison of Estimated Excess Deaths in New York City During the COVID-19 and 1918 Influenza Pandemics," *JAMA Network Open* 3, no. 8 (2020), https://jamanetwork.com/journals/jamanetworkopen/fullarticle/2769236.
50. Edgar Jones, "The Psychology of Protecting the UK Public Against External Threat: COVID-19 and the Blitz Compared," *Lancet*, August 27, 2020, https://doi.org/10.1016/S2215-0366(20)30342-4.

Chapter 2: Cycles and Tragedies

1. Lucretius, *On the Nature of the Universe*, trans. R. E. Latham, rev. ed. (Harmondsworth, UK: Penguin, 1994), pp. 64ff.
2. Herbert Butterfield, *The Origins of History*, ed. J. H. Adam Watson (London: Eyre Methuen, 1981), p. 207.
3. Polybius, *The Rise of the Roman Empire*, trans. Ian Scott-Kilvert (Harmondsworth, UK: Penguin, 1979), pp. 41, 44; Tacitus, *The Histories*, trans. Kenneth Wellesley (Harmondsworth, UK: Penguin, 1975), p. 17.
4. Butterfield, *Origins of History*, p. 125.
5. Michael Puett, "Classical Chinese Historical Thought," in *A Companion to Global Historical Thought*, ed. Prasenjit Duara, Viren Murthy, and Andrew Sartori (Hoboken, NJ: John Wiley, 2014), pp. 34–46. See also Edwin O. Reischauer, "The Dynastic Cycle," in *The Pattern of Chinese History*, ed. John Meskill (Lexington, KY: D. C. Heath, 1965), pp. 31–33.
6. Giambattista Vico, "The New Science," in *Theories of History*, ed. Patrick Gardiner (New York: Free Press, 1959), pp. 18f.
7. Pieter Geyl and Arnold Toynbee, "Can We Know the Pattern of the Past? A Debate," in *Theories of History*, ed. Patrick Gardiner (New York: Free Press, 1959), p. 308ff. On Toynbee's monumental, briefly influential, and now almost entirely unread *A Study of History*, see Arthur Marwick, *The Nature of History*, 3rd ed. (London: Palgrave Macmillan, 1989), pp. 287f.
8. Karl Marx, *Das Kapital: A Critique of Political Economy*, trans. Serge L. Levitsky (New York: Simon & Schuster, 2012), vol. I, chapter 32.
9. David C. Baker, "The Roman Dominate from the Perspective of Demographic-Structure Theory," *Cliodynamics* 2, no. 2 (2011), pp. 217–51.
10. Leonid Grinin, "State and Socio-Political Crises in the Process of Modernization," *Cliodynamics* 3, no. 1 (2012), pp. 124–57.
11. A. Korotayev et al., "A Trap at the Escape from the Trap? Demographic-Structural Factors of Political Instability in Modern Africa and West Asia," *Cliodynamics* 2, no. 2 (2011), p. 289.
12. H. Urdal, "People vs. Malthus: Population Pressure, Environmental Degradation, and Armed Conflict Revisited," *Journal of Peace Research* 42, no. 4 (July 2005), p. 430; H. Urdal, "A Clash of Generations? Youth Bulges and Political Violence," *International Studies Quarterly* 50 (September 2006), pp. 617, 624.
13. Jack A. Goldstone et al., "A Global Model for Forecasting Political Instability," *American Journal of Political Science* 54, no. 1 (January 2010), pp. 190–208. See also J. A. Goldstone, *Revolution and Rebellion in the Early Modern World* (Berkeley: University of California Press, 1991).
14. Arthur M. Schlesinger Jr., *The Cycles of American History* (New York: Houghton Mifflin Harcourt, 1986).

15. William Strauss and Neil Howe, *The Fourth Turning: What the Cycles of History Tell Us About America's Next Rendezvous with Destiny* (New York: Three Rivers Press, 2009 [1997]).

16. Robert Huebscher, "Neil Howe—The Pandemic and the Fourth Turning," Advisor Perspectives, May 20, 2020, https://www.advisorperspectives.com/articles/2020/05/20/neil-howe-the-pandemic-and-the-fourth-turning.

17. See, e.g., W. R. Thompson, "Synthesizing Secular, Demographic-Structural, Climate, and Leadership Long Cycles: Moving Toward Explaining Domestic and World Politics in the Last Millennium," *Cliodynamics* 1, no. 1 (2010), pp. 26–57.

18. Ian Morris, "The Evolution of War," *Cliodynamics* 3, no. 1 (2012), pp. 9–37. See also S. Gavrilets, David G. Anderson, and Peter Turchin, "Cycling in the Complexity of Early Societies," *Cliodynamics* 1, no. 1 (2010), pp. 58–80.

19. Qiang Chen, "Climate Shocks, Dynastic Cycles, and Nomadic Conquests: Evidence from Historical China," School of Economics, Shandong University (October 2012).

20. See, e.g., Michael J. Storozum et al., "The Collapse of the North Song Dynasty and the AD 1048–1128 Yellow River Floods: Geoarchaeological Evidence from Northern Henan Province, China," *Holocene* 28, no. 11 (2018), https://doi.org/10.1177/0959683618788682.

21. Peter Turchin, *Historical Dynamics: Why States Rise and Fall* (Princeton, NJ: Princeton University Press, 2003), p. 93.

22. Peter Turchin, *War and Peace and War: The Rise and Fall of Empires* (New York: Plume, 2006), p. 163.

23. Peter Turchin and Sergey A. Nefedov, *Secular Cycles* (Princeton, NJ: Princeton University Press, 2009).

24. Turchin and Nefedov, *Secular Cycles*, p. 314.

25. Peter Turchin, "Arise 'Cliodynamics,'" *Nature* 454 (2008), pp. 34–35.

26. Peter Turchin, *Ages of Discord: A Structural-Demographic Analysis of American History* (Chaplin, CT: Beresta Books, 2016), p. 11.

27. Peter Turchin et al., "Quantitative Historical Analysis Uncovers a Single Dimension of Complexity That Structures Global Variation in Human Social Organization," *PNAS* 115, no. 2 (2018), pp. E144–E151.

28. Jaeweon Shin et al., "Scale and Information-Processing Thresholds in Holocene Social Evolution," *Nature Communications* 11, no. 2394 (2020), pp. 1–8, https://doi.org/10.1038/s41467-020-16035-9.

29. Shin, "Scale and Information-Processing Thresholds," p. 7.

30. Turchin and Nefedov, *Secular Cycles*.

31. Turchin, *Ages of Discord*, pp. 243f. See also Peter Turchin, "Dynamics of Political Instability in the United States, 1780–2010," *Journal of Peace Research* 49, no. 4 (July 2012), p. 12. See also Laura Spinney, "History as Science," *Nature*, August 2, 2012.

32. Turchin, *Ages of Discord*, pp. 72ff., 86ff., 91, 93, 104ff., 109f., 201–39.

33. Turchin, *Ages of Discord*, fig. 6.1.

34. Ray Dalio, "The Changing World Order: Introduction," *Principles* (blog), https://www.principles.com/the-changing-world-order/#introduction.

35. Dalio, "Changing World Order."

36. Michael Sheetz, "Ray Dalio Says 'Cash Is Trash' and Advises Investors Hold a Global, Diversified Portfolio," CNBC, January 21, 2020, https://www.cnbc.com/2020/01/21/ray-dalio-at-davos-cash-is-trash-as-everybody-wants-in-on-the-2020-market.html.

37. Andrea Saltelli et al., "Five Ways to Ensure That Models Serve Society: A Manifesto," *Nature*, June 24, 2020. See also D. Sarewitz, R. A. Pielke, and R. Byerly, *Prediction: Science, Decision Making, and the Future of Nature* (Washington, D.C.: Island Press, 2000).

38. Jared Diamond, *Collapse: How Societies Choose to Fall or Survive* (London: Penguin, 2011), p. 11.

39. Diamond, *Collapse*, p. 509.

40. Diamond, *Collapse*, pp. 118f.

41. Benny Peiser, "From Genocide to Ecocide: The Rape of Rapa Nui," *Energy and Environment* 16, nos. 3–4 (2005); Terry L. Hunt and Carl P. Lipo, "Late Colonization of Easter Island," *Science*, March 9, 2006; Hunt and Lipo, *The Statues That Walked: Unraveling the Mystery of Easter Island* (Berkeley, CA: Counterpoint Press, 2012). For Diamond's response, see Mark Lynas, "The Myths of Easter Island—Jared Diamond Responds," September 22, 2011, *Mark Lynas* (blog), https://www.marklynas.org/2011/09/the-myths-of-easter-island-jared-diamond-responds/. See also Paul Bahn and John Flenley, "Rats, Men—or Dead Ducks?," *Current World Archaeology* 49 (2017), pp. 8f.

42. Catrine Jarman, "The Truth About Easter Island," *The Conversation*, October 12, 2017, https://theconversation.com/the-truth-about-easter-island-a-sustainable-society-has-been-falsely-blamed-for-its-own-demise-85563.

43. Jared Diamond, *Upheaval: How Nations Cope with Crisis and Change* (London: Allen Lane, 2019).

44. David Mamet, "The Code and the Key," *National Review*, May 14, 2020, https://www.nationalreview.com/magazine/2020/06/01/the-code-and-the-key/.

45. Aeschylus, *Agamemnon*, in *The Oresteia*, trans. Ian Johnston (Arlington, VA: Richer Resources, 2007), loc. 599, Kindle.

46. Aeschylus, *Agamemnon*, loc. 599, 617.

47. Aeschylus, *Agamemnon*, loc. 689.

48. Aeschylus, *Agamemnon*, loc. 727, 748.

49. Aeschylus, *The Libation Bearers,* in *The Oresteia,* trans. Ian Johnston (Arlington, VA: Richer Resources, 2007), loc. 1074, Kindle.

50. Aeschylus, *The Kindly Ones,* in *The Oresteia,* trans. Ian Johnston (Arlington, VA: Richer Resources, 2007), loc. 2029, Kindle.

51. Sophocles, *Oedipus Rex,* trans. Francis Storr (London: Heinemann, 1912).

52. Richard A. Clarke and R. P. Eddy, *Warnings: Finding Cassandras to Stop Catastrophes* (New York: HarperCollins, 2018).

53. Clarke and Eddy, *Warnings,* pp. 171–76.

54. Clarke and Eddy, *Warnings,* pp. 177–81.

55. Nick Bostrom, *Anthropic Bias: Observation Selection Effects in Science and Philosophy* (New York: Routledge, 2002); Charles S. Taber and Milton Lodge, "Motivated Skepticism in the Evaluation of Political Beliefs," *American Journal of Political Science* 50, no. 3 (2006), pp. 755–69.

56. Frank H. Knight, *Risk, Uncertainty and Profit* (Boston: Houghton Mifflin, 1921). See also John A. Kay and Mervyn A. King, *Radical Uncertainty: Decision-Making Beyond the Numbers* (New York: W. W. Norton, 2020).

57. John Maynard Keynes, "The General Theory of Employment," *Quarterly Journal of Economics* 51, no. 2 (1937), p. 214.

58. Daniel Kahneman and Amos Tversky, "Prospect Theory: An Analysis of Decision Under Risk," *Econometrica* 47, no. 2 (March 1979), pp. 263–92.

59. Eliezer Yudkowsky, "Cognitive Biases Potentially Affecting Judgement of Global Risks," in *Global Catastrophic Risks,* ed. Nick Bostrom and Milan M. Ćirković (Oxford: Oxford University Press, 2008), pp. 91–119.

60. Leon Festinger, *A Theory of Cognitive Dissonance* (Stanford, CA: Stanford University Press, 1957), pp. 2f.

61. Gilbert Ryle, *The Concept of Mind* (Chicago: University of Chicago Press, 1949), p. 17.

62. Ryle, *Concept of Mind,* pp. 15f.

63. Keith Thomas, *Religion and the Decline of Magic: Studies in Popular Beliefs in Sixteenth and Seventeenth Century England* (London: Weidenfeld & Nicolson, 1971).

64. Thomas S. Kuhn, *The Structure of Scientific Revolutions* (Chicago: University of Chicago Press, 2006 [1962]).

65. See, e.g., R. M. Szydlo, I. Gabriel, E. Olavarria, and J. Apperley, "Sign of the Zodiac as a Predictor of Survival for Recipients of an Allogeneic Stem Cell Transplant for Chronic Myeloid Leukaemia (CML): An Artificial Association," *Transplantation Proceedings* 42 (2010), pp. 3312–15.

66. Philip W. Tetlock and Dan Gardiner, *Superforecasting: The Art and Science of Prediction* (New York: Crown, 2015).

67. Scott Alexander, *Slate Star Codex* (blog), April 14, 2020, https://slatestarcodex.com/2020/04/14/a-failure-but-not-of-prediction/.

68. Edward Verrall Lucas, *The Vermilion Box* (New York: George H. Doran Company, 1916), p. 343.

69. Lucas, *Vermilion Box,* pp. 342f.

70. Lucas, *Vermilion Box,* p. 346.

71. Carl Werthman, "The Police as Perceived by Negro Boys," in *The American City: A Source Book of Urban Imagery,* ed. Anselm L. Strauss (Chicago: Aldine, 1968), p. 285.

Chapter 3: Gray Rhinos, Black Swans, and Dragon Kings

1. Kevin Rawlinson, "'This Enemy Can Be Deadly': Boris Johnson Invokes Wartime Language," *Guardian,* March 17, 2020; Donald J. Trump (@realDonaldTrump), "The Invisible Enemy will soon be in full retreat!" Twitter, April 10, 2020, 9:15 a.m., https://twitter.com/realdonaldtrump/status/1248630671754563585.

2. Lawrence Freedman, "Coronavirus and the Language of War," *New Statesman,* April 11, 2020, https://www.newstatesman.com/science-tech/2020/04/coronavirus-and-language-war; Karl Eikenberry and David Kennedy Tuesday, "World War COVID-19: Who Bleeds, Who Pays?," *Lawfare* (blog), April 28, 2020, https://www.lawfareblog.com/world-war-covid-19-who-bleeds-who-pays.

3. Anne Curry, *The Hundred Years War,* 2nd ed. (Basingstoke, UK: Palgrave Macmillan, 2003), p. 5.

4. Izabella Kaminska, "Man Group's Draaisma Notes Inflation Paradigm Shift Is Possible," *Financial Times,* March 20, 2020, https://ftalphaville.ft.com/2020/03/20/1584698846000/Man-Group-s-Draaisma-notes-inflation-paradigm-shift-is-possible/.

5. John Authers, "And Now for Something Completely Different," Bloomberg, March 19, 2020, https://www.bloomberg.com/opinion/articles/2020-03-19/lagarde-s-ecb-bazooka-needs-fiscal-support-from-governments.

6. "Coronavirus Tracked," *Financial Times,* July 10, 2020, https://www.ft.com/content/a26fbf7e-48f8-11ea-aeb3-955839e06441. See also Giuliana Viglione, "How Many People Has the Coronavirus Killed?," *Nature* 585 (September 1, 2020), pp. 22–24, https://www.nature.com/articles/d41586-020-02497-w.

7. Patrick G. T. Walker et al., "The Global Impact of COVID-19 and Strategies for Mitigation and Suppression," Imperial College COVID-19 Response Team Report 12 (March 26, 2020), https://doi.org/10.25561/77735.

8. Michele Wucker, *The Gray Rhino: How to Recognize and Act on the Obvious Dangers We Ignore* (New York: Macmillan, 2016).

9. Nassim Nicholas Taleb, *The Black Swan: The Impact of the Highly Improbable* (London: Penguin/Allen Lane, 2007).

10. Peter Taylor, "Catastrophes and Insurance," in *Global Catastrophic Risks,* ed. Nick Bostrom and Milan M. Ćirković (Oxford: Oxford University Press, 2008), p. 181. See also Didier Sornette, *Critical Phenomena in Natural Sciences: Chaos, Fractals, Self-Organization and Disorder: Concepts and Tools,* 2nd ed. (Berlin: Springer, 2004).

11. Mark Buchanan, *Ubiquity: Why Catastrophes Happen* (New York: Crown, 2002).

12. Brian Hayes, "Statistics of Deadly Quarrels," *American Scientist* 90 (January–February 2002), pp. 10–15.

13. Céline Cunen, Nils Lid Hjort, and Håvard Mokleiv Nygård, "Statistical Sightings of Better Angels: Analysing the Distribution of Battle-Deaths in Interstate Conflict Over Time," *Journal of Peace Research* 57, no. 2 (2020), pp. 221–34.

14. Edward D. Lee et al., "A Scaling Theory of Armed Conflict Avalanches," April 29, 2020, arXiv:2004.14311v1.

15. Didier Sornette, "Dragon Kings, Black Swans and the Prediction of Crises," Swiss Finance Institute Research Paper Series 09-36 (2009), available at SSRN, http://ssrn.com/abstract=1470006.

16. Edward Lorenz, "Deterministic Nonperiodic Flow," *Journal of the Atmospheric Sciences* 20 (1963), pp. 130, 141.

17. Edward Lorenz, "Predictability: Does the Flap of a Butterfly's Wings in Brazil Set Off a Tornado in Texas?," presented before the American Association for the Advancement of Science, December 29, 1972.

18. Simon Kennedy and Peter Coy, "Why Are Economists So Bad at Forecasting Recessions?," *Bloomberg Businessweek,* March 27, 2019, https://www.bloomberg.com/news/articles/2019-03-28/economists-are-actually-terrible-at-forecasting-recessions.

19. Christopher G. Langton, "Computation at the Edge of Chaos: Phase Transitions and Emergent Computation," *Physica D: Nonlinear Phenomena* 42, nos. 1–3 (1990), pp. 12–37.

20. Taleb, *Black Swan,* pp. 62–84.

21. Lawrence Wright, *The Looming Tower: Al-Qaeda and the Road to 9/11* (New York: Alfred A. Knopf, 2006).

22. Paul Krugman, "Disaster and Denial," *New York Times,* December 13, 2009.

23. Melanie Mitchell, *Complexity: A Guided Tour* (New York: Oxford University Press, 2009).

24. M. Mitchell Waldrop, *Complexity: The Emerging Science at the Edge of Chaos* (New York: Simon & Schuster, 1992).

25. See John H. Holland, *Hidden Order: How Adaptation Builds Complexity* (New York: Perseus, 1995).

26. See, e.g., Stuart Kauffman, *At Home in the Universe: The Search for the Laws of Self-Organization and Complexity* (New York: Oxford University Press, 1995), p. 5.

27. Holland, *Hidden Order,* p. 5. See also John H. Holland, *Emergence: From Chaos to Order* (Reading, MA: Perseus, 1998).

28. Nassim Nicholas Taleb, "The Fourth Quadrant: A Map of the Limits of Statistics," *Edge,* September 15, 2008.

29. Niall Ferguson, *The Ascent of Money: A Financial History of the World* (New York: Penguin Press, 2008).

30. Yacov Haimes, "Systems-Based Risk Analysis," in *Global Catastrophic Risks,* ed. Nick Bostrom and Milan M. Ćirković (Oxford: Oxford University Press, 2008), pp. 161f.

31. D. C. Krakauer, "The Star Gazer and the Flesh Eater: Elements of a Theory of Metahistory," *Cliodynamics* 2, no. 1 (2011), pp. 82–105; Peter J. Richerson, "Human Cooperation Is a Complex Problem with Many Possible Solutions: Perhaps All of Them Are True!," *Cliodynamics* 4, no. 1 (2013), pp. 139–52.

32. W. R. Thompson, "Synthesizing Secular, Demographic-Structural, Climate, and Leadership Long Cycles: Explaining Domestic and World Politics in the Last Millennium," Annual Meeting of the International Studies Association, San Francisco (2008).

33. "The World Should Think Better About Catastrophic and Existential Risks," *Economist,* June 25, 2020, https://www.economist.com/briefing/2020/06/25/the-world-should-think-better-about-catastrophic-and-existential-risks.

34. John A. Eddy, "The Maunder Minimum," *Science* 192, no. 4245 (June 1976), pp. 1189–202, https://doi:10.1126/science.192.4245.1189.

35. William Napier, "Hazards from Comets and Asteroids," in *Global Catastrophic Risks,* ed. Nick Bostrom and Milan M. Ćirković (Oxford: Oxford University Press, 2008), pp. 230–35.

36. Michael M. Rampino, "Super-Volcanism and Other Geophysical Processes of Catastrophic Import," in *Global Catastrophic Risks,* ed. Nick Bostrom and Milan M. Ćirković (Oxford: Oxford University Press, 2008), pp. 214f.

37. Joseph R. McConnell et al., "Extreme Climate After Massive Eruption of Alaska's Okmok Volcano in 43 BCE and Effects on the Late Roman Republic and Ptolemaic Kingdom," *PNAS* 117, no. 27 (2020), pp. 15443–49, https://doi.org/10.1073/pnas.2002722117.
38. Giuseppe Mastrolorenzo et al., "The Avellino 3780-yr-B.P. Catastrophe as a Worst-Case Scenario for a Future Eruption at Vesuvius," *PNAS* 103, no. 12 (March 21, 2006), pp. 4366–70, https://doi.org/10.1073 /pnas.0508697103.
39. "Two Letters Written by Pliny the Younger About the Eruption of Vesuvius," Pompeii Tours, http:// www.pompeii.org.uk/s.php/tour-the-two-letters-written-by-pliny-the-elder-about-the-eruption-of -vesuvius-in-79-a-d-history-of-pompeii-en-238-s.htm.
40. Catherine Connors, "In the Land of the Giants: Greek and Roman Discourses on Vesuvius and the Phlegraean Fields," *Illinois Classical Studies* 40, no. 1 (2015), pp. 121–37. See also Andrew Wallace-Hadrill, "Pompeii—Portents of Disaster," BBC History, last updated March 29, 2011, http://www.bbc .co.uk/history/ancient/romans/pompeii_portents_01.shtml.
41. "Two Letters Written by Pliny the Younger About the Eruption of Vesuvius."
42. "Two Letters Written by Pliny the Younger About the Eruption of Vesuvius."
43. Giuseppe Mastrolorenzo et al., "Herculaneum Victims of Vesuvius in AD 79," *Nature* 410, no. 6830 (April 12, 2001), pp. 769–70, https://doi.org/10.1038/35071167.
44. Boris Behncke, "The Eruption of 1631," Geological and Mining Engineering and Sciences, Michigan Tech, January 14, 1996, http://www.geo.mtu.edu/volcanoes/boris/mirror/mirrored_html/VESUVIO _1631.html.
45. Catherine Edwards, "Italy Puzzles Over How to Save 700,000 People from Wrath of Vesuvius," *The Local,* October 13, 2016, https://www.thelocal.it/20161013/evacuation-plan-for-vesuvius-eruption -naples-campania-will-be-ready-by-october.
46. F. Lavigne et al., "Source of the Great A.D. 1257 Mystery Eruption Unveiled, Samalas Volcano, Rinjani Volcanic Complex, Indonesia," *PNAS* 110, no. 42 (2013), pp. 16742–47, https://doi.org/10.1073/pnas .1307520110.
47. Aatish Bhatia, "The Sound So Loud That It Circled the Earth Four Times," *Nautilus,* September 29, 2014, http://nautil.us/blog/the-sound-so-loud-that-it-circled-the-earth-four-times.
48. Tom Simkin and Richard S. Fiske, *Krakatau 1883: The Volcanic Eruption and Its Effects* (Washington, D.C.: Smithsonian Institution Press, 1983).
49. I. Yokoyama, "A Geophysical Interpretation of the 1883 Krakatau Eruption," *Journal of Volcanology and Geothermal Research* 9, no. 4 (March 1981), p. 359, https://doi.org/10.1016/0377-0273(81)90044-5. See also Simon Winchester, *Krakatoa: The Day the World Exploded* (London: Penguin, 2004); Benjamin Reilly, *Disaster and Human History: Case Studies in Nature, Society and Catastrophe* (Jefferson, NC, and London: McFarland, 2009), pp. 44f.
50. Reilly, *Disaster and Human History,* pp. 44f.
51. K. L. Verosub and J. Lippman, "Global Impacts of the 1600 Eruption of Peru's Huaynaputina Volcano," *Eos* 89, no. 15 (2008), pp. 141–48.
52. William S. Atwell, "Volcanism and Short-Term Climatic Change in East Asian and World History, c.1200–1699," *Journal of World History* 12, no. 1 (2001), pp. 29–98.
53. T. De Castella, "The Eruption That Changed Iceland Forever," BBC News, April 16, 2010, http://news .bbc.co.uk/1/hi/8624791.stm; J. Grattan et al., "Volcanic Air Pollution and Mortality in France 1783–1784," *C. R. Geoscience* 337, no. 7 (2005), pp. 641–51.
54. B. de Jong Boers, "Mount Tambora in 1815: A Volcanic Eruption in Indonesia and Its Aftermath," *Indonesia* 60 (1995), pp. 37–60.
55. Raymond S. Bradley, "The Explosive Volcanic Eruption Signal in Northern Hemisphere Continental Temperature Records," *Climatic Change* 12 (1988), pp. 221–43, http://www.geo.umass.edu/faculty /bradley/bradley1988.pdf.
56. Mary Bagley, "Krakatoa Volcano: Facts About 1883 Eruption," *LiveScience,* September 15, 2017, https:// www.livescience.com/28186-krakatoa.html; Stephen Self and Michael R. Rampino, "The 1883 Eruption of Krakatau," *Nature* 294 (December 24, 1981), p. 699, https://doi.org/10.1038/294699a0.
57. Alexander Koch et al., "Earth System Impacts of the European Arrival and Great Dying in the Americas After 1492," *Quaternary Science Reviews* 207 (2019), pp. 13–36. For a scathing critique, see Alberto Borettia, "The European Colonization of the Americas as an Explanation of the Little Ice Age," *Journal of Archaeological Science: Reports* 29 (February 2020).
58. John A. Matthews and Keith R. Briffa, "The 'Little Ice Age': Re-Evaluation of an Evolving Concept," *Geografiska Annaler* 87 (2005), pp. 17–36.
59. M. Kelly and Cormac Ó Gráda, "The Economic Impact of the Little Ice Age," UCD School of Economics Working Paper Series, WP10/14 (2010), pp. 1–20. See Tom de Castella, "Frost Fair: When an Elephant Walked on the Frozen River Thames," *BBC News Magazine,* January 28, 2014, https://www.bbc.com /news/magazine-25862141.
60. Atwell, "Volcanism," pp. 53, 69; Verosub and Lippman, "Global Impacts."
61. G. Neale, "How an Icelandic Volcano Helped Spark the French Revolution," *Guardian,* April 15, 2010, http://www.guardian.co.uk/world/2010/apr/15/iceland-volcano-weather-french-revolution/print.

62. De Jong Boers, "Mount Tambora in 1815."

63. Robert Coontz, "Comparing Earthquakes, Explained," *Science,* March 15, 2011, https://www.sciencemag .org/news/2011/03/comparing-earthquakes-explained.

64. U.S. Geological Survey, "Preferred Magnitudes of Selected Significant Earthquakes," June 24, 2013, https://earthquake.usgs.gov/data/sign_eqs.pdf.

65. Eduard G. Reinhardt et al., "The Tsunami of 13 December A.D. 115 and the Destruction of Herod the Great's Harbor at Caesarea Maritima, Israel," *Geology* 34, no. 12 (December 2006), pp. 1061–64, https://doi.org/10.1130/G22780A.1.

66. Mohamed Reda Sbeinati, Ryad Darawcheh, and Mikhail Mouty, "The Historical Earthquakes of Syria: An Analysis of Large and Moderate Earthquakes from 1365 B.C. to 1900 A.D.," *Annals of Geophysics* 48 (June 2005), p. 355, https://www.earth-prints.org/bitstream/2122/908/1/01Sbeinati.pdf.

67. H. Serdar Akyuz et al., "Historical Earthquake Activity of the Northern Part of the Dead Sea Fault Zone, Southern Turkey," *Tectonophysics* 426, nos. 3–4 (November 2006), p. 281.

68. Mischa Meier, "Natural Disasters in the Chronographia of John Malalas: Reflections on Their Function—An Initial Sketch," *Medieval History Journal* 10, nos. 1–2 (October 2006), p. 242, https:// doi.org/10.1177/097194580701000209.

69. Lee Mordechai, "Antioch in the Sixth Century: Resilience or Vulnerability?," in *Environment and Society in the Long Late Antiquity,* ed. Adam Izdebski and Michael Mulryan (Leiden: Koninklijke Brill, 2018), pp. 25–41.

70. G. Magri and D. Molin, *Il terremoto del dicembre 1456 nell'Appeninno centro-meridionale* (Rome: Energia Nucleare ed Energie Alternative [ENEA], 1983), pp. 1–180.

71. Umberto Fracassi and Gianluca Valensise, "Frosolone Earthquake of 1456," *Istituto Nazionale di Geofisica e Vulcanologia (INGV) Database of Individual Seismogenic Sources,* August 4, 2006, p. 20. See also C. Meletti et al., "Il terremoto del 1456 e la sua interpretazione nel quadro sismotettonico dell'Appennino Meridionale," in *Il terremoto del 1456. Osservatorio Vesuviano, storia e scienze della terra,* ed. B. Figliuolo (1998), pp. 71–108; Gruppo di Lavoro CPTI, "Catalogo Parametrico dei Terremoti Italiani, versione 2004 (CPTI04)," Istituto Nazionale di Geofisica e Vulcanologia (2004), http:// emidius.mi.ingv.it/CPTI; Enzo Boschi et al., "Catalogue of Strong Italian Earthquakes from 461 B.C. to 1997," *Annals of Geophysics* 43, no. 4 (2000), pp. 609–868, https://doi.org/10.4401/ag-3668.

72. C. Nunziata and M. R. Costanzo, "Ground Shaking Scenario at the Historical Center of Napoli (Southern Italy) for the 1456 and 1688 Earthquakes," *Pure and Applied Geophysics* 177 (January 2020), pp. 3175–90, https://doi.org/10.1007/s00024-020-02426-y.

73. A. Amoruso et al., "Spatial Reaction Between the 1908 Messina Straits Earthquake Slip and Recent Earthquake Distribution," *Geophysical Research Letters* 33, no. 17 (September 2006), p. 4, https://doi.org /10.1029/2006GL027227.

74. Giuseppe Restifo, "Local Administrative Sources on Population Movements After the Messina Earthquake of 1908," *Istituto Nazionale di Geofisica e Vulcanologia (INGV) Annals of Geophysics* 38, nos. 5–6 (November–December 1995), pp. 559–66, https://doi.org/10.4401/ag-4058; Heather Campbell, "Messina Earthquake and Tsunami of 1908," *Encyclopaedia Britannica,* January 29, 2020, https://www .britannica.com/event/Messina-earthquake-and-tsunami-of-1908.

75. Emanuela Guidoboni, "Premessa a terremoti e storia," *Quaderni Storici* 20, no. 60 (3) (December 1985), pp. 653–64, https://www.jstor.org/stable/43777325.

76. Giacomo Parrinello, "Post-Disaster Migrations and Returns in Sicily: The 1908 Messina Earthquake and the 1968 Belice Valley Earthquake," *Global Environment* 9 (2012), pp. 26–49, http://www.environmentandsociety.org/sites/default/files/key_docs/ge9_parrinello.pdf.

77. A. S. Pereira, "The Opportunity of a Disaster: The Economic Impact of the 1755 Lisbon Earthquake," *Journal of Economic History* 69, no. 2 (June 2009), pp. 466–99.

78. Pereira, "Opportunity of a Disaster," pp. 487f.

79. Gregory Clancey, "The Meiji Earthquake: Nature, Nation, and the Ambiguities of Catastrophe," *Modern Asian Studies* 40, no. 4 (2006), p. 920.

80. Gregory Clancey, "Japanese Seismicity and the Limits of Prediction," *Journal of Asian Studies* 71, no. 2 (May 2012), p. 335.

81. Christopher Sholz, "What Ever Happened to Earthquake Prediction?," *Geotimes* 17 (1997), pp. 16–19.

82. Ishibashi Katsuhiko, "Why Worry? Japan's Nuclear Plans at Growing Risk from Quake Damage," *International Herald Tribune,* August 11, 2007, reposted on *Asia-Pacific Journal: Japan Focus,* http://www .japanfocus.org/-Ishibashi-Katsuhiko/2495.

83. Richard A. Clarke and R. P. Eddy, *Warnings: Finding Cassandras to Stop Catastrophes* (New York: HarperCollins, 2018), pp. 76ff., 92, 96f.

84. Peter Symonds, "The Asian Tsunami: Why There Were No Warnings," World Socialist website, January 3, 2005, https://www.wsws.org/en/articles/2005/01/warn-j03.html.

85. "Scientist Who Warned of Tsunamis Finally Heard," NBC News, November 1, 2005, https://www .nbcnews.com/id/wbna6813771. See also Natalie Muller, "Tsunami Warning: Why Prediction Is So Hard," *Australian Geographic,* May 11, 2012, https://www.australiangeographic.com.au/topics/science -environment/2012/05/tsunami-warning-why-prediction-is-so-hard/.

86. Becky Oskin, "Two Years Later: Lessons from Japan's Tohoku Earthquake," *LiveScience,* March 10, 2013, https://www.livescience.com/27776-tohoku-two-years-later-geology.html.

87. Clarke and Eddy, *Warnings,* pp. 81–82.

88. Ari M. Beser, "One Man's Harrowing Story of Surviving the Japan Tsunami," *National Geographic,* March 23, 2016, https://blog.nationalgeographic.org/2016/03/23/exclusive-one-mans-harrowing-story -of-surviving-the-japan-tsunami/.

89. Clancey, "Japanese Seismicity," p. 333.

90. Harrison Salisbury, *The Great Black Dragon Fire* (New York: Little, Brown, 1989).

91. Rev. Peter Pernin and Stephen J. Pyne, *The Great Peshtigo Fire: An Eyewitness Account* (Madison: Wisconsin Historical Society Press, 1999), loc. 273–75, Kindle. The largest of the 2020 California wildfires, the "August Complex," is estimated to have burned just over one million acres, not quite matching Peshtigo.

92. Erin Blakemore, "Why America's Deadliest Wildfire Is Largely Forgotten Today," *History,* August 4, 2017 (updated September 1, 2018), https://www.history.com/news/why-americas-deadliest-wildfire-is -largely-forgotten-today.

93. Pernin and Pyne, *Great Peshtigo Fire,* loc. 273–75.

94. Pernin and Pyne, *Great Peshtigo Fire,* loc. 413–14.

95. Pernin and Pyne, *Great Peshtigo Fire,* loc. 437–47. See also Tom Hultquist, "The Great Midwest Fire of 1871," https://www.weather.gov/grb/peshtigofire2.

96. A. Korotayev et al., "A Trap at the Escape from the Trap? Demographic-Structural Factors of Political Instability in Modern Africa and West Asia," *Cliodynamics* 2, no. 2 (2011), pp. 276–303.

97. Thayer Watkins, "The Catastrophic Dam Failures in China in August 1975," San José State University Department of Economics, n.d., https://www.sjsu.edu/faculty/watkins/aug1975.htm.

98. Yi Si, "The World's Most Catastrophic Dam Failures: The August 1975 Collapse of the Banqiao and Shimantan Dams," in *The River Dragon Has Come!,* ed. Dai Qing (New York: M. E. Sharpe, 1998).

99. Eric Fish, "The Forgotten Legacy of the Banqiao Dam Collapse," *Economic Observer,* February 8, 2013, http://www.eeo.com.cn/ens/2013/0208/240078.shtml; Justin Higginbottom, "230,000 Died in a Dam Collapse That China Kept Secret for Years," *Ozy,* February 17, 2019, https://www.ozy.com/true-and -stories/230000-died-in-a-dam-collapse-that-china-kept-secret-for-years/91699/; Kenneth Pletcher and Gloria Lotha, "Typhoon Nina—Banqiao Dam Failure," *Encyclopaedia Britannica* (2014), https://www .britannica.com/event/Typhoon-Nina-Banqiao-dam-failure. See also N. H. Ru and Y. G. Niu, *Embankment Dam—Incidents and Safety of Large Dams* (Beijing: Water Power Press, 2001) (in Chinese).

100. Yi, "World's Most Catastrophic Dam Failures."

101. "The Three Gorges Dam in China: Forced Resettlement, Suppression of Dissent and Labor Rights Concerns," *Human Rights Watch* 7, no. 1 (February 1995), https://www.hrw.org/reports/1995/China1 .htm.

102. David Schoenbrod, "The Lawsuit That Sank New Orleans," *Wall Street Journal,* September 26, 2005, http://online.wsj.com/article/SB112769984088951774.html.

103. Lawrence H. Roth, "The New Orleans Levees: The Worst Engineering Catastrophe in US History— What Went Wrong and Why," seminar given at Auburn University College of Engineering, April 5, 2007, https://web.archive.org/web/20071015234208/http://eng.auburn.edu/admin/marketing/semi nars/2007/l-roth.html.

104. Rawle O. King, "Hurricane Katrina: Insurance Losses and National Capacities for Financing Disaster Risks," Congressional Research Service Report for Congress, January 31, 2008, table 1.

105. John Schwartz, "One Billion Dollars Later, New Orleans Is Still at Risk," *New York Times,* August 17, 2007; Michael Lewis, "In Nature's Casino," *New York Times Magazine,* August 26, 2007.

106. Clarke and Eddy, *Warnings,* pp. 41–45.

107. Louise K. Comfort, "Cities at Risk: Hurricane Katrina and the Drowning of New Orleans," *Urban Affairs Review* 41, no. 4 (March 2006), pp. 501–16.

108. Clarke and Eddy, *Warnings,* pp. 47–54.

109. U.S. House of Representatives, *A Failure of Initiative: Final Report of the Select Bipartisan Committee to Investigate the Preparation for and Response to Hurricane Katrina* (Washington, D.C.: U.S. Government Printing Office, 2006), https://www.nrc.gov/docs/ML1209/ML12093A081.pdf.

110. Neil L. Frank and S. A. Husain, "The Deadliest Tropical Cyclone in History?," *Bulletin of the American Meteorological Society* 52, no. 6 (June 1971), p. 441.

111. "A Brief History of the Deadliest Cyclones in the Bay of Bengal," *Business Standard,* May 19, 2020, https://tbsnews.net/environment/brief-history-deadliest-cyclones-bay-bengal-83323.

112. Frank and Husain, "Deadliest Tropical Cyclone," p. 443.

113. Jack Anderson, "Many Pakistan Flood Victims Died Needlessly," *Lowell Sun,* January 31, 1971, https:// www.newspapers.com/clip/2956402/many-pakistan-flood-victims-died/.

114. N. D. Kondratieff and W. F. Stolper, "The Long Waves in Economic Life," *Review of Economics and Statistics* 17, no. 6 (November 1935), pp. 105–15.

115. Paul Schmelzing, "Eight Centuries of Global Real Rates, R-G, and the 'Suprasecular Decline,' 1311– 2018" (PhD diss., Harvard University, August 2019). See, for a summary, Paul Schmelzing, "Eight Centuries of Global Real Interest Rates, R-G, and the 'Suprasecular' Decline, 1311–2018," Bank of England

Staff Working Paper No. 845 (January 2020), https://www.bankofengland.co.uk/working-paper
/2020/eight-centuries-of-global-real-interest-rates-r-g-and-the-suprasecular-decline-1311-2018.

Chapter 4: Networld

1. George R. Havens, "The Conclusion of Voltaire's Poème sur le désastre de Lisbonne," *Modern Language Notes* 56 (June 1941), pp. 422–26. See also Peter Gay, *The Enlightenment: An Interpretation,* vol. I (New York: W. W. Norton, 1995), pp. 51f.

2. Voltaire, "The Lisbon Earthquake," in *Candide, or Optimism,* trans. Tobias Smollett (London: Penguin, 2005).

3. John T. Scott, "Pride and Providence: Religion in Rousseau's Lettre à Voltaire sur la providence," in *Rousseau and l'Infâme: Religion, Toleration, and Fanaticism in the Age of Enlightenment,* ed. Ourida Mostefai and John T. Scott (Amsterdam and New York: Editions Rodopi, 2009), pp. 116–32.

4. Catriona Seth, "Why Is There an Earthquake in Candide?," Oxford University, https://bookshelf.mml
.ox.ac.uk/2017/03/29/why-is-there-an-earthquake-in-candide/.

5. Maria Teodora et al., "The French Enlightenment Network," *Journal of Modern History* 88, no. 3 (September 2016), pp. 495–534.

6. Julie Danskin, "The 'Hotbed of Genius': Edinburgh's Literati and the Community of the Scottish Enlightenment," *eSharp,* special issue 7: *Real and Imagined Communities* (2013), pp. 1–16.

7. Adam Smith, *The Theory of Moral Sentiments* (Los Angeles: Enhanced Media Publishing, 2016 [1759]), p. 157.

8. Claud Cockburn, *In Time of Trouble: An Autobiography* (London: Hart-Davis, 1957), p. 125.

9. "'Times' Not Amused by Parody Issue," *New York,* July 30, 1979, p. 8.

10. Geoffrey West, *Scale: The Universal Laws of Growth, Innovation, Sustainability, and the Pace of Life in Organisms, Cities, Economies, and Companies* (New York: Penguin Press, 2017).

11. Steven H. Strogatz, "Exploring Complex Networks," *Nature* 410 (March 8, 2001), pp. 268–76.

12. Duncan J. Watts, "Networks, Dynamics, and the Small-World Phenomenon," *American Journal of Sociology* 105, no. 2 (1999), p. 515.

13. Geoffrey West, "Can There Be a Quantitative Theory for the History of Life and Society?," *Cliodynamics* 2, no. 1 (2011), pp. 211f.

14. Guido Caldarelli and Michele Catanzaro, *Networks: A Very Short Introduction* (Oxford: Oxford University Press, 2011), pp. 23f.

15. Joseph Henrich, *The Secret of Our Success: How Culture Is Driving Human Evolution, Domesticating Our Species, and Making Us Smarter* (Princeton, NJ: Princeton University Press, 2016), p. 5.

16. R. I. M. Dunbar, "Coevolution of Neocortical Size, Group Size and Language in Humans," *Behavioral and Brain Sciences* 16, no. 4 (1993), pp. 681–735.

17. Nicholas A. Christakis and James H. Fowler, *Connected: The Surprising Power of Our Social Networks and How They Shape Our Lives* (New York: Little, Brown (2009), p. 239.

18. Michael Tomasello et al., "Two Key Steps in the Evolution of Human Cooperation: The Interdependence Hypothesis," *Current Anthropology* 53, no. 6 (2012), pp. 673–92.

19. Douglas S. Massey, "A Brief History of Human Society: The Origin and Role of Emotion in Social Life," *American Sociological Review* 67, no. 1 (2002), pp. 3–6.

20. J. R. McNeill and William McNeill, *The Human Web: A Bird's-Eye View of Human History* (New York and London: W. W. Norton, 2003).

21. Niall Ferguson, *The Square and the Tower: Networks and Power from the Freemasons to Facebook* (New York: Penguin Press, 2018).

22. Shin-Kap Han, "The Other Ride of Paul Revere: The Brokerage Role in the Making of the American Revolution," *Mobilization: An International Quarterly* 14, no. 2 (2009), pp. 143–62.

23. Duncan J. Watts, *Six Degrees: The Science of a Connected Age* (London: Vintage, 2004), p. 134.

24. Albert-László Barabási, *Linked: How Everything Is Connected to Everything Else and What It Means for Business, Science, and Everyday Life* (New York: Basic Books, 2014), p. 29.

25. Miller McPherson, Lynn Smith-Lovin, and James M. Cook, "Birds of a Feather: Homophily in Social Networks," *Annual Review of Sociology* 27 (2001), p. 419.

26. Mark Granovetter, "The Strength of Weak Ties," *American Journal of Sociology* 78, no. 6 (1973), pp. 1360–80.

27. Mark Granovetter, "The Strength of Weak Ties: A Network Theory Revisited," *Sociological Theory* 1 (1983), p. 202.

28. Andreas Tutic and Harald Wiese, "Reconstructing Granovetter's Network Theory," *Social Networks* 43 (2015), pp. 136–48.

29. Duncan J. Watts and Steven H. Strogatz, "Collective Dynamics of 'Small-World' Networks," *Nature* 393 (June 4, 1998), pp. 400–42.

30. Watts, "Networks, Dynamics, and the Small-World Phenomenon," p. 522.

31. Christakis and Fowler, *Connected,* p. 97.

32. Eugenia Roldán Vera and Thomas Schupp, "Network Analysis in Comparative Social Sciences," *Comparative Education* 43, no. 3, pp. 418f.

33. Matthew O. Jackson, "Networks in the Understanding of Economic Behaviors," *Journal of Economic Perspectives* 28, no. 4 (2014), p. 8.
34. Alison L. Hill et al., "Emotions as Infectious Diseases in a Large Social Network: The SISa Model," *Proceedings of the Royal Society B: Biological Sciences* (2010), pp. 1–9.
35. Peter Dolton, "Identifying Social Network Effects," *Economic Report* 93, supp. S1 (2017), pp. 1–15.
36. Christakis and Fowler, *Connected*, p. 22.
37. Charles Kadushin, *Understanding Social Networks: Theories, Concepts, and Findings* (New York: Oxford University Press, 2012), pp. 209f.
38. Karine Nahon and Jeff Hemsley, *Going Viral* (Cambridge, UK: Polity, 2013).
39. Damon Centola and Michael Macy, "Complex Contagions and the Weakness of Long Ties," *American Journal of Sociology* 113, no. 3 (2007), pp. 702–34.
40. Watts, *Six Degrees*, p. 249.
41. Sherwin Rosen, "The Economics of Superstars," *American Economic Review* 71, no. 5 (1981), pp. 845–58.
42. Albert-László Barabási and Réka Albert, "Emergence of Scaling in Random Networks," *Science* 286, no. 5439 (1999), pp. 509–12.
43. Barabási, *Linked*, pp. 33–34, 66, 68f., 204.
44. Barabási, *Linked*, p. 221.
45. Barabási, *Linked*, p. 103, 221. For an important critique of Barabási and Albert's central claim that scale-free networks are common, see Anna D. Broido and Aaron Clauset, "Scale-Free Networks Are Rare," January 9, 2018, arXiv:1801.03400v1.
46. Vittoria Colizza, Alain Barrat, Marc Barthélemy, and Alessandro Vespignani, "The Role of the Airline Transportation Network in the Prediction and Predictability of Global Epidemics," *PNAS* 103, no. 7 (2006), pp. 2015–20.
47. Dolton, "Identifying Social Network Effects."
48. Romualdo Pastor-Satorras and Alessandro Vespignani, "Immunization of Complex Networks," Abdus Salam International Centre for Theoretical Physics, February 1, 2008.
49. Strogatz, "Exploring Complex Networks."
50. Niall Ferguson, "Complexity and Collapse: Empires on the Edge of Chaos," *Foreign Affairs* 89, no. 2 (March/April 2010), pp. 18–32.
51. Barabási, *Linked*, pp. 113–18.
52. Barabási, *Linked*, p. 135.
53. Dorothy H. Crawford, *Deadly Companions: How Microbes Shaped Our History* (Oxford: Oxford University Press, 2007).
54. Angus Deaton, *The Great Escape: Health, Wealth, and the Origins of Inequality* (Princeton, NJ: Princeton University Press, 2015).
55. Edward Jenner, *An Inquiry into the Causes and Effects of the Variolae Vaccinae* (1798), quoted in Daniel J. Sargent, "Strategy and Biosecurity: An Applied History Perspective," paper prepared for the Hoover History Working Group, June 18, 2020.
56. Crawford, *Deadly Companions*, pp. 13f.
57. M. B. A. Oldstone, *Viruses, Plagues, and History: Past, Present, and Future* (Oxford and New York: Oxford University Press, 2010).
58. M. B. A. Oldstone and J. C. De La Torre, "Viral Diseases of the Next Century," *Transactions of the American Clinical and Climatological Association* 105 (1994), pp. 62–68.
59. A. Moya et al., "The Population Genetics and Evolutionary Epidemiology of RNA Viruses," *Nature Reviews* 2 (2004), pp. 279–88; P. Simmonds, "Virus Evolution," *Microbiology Today* (May 2009), pp. 96–99; R. Ehrenberg, "Enter the Viros: As Evidence of the Influence of Viruses Escalates, Appreciation of These Master Manipulators Grows," *Science News* 176, no. 8 (October 10, 2009), pp. 22–25; G. Hamilton, "Viruses: The Unsung Heroes of Evolution," *New Scientist* 2671 (August 2008), pp. 38–41, http://www.newscientist.com/article/mg19926711.600-viruses-the-unsung-heroes-of-evolution.html.
60. Crawford, *Deadly Companions*, pp. 25, 43.
61. M. Achtman et al., "*Yersinia pestis*, the Cause of Plague, Is a Recently Emerged Clone of *Yersinia pseudotuberculosis*," *PNAS* 96, no. 24 (1999), pp. 14043–48. See also G. Morelli et al., "*Yersinia pestis* Genome Sequencing Identifies Patterns of Global Phylogenetic Diversity," *Nature Genetics* 42, no. 12 (2010), pp. 1140–43.
62. Crawford, *Deadly Companions*, pp. 96f. See also Richard E. Lenski, "Evolution of the Plague Bacillus," *Nature* 334 (August 1988), pp. 473f.; Stewart T. Cole and Carmen Buchrieser, "A Plague o' Both Your Hosts," *Nature* 413 (2001), pp. 467ff.; Thomas V. Inglesby et al., "Plague as a Biological Weapon," *Journal of the American Medical Association* 283, no. 17 (2000), pp. 2281–90.
63. R. Rosqvist, Mikael Skurnik, and Hans Wolf-Watz, "Increased Virulence of *Yersinia pseudotuberculosis* by Two Independent Mutations," *Nature* 334 (August 1988), pp. 522–25.
64. S. Ayyadurai et al., "Body Lice, *Yersinia pestis* Orientalis, and Black Death," *Emerging Infectious Diseases* 16, no. 5 (2010), pp. 892–93.
65. Stephen M. Kaciv, Eric J. Frehm, and Alan S. Segal, "Case Studies in Cholera: Lessons in Medical History and Science," *Yale Journal of Biology and Medicine* 72 (1999), pp. 393–408.
66. Crawford, *Deadly Companions*, pp. 96f., 109.

67. World Health Organization, "Yellow Fever Fact Sheet No. 100" (May 2013), http://www.who.int/me diacentre/factsheets/fs100/en/.

68. Alice F. Weissfeld, "Infectious Diseases and Famous People Who Succumbed to Them," *Clinical Microbiology Newsletter* 31, no. 22 (2009), pp. 169–72.

69. Nathan D. Wolfe et al., "Origins of Major Human Infectious Diseases," *Nature* 447, no. 7142 (2007), pp. 279–83, http://www.ncbi.nlm.nih.gov/books/NBK114494/; Robin A. Weiss, "The Leeuwenhoek Lecture, 2001: Animal Origins of Human Infectious Diseases," *Philosophical Transactions of the Royal Society Biological Sciences* 356 (2001), pp. 957–77.

70. David Quammen, *Spillover: Animal Infections and the Next Human Pandemic* (New York: W. W. Norton, 2012).

71. L. Dethlefsen et al., "An Ecological and Evolutionary Perspective on Human-Microbe Mutualism and Disease," *Nature* 449 (October 2007), pp. 811–18.

72. Thucydides, *The History of the Peloponnesian War,* trans. Richard Crawley (Project Gutenberg, 2009), book I, chap. 1.

73. Kyle Harper, *The Fate of Rome: Climate, Disease, and the End of an Empire* (Princeton, NJ: Princeton University Press, 2017).

74. Edward Gibbon, *The Decline and Fall of the Roman Empire* (New York: Harper & Bros., 1836), vol. I, chap. 10, part IV.

75. Guido Alfani and Tommy E. Murphy, "Plague and Lethal Epidemics in the Pre-Industrial World," *Journal of Economic History* 77, no. 1 (March 2017), pp. 316f.

76. R. P. Duncan-Jones, "The Impact of the Antonine Plague," *Journal of Roman Archaeology* 9 (1996), pp. 108–36, https://doi:10.1017/S1047759400016524; R. P. Duncan-Jones, "The Antonine Plague Revisited," *Arctos* 52 (2018), pp. 41–72.

77. Rodney Stark, "Epidemics, Networks, and the Rise of Christianity," *Semeia* 56 (1992), pp. 159–75.

78. Gibbon, *Decline and Fall,* vol. IV, chap. 43, part IV.

79. Gibbon, *Decline and Fall.*

80. Lee Mordechai et al., "The Justinianic Plague: An Inconsequential Pandemic?," *PNAS* 116, no. 51 (2019), pp. 25546–54, https://doi.org/10.1073/pnas.1903797116.

81. Elizabeth Kolbert, "Pandemics and the Shape of Human History," *New Yorker,* March 30, 2020, https://www.newyorker.com/magazine/2020/04/06/pandemics-and-the-shape-of-human-history.

82. Gibbon, *Decline and Fall,* vol. IV, chap. 43, part IV.

83. Matthew O. Jackson, Brian W. Rogers, and Yves Zenou, "Connections in the Modern World: Network-Based Insights," *VoxEU & CEPR,* March 6, 2015, https://voxeu.org/article/network-based-insights -economists.

84. J. Theilmann and Frances Cate, "A Plague of Plagues: The Problem of Plague Diagnosis in Medieval England," *Journal of Interdisciplinary History* 37, no. 3 (2007), pp. 371–93.

85. M. Drancourt et al., "*Yersinia pestis* Orientalis in Remains of Ancient Plague Patients," *Emerging Infectious Diseases* 13, no. 2 (2007), pp. 332–33; S. Haensch et al., "Distinct Clones of *Yersinia pestis* Caused the Black Death," *PLOS Pathogens* 6, no. 10 (2010), pp. 1–8.

86. Manny Rincon Cruz, "Contagion, Borders, and Scale: Lessons from Network Science and History," Hoover History Working Group, June 24, 2020.

87. Mark Bailey, "After the Black Death: Society, Economy and the Law in Fourteenth-Century England," James Ford Lectures, 2019, Lecture 1: "Old Problems, New Approaches," https://www.history.ox.ac .uk/event/the-james-ford-lectures-old-problems-new-approaches.

88. Mark Bailey, "After the Black Death," Lecture 2: "Reaction and Regulation," https://www.history.ox .ac.uk/event/the-james-ford-lectures-reaction-and-regulation.

89. N. C. Stenseth et al., "Plague Dynamics Are Driven by Climate Variation," *PNAS* 103, no. 35 (2006), pp. 13110–15.

90. Mark R. Welford and Brian H. Bossak, "Validation of Inverse Seasonal Peak Mortality in Medieval Plagues, Including the Black Death, in Comparison to Modern *Yersinia pestis*-Variant Diseases," *PLOS One* 4, no. 12 (2009), pp. 1–6.

91. Stenseth et al., "Plague Dynamics."

92. Stenseth et al., "Plague Dynamics." See also Ayyadurai et al., "Body Lice."

93. Ferguson, *Square and the Tower,* p. 431.

94. Rincon Cruz, "Contagion, Borders, and Scale." See also Mark Koyama, Remi Jedwab, and Noel Johnson, "Pandemics, Places, and Populations: Evidence from the Black Death," Centre for Economic Policy Research Discussion Paper No. 13523 (2019).

95. Maarten Bosker, Steven Brakman, Harry Garretsen, Herman De Jong, and Marc Schramm, "Ports, Plagues and Politics: Explaining Italian City Growth 1300–1861," *European Review of Economic History* 12, no. 1 (2008), pp. 97–131, https://doi.org/10.1017/S1361491608002128.

96. Ricardo A. Olea and George Christakos, "Duration of Urban Mortality for the 14th-Century Black Death Epidemic," *Human Biology* 77, no. 3 (2005), pp. 291–303, https://doi.org/10.1353/hub.2005.0051.

97. José M. Gómez and Miguel Verdú, "Network Theory May Explain the Vulnerability of Medieval Human Settlements to the Black Death Pandemic," *Nature Scientific Reports,* March 6, 2017, https://www.nature .com/articles/srep43467.

98. Oscar Jorda, Sanjay R. Singh, and Alan M. Taylor, "Longer-Run Economic Consequences of Pandemics," Federal Reserve Bank of San Francisco Working Paper 2020-09 (March 2020).
99. Gregory Clark, *A Farewell to Alms: A Brief Economic History of the World* (Princeton, NJ: Princeton University Press, 2007). See also Paul Schmelzing, "Eight Centuries of Global Real Rates, R-G, and the 'Suprasecular Decline,' 1311–2018" (PhD diss., Harvard University, August 2019).
100. Mark Bailey, "A Mystery Within an Enigma: The Economy, 1355–1375," Ford Lectures 2019, Lecture 3, https://www.history.ox.ac.uk/event/the-james-ford-lectures-a-mystery-within-an-enigma-the-economy-1355-75.
101. Mark Bailey, "The End of Serfdom and the Rise of the West," Ford Lectures 2019, Lecture 6, https://www.history.ox.ac.uk/event/the-james-ford-lectures-the-end-of-serfdom-and-the-rise-of-the-west.
102. Mark Bailey, "Injustice and Revolt," Ford Lectures 2019, Lecture 4, https://www.history.ox.ac.uk/event/the-james-ford-lectures-injustice-and-revolt.
103. Mark Bailey, "A New Equilibrium," Ford Lectures 2019, Lecture 5, https://www.history.ox.ac.uk/event/the-james-ford-lectures-a-new-equilibrium-c.1375-1400.
104. Bailey, "The End of Serfdom," Ford Lectures 2019, Lecture 6.
105. Alexander Lee, "What Machiavelli Knew About Pandemics," *New Statesman,* June 3, 2020, https://www.newstatesman.com/2020/06/what-machiavelli-knew-about-pandemics; Eleanor Russell and Martin Parker, "How Pandemics Past and Present Fuel the Rise of Mega-Corporations," *The Conversation,* June 3, 2020, https://theconversation.com/how-pandemics-past-and-present-fuel-the-rise-of-mega-corporations-137732; Paula Findlen, "What Would Boccaccio Say About COVID-19?," *Boston Review,* April 24, 2020, http://bostonreview.net/arts-society/paula-findlen-what-would-boccaccio-say-about-covid-19.
106. Richard Trexler, *Public Life in Renaissance Florence* (New York: Academic Press, 1980), p. 362.
107. Norman Cohn, *The Pursuit of the Millennium* (New York: Oxford University Press, 1961 [1957]), pp. 132f.
108. Nico Voigtlander and Hans-Joachim Voth, "Persecution Perpetuated: The Medieval Origins of Anti-Semitic Violence in Nazi Germany," *Quarterly Journal of Economics* 127, no. 3 (August 2012), pp. 1339–92, https://www.jstor.org/stable/23251987.
109. Samuel K. Cohn Jr., "The Black Death and the Burning of Jews," *Past and Present* 196 (August 2007), pp. 3–36.
110. Cohn, "The Black Death," pp. 87, 136–40.
111. M. W. Flinn, "Plague in Europe and the Mediterranean Countries," *Journal of European Economic History* 8, no. 1 (1979), pp. 134–47.
112. Stephen Greenblatt, "What Shakespeare Actually Wrote About the Plague," *New Yorker,* May 7, 2020.
113. Daniel Defoe, *A Journal of the Plague Year* (London: Penguin, 2003 [1722]).
114. Charles F. Mullett, "The English Plague Scare of 1720–30," *Osiris* 2 (1936), pp. 484–516.
115. Defoe, *Journal,* pp. 18f.
116. Defoe, *Journal,* p. 172.
117. Defoe, *Journal,* p. 66.
118. Gibbon, *Decline and Fall,* vol. IV, chap. 43, part IV.
119. Defoe, *Journal,* p. 9.
120. Defoe, *Journal,* pp. 40f.

Chapter 5: The Science Delusion

1. Quoted in Roy MacLeod and M. Lewis, eds., *Disease, Medicine and Empire: Perspectives on Western Medicine and the Experience of European Expansion* (London and New York: Routledge, 1988), p. 7.
2. Niall Ferguson, *Civilization: The West and the Rest* (New York: Penguin Press, 2011).
3. John Jennings White III, "Typhus: Napoleon's Tragic Invasion of Russia, the War of 1812," in *Epidemics and War: The Impact of Disease on Major Conflicts in History,* ed. Rebecca M. Seaman (Santa Barbara, CA: ABC-CLIO, 2018), pp. 74f.
4. Richard Bonney, *The Thirty Years' War 1618–1648* (New York: Bloomsbury, 2014).
5. T. Nguyen-Hieu et al., "Evidence of a Louse-Borne Outbreak Involving Typhus in Douai, 1710–1712 During the War of the Spanish Succession," *PLOS One* 5, no. 10 (2010), pp. 1–8. See, in general, Joseph M. Conlon, "The Historical Impact of Epidemic Typhus" (2009), www.entomology.montana.edu/history bug/TYPHUS-Conlon.pdf.
6. Dominic Lieven, *Russia Against Napoleon: The True Story of the Campaigns of War and Peace* (New York: Viking, 2010).
7. D. Raoult et al., "Evidence for Louse-Transmitted Diseases in Soldiers of Napoleon's Grand Army in Vilnius," *Journal of Infectious Diseases* 193 (2006), pp. 112–20.
8. Alfred W. Crosby, *Ecological Imperialism: The Biological Expansion of Europe, 900–1900* (New York: Cambridge University Press, 1993); Noble David Cook, *Born to Die: Disease and New World Conquest, 1492–1650* (New York: Cambridge University Press, 1998). For a critique of the "virgin soil" framework, stressing the effects of exploitation and enslavement on indigenous mortality, see David S. Jones, "Virgin Soils Revisited," *William and Mary Quarterly* 60, no. 4 (2003), pp. 703–42.

9. Angus Chen, "One of History's Worst Epidemics May Have Been Caused by a Common Microbe," *Science,* January 16, 2018, https://doi.org/10.1126/science.aat0253.

10. Niall Ferguson, *Empire: How Britain Made the Modern World* (London: Penguin, 2003), p. 65.

11. John E. Lobdell and Douglas Owsley, "The Origin of Syphilis," *Journal of Sex Research* 10, no. 1 (1974), pp. 76–79; Bruce M. Rothschild et al., "First European Exposure to Syphilis: The Dominican Republic at the Time of Columbian Contact," *Clinical Infectious Diseases* 31, no. 4 (2000), pp. 936–41; Robert M. May et al., "Infectious Disease Dynamics: What Characterizes a Successful Invader?," *Philosophical Transactions of the Royal Society* 356 (2001), pp. 901–10; Bruce M. Rothschild, "History of Syphilis," *Clinical Infectious Diseases* 40, no. 10 (2005), pp. 1454–63; George J. Armelagos et al., "The Science Behind Pre-Columbian Evidence of Syphilis in Europe: Research by Documentary," *Evolutionary Anthropology* 21 (2012), pp. 50–57.

12. Dorothy H. Crawford, *Deadly Companions: How Microbes Shaped Our History* (Oxford: Oxford University Press, 2007), pp. 129ff.

13. J. R. McNeill, *Mosquito Empires: Ecology and War in the Greater Caribbean, 1620–1914* (New York: Cambridge University Press, 2010); Jason Sharman, *Empires of the Weak: The Real Story of European Expansion and the Creation of the New World Order* (Princeton, NJ: Princeton University Press, 2019).

14. M. B. A. Oldstone, *Viruses, Plagues, and History: Past, Present, and Future* (Oxford and New York: Oxford University Press, 2010), p. 103. See also J. R. McNeill, "Yellow Jack and Geopolitics: Environment, Epidemics, and the Struggles for Empire in the American Tropics, 1650–1825," *OAH Magazine of History,* April 2004, pp. 9–13.

15. McNeill, "Yellow Jack."

16. Emmanuel Le Roy Ladurie, "A Concept: The Unification of the Globe by Disease," in *The Mind and Method of the Historian* (Chicago: University of Chicago Press, 1981), pp. 28–91.

17. Ferguson, *Empire,* pp. 70, 170.

18. Ferguson, *Civilization,* p. 168.

19. Louis-Ferdinand Céline, *Journey to the End of the Night,* trans. Ralph Manheim (New York: New Directions, 2006 [1934]), p. 126.

20. Ferguson, *Empire,* pp. 167–70.

21. Disappointingly overlooked in William Dalrymple, *The Anarchy: The East India Company, Corporate Violence and the Pillage of an Empire* (New York: Bloomsbury, 2019).

22. Stephen M. Kaciv, Eric J. Frehm, and Alan S. Segal, "Case Studies in Cholera: Lessons in Medical History and Science," *Yale Journal of Biology and Medicine* 72 (1999), pp. 393–408. See also Jim Harris, "Pandemics: Today and Yesterday," *Origins* 13, no. 10 (2020).

23. R. E. McGrew, "The First Cholera Epidemic and Social History," *Bulletin of the History of Medicine* 34, no. 1 (January–February 1960), pp. 61–73.

24. Richard J. Evans, *Death in Hamburg: Society and Politics in the Cholera Years, 1830–1910* (Oxford: Oxford University Press, 1987), p. 313.

25. M. Echenberg, "Pestis Redux: The Initial Years of the Third Bubonic Plague Pandemic, 1894–1901," *Journal of World History* 13, no. 2 (2002), pp. 429–49.

26. Ballard C. Campbell, *Disasters, Accidents, and Crises in American History: A Reference Guide to the Nation's Most Catastrophic Events* (New York: Facts on File, 2008), pp. 182–84.

27. Sarah F. Vanneste, "The Black Death and the Future of Medicine" (unpublished master's thesis, Wayne State University, 2010), pp. 41, 77.

28. Alexander Lee, "What Machiavelli Knew About Pandemics," *New Statesman,* June 3, 2020, https://www.newstatesman.com/2020/06/what-machiavelli-knew-about-pandemics.

29. Nancy G. Siraisi, *Medieval and Early Renaissance Medicine: An Introduction to Knowledge and Practice* (Chicago: University of Chicago Press, 1990); Ismail H. Abdalla, "Diffusion of Islamic Medicine into Hausaland," in *The Social Basis of Health and Healing in Africa,* ed. Steven Feierman and John M. Janzen (Berkeley: University of California Press, 1992).

30. Richard Palmer, "The Church, Leprosy, and Plague in Medieval and Early Modern Europe," in *The Church and Healing,* ed. W. J. Shiels (Oxford: Basil Blackwell, 1982), p. 96.

31. S. White, "Rethinking Disease in Ottoman History," *International Journal of Middle East Studies* 42 (2010), p. 554.

32. Manny Rincon Cruz, "Contagion, Borders, and Scale: Lessons from Network Science and History," Hoover History Working Group, June 24, 2020.

33. Gianfranco Gensini, Magdi H. Yacoub, and Andrea A. Conti, "The Concept of Quarantine in History: From Plague to SARS," *Journal of Infection* 49, no. 4 (November 1, 2004), pp. 257–61; Eugenia Tognotti, "Lessons from the History of Quarantine, from Plague to Influenza A," *Emerging Infectious Diseases* 19, no. 2 (February 2013), pp. 254–59.

34. Frank M. Snowden, *Epidemics and Society: From the Black Death to the Present* (New Haven, CT: Yale University Press, 2019), p. 70.

35. See John Henderson, *Florence Under Siege: Surviving Plague in an Early Modern City* (New Haven, CT: Yale University Press, 2019).

36. Rincon Cruz, "Contagion, Borders, and Scale."

37. Alexander William Kinglake, *Eothen, or Traces of Travel Brought Home from the East* (New York: D. Appleton, 1899 [1844]), p. 1.

38. A. Wess Mitchell and Charles Ingrao, "Emperor Joseph's Solution to Coronavirus," *Wall Street Journal,* April 6, 2020, https://www.wsj.com/articles/emperor-josephs-solution-to-coronavirus-11586214561; Snowden, *Epidemics and Society,* pp. 72–73; Gunther Rothenberg, "The Austrian Sanitary Cordon and the Control of the Bubonic Plague: 1710–1871," *Journal of the History of Medicine and Allied Sciences* 28, no. 1 (1973), pp. 15–23.

39. Simon Schama, "Plague Time: Simon Schama on What History Tells Us," *Financial Times,* April 10, 2020, https://www.ft.com/content/279dee4a-740b-11ea-95fe-fcd274e920ca.

40. Norman Howard-Jones, "Fracastoro and Henle: A Re-appraisal of Their Contribution to the Concept of Communicable Diseases," *Medical History* 21, no. 1 (1977), pp. 61–68, https://doi.org/10.1017/S0025727300037170; V. Nutton, "The Reception of Fracastoro's Theory of Contagion: The Seed That Fell Among Thorns?," *Osiris* 6 (1990), pp. 196–234.

41. Ferguson, *Empire,* p. 9.

42. Cary P. Gross and Kent A. Sepkowitz, "The Myth of the Medical Breakthrough: Smallpox, Vaccination, and Jenner Reconsidered," *International Journal of Infectious Disease* 3 (1998), pp. 54–60; S. Riedel, "Edward Jenner and the History of Smallpox and Vaccination," *Baylor University Medical Center Proceedings* 18 (2005), pp. 21–25.

43. John D. Burton, "'The Awful Judgements of God upon the Land': Smallpox in Colonial Cambridge, Massachusetts," *New England Quarterly* 74, no. 3 (2001), pp. 495–506. See also Elizabeth A. Fenn, *Pox Americana: The Great Smallpox Epidemic of 1775–82* (New York: Farrar, Straus and Giroux, 2002).

44. Gross and Sepkowitz, "Myth of the Medical Breakthrough," p. 57.

45. Burton, "'Awful Judgements of God,'" p. 499.

46. Edward Edwardes, *A Concise History of Small-pox and Vaccination in Europe* (London: H. K. Lewis, 1902).

47. Charles E. Rosenberg, *The Cholera Years: The United States in 1832, 1849, and 1866* (Chicago and London: University of Chicago Press, 1987), pp. 66f.

48. Dona Schneider and David E. Lilienfeld, "History and Scope of Epidemiology," in *Lilienfeld's Foundations of Epidemiology,* 4th ed. (Oxford: Oxford University Press, 2015), pp. 1–53.

49. V. Curtis, "Dirt, Disgust and Disease: A Natural History of Hygiene," *Journal of Epidemiology and Community Health* 61 (2007), pp. 660–64; M. Best and D. Neuhauser, "Ignaz Semmelweis and the Birth of Infection Control," *Quality and Safety in Health Care* 13 (2004), pp. 233–34; K. Codell Carter, "Ignaz Semmelweis, Carl Mayrhofer, and the Rise of Germ Theory," *Medical History* 29 (1985), pp. 33–53; K. Codell Carter, "Koch's Postulates in Relation to the Work of Jacob Henle and Edwin Klebs," *Medical History* 29 (1985), pp. 353–74.

50. Muhammad H. Zaman, *Biography of Resistance: The Epic Battle Between People and Pathogens* (New York: HarperWave, 2020).

51. Sheldon Watts, *Epidemics and History* (New Haven, CT: Yale University Press, 1997), p. xii.

52. A. Lustig and A. J. Levine, "One Hundred Years of Virology," *Journal of Virology* 66, no. 2 (1992), pp. 4629–31.

53. J. Erin Staples and Thomas P. Monath, "Yellow Fever: 100 Years of Discovery," *Journal of the American Medical Association* 300, no. 8 (2008), pp. 960–62.

54. J. Gordon Frierson, "The Yellow Fever Vaccine: A History," *Yale Journal of Biological Medicine* 83, no. 2 (June 2010), pp. 77–85.

55. Ferguson, *Civilization,* p. 147.

56. Ferguson, *Civilization,* pp. 169f., 174.

57. Frierson, "Yellow Fever Vaccine."

58. McGrew, "First Cholera Epidemic," p. 72.

59. Theodore H. Friedgut, "Labor Violence and Regime Brutality in Tsarist Russia: The Iuzovka Cholera Riots of 1892," *Slavic Review* 46, no. 2 (Summer 1987), pp. 245–65.

60. Richard L. Stefanik, "The Smallpox Riots of 1894," *Milwaukee County Historical Society Historical Messenger* 26, no. 4 (December 1970), pp. 1–4.

61. Echenberg, "Pestis Redux," p. 443f.

62. Valeska Huber, "The Unification of the Globe by Disease? The International Sanitary Conferences on Cholera, 1851–1894," *Historical Journal* 49, no. 2 (2006), pp. 453–76. See also Andrew Ehrhardt, "Disease and Diplomacy in the 19th Century," *War on the Rocks* (blog), April 30, 2020, https://warontherocks.com/2020/04/disease-and-diplomacy-in-the-nineteenth-century/.

63. Peter Baldwin, *Contagion and the State in Europe, 1830–1930* (Cambridge: Cambridge University Press, 1999).

64. Echenberg, "Pestis Redux," pp. 443f.

65. Mahatma Gandhi, *Hind Swaraj* (New Delhi: Rajpal & Sons, 2010), p. 30.

66. Ferguson, *Civilization,* p. 146.

67. Ferguson, *Civilization,* pp. 171f., 175.

68. William H. McNeill, *Plagues and Peoples* (Garden City, NY: Anchor, 1998 [1976]), p. 182.

69. James C. Riley, "Insects and the European Mortality Decline," *American Historical Review* 91, no. 4 (October 1986), pp. 833–58.
70. Rosenberg, *Cholera Years,* pp. 206–10.
71. David Cutler and Grant Miller, "The Role of Public Health Improvements in Health Advances: The 20th Century United States," NBER Working Paper No. 10511 (May 2004).
72. George Bernard Shaw, *The Doctor's Dilemma* (London: Penguin, 1946), pp. 64f.
73. Ian Gazeley and Andrew Newell, "Urban Working-Class Food Consumption and Nutrition in Britain in 1904," *Economic History Review* 68, no. 1 (February 2015), p. 17.
74. Andrew T. Newell and Ian Gazeley, "The Declines in Infant Mortality and Fertility: Evidence from British Cities in Demographic Transition," IZA Discussion Paper No. 6855 (October 2012), p. 17.
75. Huber, "The Unification of the Globe by Disease?," pp. 466f.
76. Nigel Jones, *Rupert Brooke: Life, Death and Myth* (London: Head of Zeus, 2015), p. 60.
77. Victoria Y. Fan, Dean T. Jamison, and Lawrence H. Summers, "Pandemic Risk: How Large Are the Expected Losses?," *Bulletin of the World Health Organization* 96 (2018), pp. 129–34, http://dx.doi.org/10.2471/BLT.17.199588.
78. Edwin D. Kilbourne, "Influenza Pandemics of the 20th Century," *Emerging Infectious Diseases* 12, no. 1 (2006), pp. 9–14.
79. Niall Ferguson, "Black Swans, Dragon Kings and Gray Rhinos: The World War of 1914–1918 and the Pandemic of 2020–?," Hoover History Working Paper 2020-1 (May 2020).
80. Christopher Clark, *The Sleepwalkers: How Europe Went to War in 1914* (New York: HarperCollins, 2012).
81. Niall Ferguson, *The War of the World: Twentieth-Century Conflict and the Descent of the West* (New York: Penguin Press, 2006).
82. Charles S. Maier, *Recasting Bourgeois Europe: Stabilization in France, Germany, and Italy in the Decade After World War I* (Princeton, NJ: Princeton University Press, 1975).
83. Barry Eichengreen, *Golden Fetters: The Gold Standard and the Great Depression, 1919–1939* (New York and Oxford: Oxford University Press, 1992).
84. Charles P. Kindleberger, *The World in Depression, 1929–1939* (Berkeley: University of California Press, 2013 [1973]).
85. Niall Philip Alan Sean Johnson, "Aspects of the Historical Geography of the 1918–19 Influenza Pandemic in Britain" (unpublished PhD diss., Cambridge University, 2001), p. 116.
86. Jeffery K. Taubenberger and David M. Morens, "1918 Influenza: The Mother of All Pandemics," *Emerging Infectious Diseases* 12, no. 1 (January 2006), pp. 15–22.
87. Kilbourne, "Influenza Pandemics of the 20th Century," pp. 9–14.
88. Alfred W. Crosby, *America's Forgotten Pandemic: The Influenza of 1918,* 2nd ed. (Cambridge: Cambridge University Press, 2003), p. 19; Eugene Opie et al., "Pneumonia at Camp Funston," *Journal of the American Medical Association* 72 (January 1919), pp. 114f.
89. Niall Ferguson, *The Pity of War: Understanding World War I* (New York: Basic Books, 1998), pp. 342f.
90. Johnson, "Aspects of the Historical Geography," pp. 177ff., 355.
91. Crosby, *America's Forgotten Pandemic,* p. 37.
92. Alexander W. Peters, "Influenza and the Press in 1918," *Concord Review* 14, no. 2 (Winter 2003), https://www.tcr.org/Influenza/.
93. Niall P. A. S. Johnson and Juergen Mueller, "Updating the Accounts: Global Mortality of the 1918–1920 'Spanish' Influenza Pandemic," *Bulletin of the History of Medicine* 76 (2002), pp. 105–15. See also Robert J. Barro, José F. Ursúa, and Joanna Weng, "The Coronavirus and the Great Influenza Pandemic: Lessons from the 'Spanish Flu' for the Coronavirus's Potential Effects on Mortality and Economic Activity," NBER Working Paper No. 26866 (March 2020).
94. Johnson, "Aspects of the Historical Geography," pp. 76, 234.
95. Carol R. Byerly, "War Losses (USA)," *International Encyclopedia of the First World War,* October 8, 2014, https://encyclopedia.1914-1918-online.net/article/war_losses_usa/2014-10-08.
96. T. A. Garrett, "Economic Effects of the 1918 Influenza Pandemic: Implications for a Modern-Day Pandemic," Federal Reserve Bank of St. Louis (November 2007).
97. Elizabeth Brainard and Mark V. Siegler, "The Economic Effects of the 1918 Influenza Epidemic," Centre for Economic Policy Research Discussion Paper No. 3791 (February 2003).
98. Katherine Anne Porter, "Pale Horse, Pale Rider," in *Pale Horse, Pale Rider: Three Short Novels* (New York: Literary Classics, 2008).
99. Johnson, "Aspects of the Historical Geography," pp. 298, 314.
100. Johnson, "Aspects of the Historical Geography," p. 423.
101. Johnson, "Aspects of the Historical Geography," pp. 258n., 269, 283.
102. Crosby, *America's Forgotten Pandemic,* pp. 64f.
103. Brainard and Siegler, "Economic Effects."
104. Garrett, "Economic Effects," tables 1 and 3, pp. 13–15.
105. Sergio Correia, Stephan Luck, and Emil Verner, "Pandemics Depress the Economy, Public Health Interventions Do Not: Evidence from the 1918 Flu," March 26, 2020, available at SSRN, https://ssrn.com/abstract=3561560; Andrew Lilley, Matthew Lilley, and Gianluca Rinaldi, "Public Health Interventions

and Economic Growth: Revisiting the Spanish Flu Evidence," May 2, 2020, available at SSRN, https://ssrn.com/abstract=3590008; Sergio Correia, Stephan Luck, and Emil Verner, "Response to Lilley, Lilley, and Rinaldi (2020)," May 15, 2020, https://almlgr.github.io/CLV_response.pdf.

106. Crosby, *America's Forgotten Pandemic,* pp. 52f.
107. Francesco Aimone, "The 1918 Influenza Epidemic in New York City: A Review of the Public Health Response," *Public Health Reports* 125, supp. 3 (2010), pp. 71–79, doi:10.1177/00333549101250S310.
108. Peters, "Influenza and the Press."
109. H. Markel et al., "Nonpharmaceutical Interventions Implemented by U.S. Cities During the 1918–1919 Influenza Pandemic," *Journal of the American Medical Association* 298, no. 6 (2007), pp. 644–54, doi:10.1001/jama.298.6.644.
110. Crosby, *America's Forgotten Pandemic,* pp. 93–119.
111. Paul Roderick Gregory, "Coronavirus and the Great Lockdown: A Non-Biological Black Swan," RealClear Markets, May 5, 2020, https://www.realclearmarkets.com/articles/2020/05/05/coronavirus_and_the_great_lockdown_a_non-biological_black_swan_490756.html.
112. Barro, Ursúa, and Weng, "Coronavirus and the Great Influenza Pandemic."
113. Dave Donaldson and Daniel Keniston, "How Positive Was the Positive Check? Investment and Fertility in the Aftermath of the 1918 Influenza in India," October 24, 2014, http://citeseerx.ist.psu.edu/viewdoc/download?doi=10.1.1.704.7779&rep=rep1&type=pdf.
114. Amanda Guimbeauy, Nidhiya Menonz, and Aldo Musacchio, "The Brazilian Bombshell? The Short and Long-Term Impact of the 1918 Influenza Pandemic the South American Way," November 21, 2019, available at SSRN, https://ssrn.com/abstract=3381800 or http://dx.doi.org/10.2139/ssrn.3381800.
115. Garrett, "Economic Effects."
116. François R. Velde, "What Happened to the U.S. Economy During the 1918 Influenza Pandemic? A View Through High-Frequency Data," Federal Reserve Bank of Chicago, April 10, 2020.
117. Christina D. Romer, "World War I and the Postwar Depression: A Reinterpretation Based on Alternative Estimates of GDP," *Journal of Monetary Economics* 22 (1988), pp. 91–115.
118. Brainard and Siegler, "Economic Effects."
119. Douglas Almond, "Is the 1918 Influenza Pandemic Over? Long-Term Effect of In Utero Influenza Exposure in the Post-1940 U.S. Population," *Journal of Political Economy* 114, no. 4 (2006), p. 673.
120. Mikko Myrskylä, Neil K. Mehta, and Virginia W. Chang, "Early Life Exposure to the 1918 Influenza Pandemic and Old-Age Mortality by Cause of Death," *American Journal of Public Health* 103, no. 7 (July 2013), pp. E83–E90.
121. Tommy Bengtsson and Jonas Helgertz, "The Long Lasting Influenza: The Impact of Fetal Stress During the 1918 Influenza Pandemic on Socioeconomic Attainment and Health in Sweden 1968–2012," IZA Discussion Paper No. 9327 (September 2015), pp. 1–40.
122. Richard E. Nelson, "Testing the Fetal Origins Hypothesis in a Developing Country: Evidence from the 1918 Influenza Pandemic," *Health Economics* 19, no 10 (October 2010), pp. 1181–92, https://onlinelibrary.wiley.com/doi/full/10.1002/hec.1544; Ming-Jen Lin and Elaine M. Liu, "Does In Utero Exposure to Illness Matter? The 1918 Influenza Epidemic in Taiwan as a Natural Experiment," NBER Working Paper No. 20166 (May 2014), https://www.nber.org/papers/w20166.pdf; Sven Neelsen and Thomas Stratmann, "Long-Run Effects of Fetal Influenza Exposure: Evidence from Switzerland," *Social Science & Medicine* 74, no. 1 (2012), pp. 58–66, https://ideas.repec.org/a/eee/socmed/v74y2012i1p58-66.html.
123. Marco Le Moglie et al., "Epidemics and Trust: The Case of the Spanish Flu," Innocenzo Gasparini Institute for Economic Research Working Paper Series No. 661 (March 2020), pp. 1–32.
124. Crosby, *America's Forgotten Pandemic,* pp. 86, 100–104.
125. Crosby, *America's Forgotten Pandemic,* pp. 12–16.
126. Johnson, "Aspects of the Historical Geography," p. 76.
127. Schama, "Plague Time."
128. George Morton-Jack, *Army of Empire: The Untold Story of the Indian Army in World War I* (New York: Basic Books, 2018).
129. Robert Skidelsky, *John Maynard Keynes: Hopes Betrayed, 1883–1920* (London: Penguin, 1986), p. 378.
130. John M. Barry, *The Great Influenza: The Story of the Deadliest Pandemic in History* (New York: Penguin, 2018), p. 386.
131. Crosby, *America's Forgotten Pandemic,* p. 175.
132. Emily Willingham, "Of Lice and Men: An Itchy History," *Scientific American,* February 14, 2011, https://blogs.scientificamerican.com/guest-blog/of-lice-and-men-an-itchy-history/.
133. Ian Kershaw, *Hitler: 1889–1936: Hubris* (New York: W. W. Norton, 1998), p. 152.
134. Adolf Hitler, *Mein Kampf,* trans. Ralph Manheim (Boston/New York: Mariner, 1999), p. 305.
135. Richard A. Koenigsberg, "Genocide as Immunology: Hitler as the Robert Koch of Germany," *Library of Social Science,* n.d., https://www.libraryofsocialscience.com/newsletter/posts/2018/2018-12-11-immunology.html.
136. Michael Burleigh and Wolfgang Wippermann, *The Racial State: Germany 1933–1945* (Cambridge: Cambridge University Press, 1991).

Chapter 6: The Psychology of Political Incompetence

1. Norman Dixon, *On the Psychology of Military Incompetence* (London: Pimlico, 1994).
2. Dixon, *Psychology of Military Incompetence,* pp. 19, 162ff., 306.
3. Dixon, *Psychology of Military Incompetence,* pp. 152–53.
4. Dixon, *Psychology of Military Incompetence,* p. 155.
5. R. Collins, "A Dynamic Theory of Battle Victory and Defeat," *Cliodynamics* 1, no. 1 (2010), pp. 3–25.
6. Leo Tolstoy, *War and Peace,* trans. Louise and Aylmer Maude (London: Wordsworth, 1993), Book IX, chap. 1.
7. Christina Boswell, *The Political Uses of Expert Knowledge: Immigration Policy and Social Research* (Cambridge: Cambridge University Press, 2009).
8. Henry Kissinger, *White House Years* (New York: Simon & Schuster), p. 43.
9. Christopher Guyver, *The Second French Republic 1848–1852: A Political Reinterpretation* (New York: Palgrave Macmillan, 2016), p. 196.
10. Amartya Sen, *Poverty and Famines: An Essay on Entitlement and Deprivation* (Oxford: Oxford University Press, 1983).
11. Amartya Sen, *Development as Freedom* (Oxford: Oxford University Press, 1999), p. 16.
12. Amartya Sen, "How Is India Doing?," *New York Review of Books,* December 16, 1982, https://www.ny books.com/articles/1982/12/16/how-is-india-doing/.
13. Adam Smith, *An Inquiry into the Nature and Causes of the Wealth of Nations,* vol. II (Oxford: Clarendon Press, 1976 [1776]), p. 102.
14. Marcel Lachiver, *Les années de misère: La famine au temps du Grand Roi* (Paris: Fayard, 1991).
15. Rajat Datta, *Society, Economy and the Market: Commercialisation in Rural Bengal, c. 1760–1800* (New Delhi: Manohar, 2000), p. 264. See William Dalrymple, *The Anarchy: The East India Company, Corporate Violence and the Pillage of an Empire* (New York: Bloomsbury, 2019), pp. 259–304.
16. Tyler Goodspeed, *Famine and Finance: Credit and the Great Famine of Ireland* (Cham, Switzerland: Palgrave Macmillan, 2017).
17. "Introduction," *The Great Irish Famine Online,* Geography Department, University College Cork and Department of Culture, Heritage and the Gaeltacht, https://dahg.maps.arcgis.com/apps/MapSeries /index.html?appid=8de2b863f4454cbf93387dacb5cb8412.
18. K. Theodore Hoppen, "The Franchise and Electoral Politics in England and Ireland 1832–1885," *History* 70, no. 299 (June 1985), pp. 202–17.
19. Angus D. Macintyre, *The Liberator: Daniel O'Connell and the Irish Party, 1830–1847* (London: Hamish Hamilton, 1965), p. 292.
20. Thomas Keneally, *Three Famines: Starvation and Politics* (New York: PublicAffairs, 2011), p. 64.
21. Niall Ferguson, *The House of Rothschild,* vol. I: *Money's Prophets: 1798–1848* (New York: Penguin, 1999), pp. 443, 449.
22. Christine Kinealy, "Peel, Rotten Potatoes and Providence: The Repeal of the Corn Laws and the Irish Famine," in *Free Trade and Its Reception, 1815–1960,* ed. Andrew Marrison (London: Routledge, 2002).
23. *The Times,* September 22, 1846.
24. Debate on the Labouring Poor (Ireland) Bill, House of Commons, February 1, 1847, *Hansard,* vol. 89, cc615-90, https://api.parliament.uk/historic-hansard/commons/1847/feb/01/labouring-poor-ireland -bill. See Tim Pat Coogan, *The Famine Plot: England's Role in Ireland's Greatest Tragedy* (New York: St. Martin's Griffin, 2012), p. 229.
25. Roman Serbyn, "The First Man-Made Famine in Soviet Ukraine, 1921–23," *Ukrainian Weekly* 56, no. 45 (November 6, 1988), http://www.ukrweekly.com/old/archive/1988/458814.shtml.
26. Anne Applebaum, *Red Famine: Stalin's War on Ukraine* (London: Penguin, 2018), pp. 67–69.
27. Applebaum, *Red Famine,* p. 166f.
28. Applebaum, *Red Famine,* pp. 229f.
29. Sergei Nefedov and Michael Ellman, "The Soviet Famine of 1931–1934: Genocide, a Result of Poor Harvests, or the Outcome of a Conflict Between the State and the Peasants?," *Europe-Asia Studies* 71, no. 6 (July 2019), pp. 1048–65.
30. Michael Ellman, "The Role of Leadership Perceptions and of Intent in the Soviet Famine of 1931–1934," *Europe-Asia Studies* 57, no. 6 (September 2005), p. 824.
31. Benjamin I. Cook, Ron L. Miller, and Richard Seager, "Amplification of the North American 'Dust Bowl' Drought Through Human-Induced Land Degradation," *PNAS* 106, no. 13 (March 31, 2009), pp. 4997–5001.
32. Ben Cook, Ron Miller, and Richard Seager, "Did Dust Storms Make the Dust Bowl Drought Worse?," Lamont-Doherty Earth Observatory, Columbia University Earth Institute, http://ocp.ldeo.columbia .edu/res/div/ocp/drought/dust_storms.shtml.
33. Timothy Egan, *The Worst Hard Time: The Untold Story of Those Who Survived the Great American Dustbowl* (Boston and New York: Mariner/Houghton Mifflin Harcourt, 2006), p. 5.
34. Robert A. McLeman et al., "What We Learned from the Dust Bowl: Lessons in Science, Policy, and Adaption," *Population and Environment* 35 (2014), pp. 417–40. See also D. Worster, *Dust Bowl: The Southern Plains in the 1930s* (New York: Oxford University Press, 1979).

35. Cook, Miller, and Seager, "Amplification of the North American 'Dust Bowl' Drought," p. 4997.
36. Egan, *Worst Hard Time,* p. 8.
37. "Honoring 85 Years of NRCS—A Brief History," Natural Resources Conservation Service, USDA, https://www.nrcs.usda.gov/wps/portal/nrcs/detail/national/about/history/?cid=nrcs143_021392.
38. Mike Davis, *Late Victorian Holocausts: El Niño Famines and the Making of the Third World* (London and New York: Verso, 2001).
39. Tirthankar Roy, *The Economic History of India, 1857–1947* (Delhi: Oxford University Press, 2000), pp. 22, 219f., 254, 285, 294. Cf. Michelle Burge McAlpin, *Subject to Famine: Food Crises and Economic Change in Western India, 1860–1920* (Princeton, NJ: Princeton University Press, 1983).
40. Christopher Bayly and Tim Harper, *Forgotten Armies: Britain's Asian Empire and the War with Japan* (London: Penguin, 2005).
41. Cormac Ó Gráda, "'Sufficiency and Sufficiency and Sufficiency': Revisiting the Great Bengal Famine, 1943–44," in *Eating People Is Wrong, and Other Essays on Famine, Its Past, and Its Future* (Princeton, NJ: Princeton University Press, 2015), p. 90.
42. Arthur Herman, *Gandhi and Churchill: The Rivalry That Destroyed an Empire and Forged Our Age* (London: Hutchinson, 2008), p. 513.
43. Keneally, *Three Famines,* p. 93.
44. Herman, *Gandhi and Churchill,* p. 515.
45. Andrew Roberts, *Churchill: Walking with Destiny* (London: Allen Lane, 2018), p. 788.
46. Keneally, *Three Famines,* p. 95.
47. Bayly and Harper, *Forgotten Armies,* pp. 284–87.
48. Frank Dikötter, *Mao's Great Famine: The History of China's Most Devastating Catastrophe, 1958–1962* (London: Bloomsbury, 2017), p. 333; Andrew G. Walder, *China Under Mao: A Revolution Derailed* (Cambridge, MA: Harvard University Press), p. 173.
49. Dali L. Yang, *Calamity and Reform in China: State, Rural Society, and Institutional Change Since the Great Leap Famine* (Stanford, CA: Stanford University Press, 1996).
50. Xin Meng, Nancy Qian, and Pierre Yared, "The Institutional Causes of China's Great Famine, 1959–61," NBER Working Paper No. 16361 (September 2010).
51. Dikötter, *Mao's Great Famine,* pp. 39f.
52. Dikötter, *Mao's Great Famine,* pp. 113f., 133.
53. Dikötter, *Mao's Great Famine,* pp. 178ff., 276, 301f.
54. Cormac Ó Gráda, "Eating People Is Wrong: Famine's Darkest Secret?," in *Eating People Is Wrong,* pp. 11–37.
55. Bengal statistics from Tim Dyson, *Population History of India: From the First Modern People to the Present Day* (Oxford: Oxford University Press, 2018), and Stephen Devereux, "Famine in the Twentieth Century," IDS Working Paper 105 (2000). Ireland statistics from Joel Mokyr, *Why Ireland Starved: A Quantitative and Analytical History of the Irish Economy, 1800–1850* (London: Allen & Unwin, 1983).
56. Theodore M. Vestal, "Famine in Ethiopia: Crisis of Many Dimensions," *Africa Today* 32, no. 4 (1984), pp. 7–28.
57. Mark R. Jury, "Climatic Determinants of March–May Rainfall Variability over Southeastern Ethiopia," *Climate Research* 66, no. 3 (December 2015), pp. 201–10.
58. Alex de Waal, *Evil Days: Thirty Years of War and Famine in Ethiopia* (New York and London: Human Rights Watch, 1991); Peter Gill, *Famine and Foreigners: Ethiopia Since Live Aid* (Oxford: Oxford University Press, 2010).
59. Keneally, *Three Famines,* p. 125.
60. David Rieff, "The Humanitarian Aid Industry's Most Absurd Apologist," *New Republic,* November 28, 2010, https://newrepublic.com/article/79491/humanitarian-aid-industrys-most-absurd-apologist-geldof.
61. Chandler Collier, "London Coal Fog of 1880," https://prezi.com/fbho-h7ba7f5/london-coal-fog-of-1880/.
62. The Hon. R. Russell, *London Fogs* (Gloucester: Dodo Press, 2009 [1880]), pp. 5–6, https://www.victorianlondon.org/weather/londonfogs.htm.
63. Christopher Klein, "The Great Smog of 1952," *History,* December 5, 2012, updated August 22, 2018, https://www.history.com/news/the-killer-fog-that-blanketed-london-60-years-ago.
64. Camila Domonoske, "Research on Chinese Haze Helps Crack Mystery of London's Deadly 1952 Fog," *The Two-Way,* NPR, November 23, 2016, https://www.npr.org/sections/thetwo-way/2016/11/23/503156414/research-on-chinese-haze-helps-crack-mystery-of-londons-deadly-1952-fog; Jane Onyanga-Omara, "Mystery of London Fog That Killed 12,000 Finally Solved," *USA Today,* December 13, 2016, https://eu.usatoday.com/story/news/world/2016/12/13/scientists-say-theyve-solved-mystery-1952-london-killer-fog/95375738/.
65. Peter Thorsheim, *Inventing Pollution: Coal, Smoke, and Culture in Britain Since 1800* (Athens: Ohio University Press, 2017), p. 161.
66. H. Ross Anderson et al., "Health Effects of an Air Pollution Episode in London, December 1991," *Thorax* 50 (1995), pp. 1188–93.

67. Winston S. Churchill, *The World Crisis, 1911–1914* (New York: Charles Scribner's Sons, 1923), p. 41.

68. David Lloyd George, *War Memoirs*, vol. I (London: Odhams Press, 1938), pp. 32, 34f.

69. Samuel Hynes, *A War Imagined: The First World War and English Culture* (London: Pimlico, 1990), p. 106.

70. Alan Clark, *The Donkeys* (London: Random House, 2011 [1961]); John Laffin, *British Butchers and Bunglers of World War One* (Stroud, UK: Sutton, 1992).

71. John Terraine, *Douglas Haig: The Educated Soldier* (London: Cassell, 1963).

72. Gary Sheffield, "An Exercise in Futility," *History Today* 66, no. 7 (2016), pp. 10–18. See also Gary Sheffield, *The Somme* (London: Cassell, 2003).

73. William Philpott, *Bloody Victory: The Sacrifice on the Somme and the Making of the Twentieth Century* (London: Abacus, 2016).

74. Gary Sheffield, *The Chief: Douglas Haig and the British Army* (London: Aurum Press, 2012), p. 166.

75. Robin Prior and Trevor Wilson, *Command on the Western Front: The Military Career of Sir Henry Rawlinson, 1914–18* (Oxford: Basil Blackwell, 1992), p. 78.

76. David French, "The Meaning of Attrition," *English Historical Review* 103, no. 407 (1986), p. 403.

77. Trevor Wilson, *The Myriad Faces of War: Britain and the Great War, 1914–1918* (Cambridge: Cambridge University Press, 1986), p. 309; Prior and Wilson, *Command on the Western Front*, pp. 150f.

78. Sheffield, "Exercise in Futility."

79. Prior and Wilson, *Command on the Western Front*, pp. 153, 163–66.

80. Ernst Jünger, *The Storm of Steel: From the Diary of a German Storm-Troop Officer on the Western Front*, trans. Basil Creighton (London: Chatto & Windus, 1929), pp. 92ff., 106f.

81. John Terraine, *The First World War* (London: Secker and Warburg, 1984), p. 172.

82. French, "Meaning of Attrition," p. 386.

83. Niall Ferguson, *The Pity of War: Understanding World War I* (New York: Basic Books, 1998), pp. 332f.

84. R. H. Tawney, "Some Reflections of a Soldier," in *The Attack and Other Papers* (London: Allen & Unwin, 1953).

85. Nicholas Reeves, "Film Propaganda and Its Audience: The Example of Britain's Official Films During the First World War," *Journal of Contemporary History* 18, no. 3 (1983), pp. 464–94.

86. Brian Bond, *British Military Policy Between the Two World Wars* (Oxford: Clarendon, 1980), p. 24.

87. James Neidpath, *The Singapore Naval Base and the Defence of Britain's Eastern Empire, 1919–1941* (Oxford: Clarendon, 1981), p. 131.

88. Bond, *British Military Policy*, p. 217.

89. For a detailed account, see Niall Ferguson, *The War of the World: Twentieth-Century Conflict and the Descent of the West* (New York: Penguin Press, 2006), pp. 312–82.

90. Winston Churchill, "The Munich Agreement," address to the House of Commons, October 5, 1938, International Churchill Society, https://winstonchurchill.org/resources/speeches/1930-1938-the-wilderness /the-munich-agreement.

91. Randolph Spencer Churchill and Martin Gilbert, *Winston S. Churchill*, vol. V: *The Prophet of Truth, 1922–1939* (New York: Houghton Mifflin, 1966), p. 1002.

92. Roberts, *Churchill*, p. 438.

93. Roberts, *Churchill*, p. 696.

94. Barnaby Crowcroft, "The End of the British Empire of Protectorates, 1945–1960" (PhD diss., Harvard University, 2019).

95. Field Marshal Lord Alanbrooke, *Alanbrooke War Diaries 1939–1945* (London: Orion, 2015), February 11 and 18, 1942.

96. "'The Buck Stops Here' Desk Sign," Harry S. Truman Library and Museum, https://www.trumanlibrary .gov/education/trivia/buck-stops-here-sign.

97. Adrian Goldsworthy, *How Rome Fell: Death of a Superpower* (New Haven, CT: Yale University Press, 2009).

98. Peter Heather, *The Fall of the Roman Empire: A New History* (London: Pan, 2006).

99. Bryan Ward-Perkins, *The Fall of Rome and the End of Civilization* (Oxford: Oxford University Press, 2005).

100. Dennis O. Flynn and Arturo Giraldez, "Arbitrage, China, and World Trade in the Early Modern Period," *Journal of the Economic and Social History of the Orient* 38, no. 4 (1995), pp. 429–48.

101. Patricia Buckley Ebrey, *The Cambridge Illustrated History of China* (Cambridge: Cambridge University Press, 1996), esp. p. 215.

102. For a good summary, see Jack Goody, *Capitalism and Modernity: The Great Debate* (Cambridge: Polity Press, 2004), pp. 103–17.

103. Hanhui Guan and Li Daokui, "A Study of GDP and Its Structure in China's Ming Dynasty," *China Economic Quarterly* 3 (2010).

104. See, e.g., L. Brandt, Debin Ma, and Thomas G. Rawski, "From Divergence to Convergence: Re-evaluating the History Behind China's Economic Boom," University of Warwick Working Paper Series No. 117 (February 2013).

105. Friedrich Percyval Reck-Malleczewen, *Diary of a Man in Despair* (Richmond, UK: Duckworth, 2000 [1947]), p. 31.

106. Stephen Kotkin, *Armageddon Averted: The Soviet Collapse, 1970–2000* (Oxford: Oxford University Press, 2008).
107. Leon Aron, "Everything You Think You Know About the Collapse of the Soviet Union Is Wrong," *Foreign Policy*, June 20, 2011, https://foreignpolicy.com/2011/06/20/everything-you-think-you-know-about -the-collapse-of-the-soviet-union-is-wrong/.
108. Charles King, "How a Great Power Falls Apart," *Foreign Affairs*, June 30, 2020, https://www.foreignaf fairs.com/articles/russia-fsu/2020-06-30/how-great-power-falls-apart.
109. See, in general, Samir Puri, *The Great Imperial Hangover: How Empires Have Shaped the World* (London: Atlantic Books, 2020).
110. Eyck Freymann, *One Belt One Road: Chinese Power Meets the World* (Cambridge, MA: Harvard University Press, 2020), pp. 42, 62, 100.
111. See his speech at the informal CIS summit, St. Petersburg, December 20, 2019, President of Russia website, http://en.kremlin.ru/events/president/news/62376; and his speech on "Shared Responsibility to History and Our Future," Moscow, June 19, 2020, President of Russia website, http://en.kremlin .ru/events/president/news/63527.
112. Manmohan Singh, speech on the acceptance of an honorary degree from Oxford University, July 8, 2005, https://archivepmo.nic.in/drmanmohansingh/speech-details.php?nodeid=140.
113. Michael Colborne and Maxim Edwards, "Erdogan Is Making the Ottoman Empire Great Again," *Foreign Policy*, June 22, 2018, https://foreignpolicy.com/2018/06/22/erdogan-is-making-the-ottoman -empire-great-again/. See also Abdullah Bozkurt, "Erdoğan's Secret Keeper Says Lausanne Treaty 'Expired,' Turkey Free to Grab Resources," *Nordic Monitor*, February 24, 2020, https://www.nordic monitor.com/2020/02/erdogans-secret-keeper-says-lausanne-treaty-invalid-turkey-free-to-grab -resources/; Sinan Baykent, "Misak-ı Millî or the 'National Oath': Turkey's New Foreign Policy Compass?," *Hurriyet Daily News*, October 31, 2016, https://www.hurriyetdailynews.com/misak-i-mill-or-the-national -oath-turkeys-new-foreign-policy-compass-105529.
114. Michael Morell, "Iran's Grand Strategy Is to Become a Regional Powerhouse," *Washington Post*, April 3, 2015, https://www.washingtonpost.com/opinions/irans-grand-strategy/2015/04/03/415ec8a8-d8a3 -11e4-ba28-f2a685dc7f89_story.html.

Chapter 7: From the Boogie Woogie Flu to Ebola in Town

1. Pasquale Cirillo and Nassim Nicholas Taleb, "Tail Risk of Contagious Diseases," *Nature Physics* 16 (2020), pp. 606–13.
2. Niall P. A. S. Johnson and Juergen Mueller, "Updating the Accounts: Global Mortality of the 1918–1920 'Spanish' Influenza Pandemic," *Bulletin of the History of Medicine* 76 (2002), pp. 105–15.
3. "Eisenhower Seeks Fund to Fight Flu," *New York Times*, August 8, 1957, https://timesmachine.nytimes .com/timesmachine/1957/08/08/90831582.html.
4. "Presidential Approval Ratings—Gallup Historical Statistics and Trends," Gallup, https://news.gallup .com/poll/116677/presidential-approval-ratings-gallup-historical-statistics-trends.aspx.
5. For the theory that the 1889 pandemic was in fact caused by a coronavirus, see Nicholas A. Christakis, *Apollo's Arrow: The Profound and Enduring Impact of Coronavirus on the Way We Live* (New York: Little, Brown Spark, 2020), pp. 309f.
6. D. A. Henderson, Brooke Courtney, Thomas V. Inglesby, Eric Toner, and Jennifer B. Nuzzo, "Public Health and Medical Responses to the 1957–58 Influenza Pandemic," *Biosecurity and Bioterrorism: Biodefense Strategy, Practice, and Science* (September 2009), pp. 265–73.
7. Cécile Viboud et al., "Global Mortality Impact of the 1957–1959 Influenza Pandemic," *Journal of Infectious Diseases* 213 (2016), pp. 738–45.
8. Viboud et al., "Global Mortality Impact," p. 744.
9. "1957–1958 Pandemic (H2N2 Virus)," Centers for Disease Control and Prevention (henceforth CDC), https://www.cdc.gov/flu/pandemic-resources/1957-1958-pandemic.html.
10. Christakis, *Apollo's Arrow*, pp. 62f. Robert J. Barro, José F. Ursúa, and Joanna Weng, "The Coronavirus and the Great Influenza Pandemic: Lessons from the 'Spanish Flu' for the Coronavirus's Potential Effects on Mortality and Economic Activity," NBER Working Paper No. 26866 (2020).
11. Elizabeth Brainard and Mark V. Siegler, "The Economic Effects of the 1918 Influenza Epidemic," Centre for Economic Policy Research Discussion Paper No. 3791 (February 2003).
12. Patrick G. T. Walker et al., "The Global Impact of COVID-19 and Strategies for Mitigation and Suppression," Imperial College COVID-19 Response Team Report 12 (March 26, 2020), https://doi.org/10.25561/77735.
13. For a survey that is somewhat more optimistic than I am about the likely IFR, see John P. A. Ioannidis, "The Infection Fatality Rate of COVID-19 Inferred from Seroprevalence Data," MedRxiv, July 14, 2020, https://doi.org/10.1101/2020.05.13.20101253.
14. Elizabeth W. Etheridge, *Sentinel for Health: A History of the Centers for Disease Control* (Berkeley: University of California Press, 1992), p. 85.
15. Robert E. Serfling, Ida L. Sherman, and William J. Houseworth, "Excess Pneumonia-Influenza Mortality by Age and Sex in Three Major Influenza A2 Epidemics, United States, 1957–58, 1960 and 1963," *American Journal of Epidemiology* 88, no. 8 (1967), pp. 433–42.

16. Eskild Petersen et al., "Comparing SARS-CoV-2 with SARS-CoV and Influenza Pandemics," *Lancet Infectious Diseases* 20, no. 9 (September 2020), table 3, https://doi.org/10.1016/S1473-3099(20)30484-9.

17. "Influenza 1957," *American Journal of Public Health and the Nation's Health* 47, no. 9 (September 1957), pp. 1141f.

18. Lina Zeldovich, "How America Brought the 1957 Influenza Pandemic to a Halt," *JSTOR Daily*, April 7, 2020, https://daily.jstor.org/how-america-brought-the-1957-influenza-pandemic-to-a-halt/.

19. Henderson et al., "Public Health and Medical Responses," p. 266.

20. Henderson et al., "Public Health and Medical Responses," p. 271.

21. Henderson et al., "Public Health and Medical Responses."

22. Edwin D. Kilbourne, "Influenza Pandemics of the 20th Century," *Emerging Infectious Diseases* 12, no. 1 (January 2006), p. 10.

23. Albert-László Barabási, *Network Science* (Cambridge: Cambridge University Press, 2016), esp. chap. 10.

24. Etheridge, *Sentinel for Health*, p. 85.

25. Etheridge, *Sentinel for Health*, p. 269.

26. Jere Housworth and Alexander D. Langmuir, "Excess Mortality from Epidemic Influenza, 1957–1966," *American Journal of Epidemiology* 100, no. 1 (1974), pp. 40–49.

27. Cécile Viboud et al., "Multinational Impact of the 1968 Hong Kong Influenza Pandemic: Evidence for a Smoldering Pandemic," *Journal of Infectious Diseases* 192 (2005), pp. 233–48; Petersen et al., "Comparing SARS-CoV-2 with SARS-CoV and Influenza," table 3.

28. Jack M. Holl, "Young Eisenhower's Fight with the 1918 Flu at Camp Colt," *Brewminate*, May 5, 2020, https://brewminate.com/young-eisenhowers-fight-with-the-1918-flu-at-camp-colt/.

29. Henderson et al., "Public Health and Medical Responses," p. 266.

30. Henderson et al., "Public Health and Medical Responses," p. 270.

31. Fred M. Davenport, "Role of the Commission on Influenza," *Studies of Epidemiology and Prevention* 73, no. 2 (February 1958), pp. 133–39.

32. Henderson et al., "Public Health and Medical Responses," p. 270.

33. "Hong Kong Battling Influenza Epidemic," *New York Times*, April 17, 1957.

34. Henderson et al., "Public Health and Medical Responses," p. 270.

35. Zeldovich, "1957 Influenza Pandemic."

36. Etheridge, *Sentinel for Health*, p. 84.

37. Henderson et al., "Public Health and Medical Responses," p. 270.

38. Kilbourne, "Influenza Pandemics," p. 10.

39. Paul A. Offit, *Vaccinated: One Man's Quest to Defeat the World's Deadliest Diseases* (Washington, D.C.: Smithsonian, 2007), pp. 128–31.

40. Milton Friedman and Anna Jacobson Schwartz, *A Monetary History of the United States, 1867–1960* (Princeton, NJ: Princeton University Press, 2008), p. 615.

41. Federal Reserve Bank of St. Louis, "The 1957–1958 Recession: Recent or Current?," *FRBSL Monthly Review* 40, no. 8 (August 1958), pp. 94–103.

42. Henderson et al., "Public Health and Medical Responses," pp. 269f.

43. U.S. Congressional Budget Office, "A Potential Influenza Pandemic: Possible Macroeconomic Effects and Policy Issues," December 8, 2005 (revised July 27, 2006), http://www.cbo.gov/ftpdocs/69xx/doc6946/12-08-BirdFlu.pdf.

44. "Democrats Widen Congress Margin," *New York Times*, November 5, 1958.

45. Heidi J. S. Tworek, "Communicable Disease: Information, Health, and Globalization in the Interwar Period," *American Historical Review*, June 2019, pp. 823, 836.

46. Tworek, "Communicable Disease," p. 838.

47. Tworek, "Communicable Disease," p. 841.

48. Frank Furedi, "Why the WHO Should Be Scrapped," *Spiked*, April 27, 2020, https://www.spiked-online.com/2020/04/27/why-the-who-should-be-scrapped/.

49. Franklin D. Roosevelt, address in Chicago, October 5, 1937, https://www.presidency.ucsb.edu/documents/address-chicago.

50. Elizabeth Borgwardt, *A New Deal for the World: America's Vision for Human Rights* (Cambridge, MA: Harvard University Press, 2005).

51. Julia Emily Johnsen, *Plans for a Post-War World* (New York: H. W. Wilson, 1942), p. 115.

52. Odd Arne Westad, *The Global Cold War: Third World Interventions and the Making of Our Times* (New York: Cambridge University Press, 2005).

53. Daniel J. Sargent, "Strategy and Biosecurity: An Applied History Perspective," paper prepared for the Hoover History Working Group, June 18, 2020.

54. Calculated from data at The Nobel Prize, http://www.nobelprize.org/prizes/.

55. S. Jayachandran, Adriana Lleras-Muney, and Kimberly V. Smith, "Modern Medicine and the 20th Century Decline in Mortality: New Evidence on the Impact of Sulfa Drugs," Online Working Paper Series, California Center for Population Research, UCLA (2008), pp. 1–48.

56. Thomas McKeown, R. G. Record, and R. D. Turner, "An Interpretation of the Decline of Mortality in England and Wales During the Twentieth Century," *Journal of Population Studies* 29, no. 3 (1975), pp. 391–422.

57. Christakis, *Apollo's Arrow*, p. 111.

58. David Cutler and Ellen Meara, "Changes in the Age Distribution of Mortality over the 20th Century," NBER Working Paper No. 8556 (October 2001).

59. J. R. Hampton, "The End of Medical History?," *Journal of the Royal College of Physicians of London* 32, no. 4 (1998), pp. 367–71.

60. Joel Slemrod, "Post-War Capital Accumulation and the Threat of Nuclear War," NBER Working Paper No. 887 (1982); Joel Slemrod, "Fear of Nuclear War and Intercountry Differences in the Rate of Saving," NBER Working Paper No. 2801 (1988); Bruce Russett and Joel Slemrod, "Diminished Expectations of Nuclear War and Increased Personal Savings: Evidence from Individual Survey Data," NBER Working Paper No. 4031 (1992).

61. John Farley, *Brock Chisholm, the World Health Organization and the Cold War* (Vancouver and Toronto: UBC Press, 2008), p. 56.

62. Meredith Reid Sarkees, "The Correlates of War Data on War: An Update to 1997," *Conflict Management and Peace Science* 18, no. 1 (2000), pp. 123–44; Therese Pettersson and Peter Wallensteen, "Armed Conflicts, 1946–2014," *Journal of Peace Research* 52, no. 4 (2015), pp. 536–50.

63. Max Roser, "War and Peace After 1945," Our World in Data (2015), http://ourworldindata.org/data /war-peace/war-and-peace-after-1945/.

64. Center for Systemic Peace, "Assessing the Qualities of Systemic Peace," https://www.systemicpeace .org/conflicttrends.html.

65. Peter J. Hotez, "Vaccines as Instruments of Foreign Policy," *European Molecular Biology Organization Reports* 2, no. 10 (2001), pp. 862–68.

66. David M. Oshinsky, *Polio: An American Story* (Oxford: Oxford University Press, 2005), pp. 252f.

67. Erez Manela, "Smallpox Eradication and the Rise of Global Governance," in *The Shock of the Global: The 1970s in Perspective*, ed. Niall Ferguson et al. (Cambridge, MA: Harvard University Press, 2010), pp. 256–57.

68. Jared Diamond, "Lessons from a Pandemic," *Financial Times*, May 25, 2020, https://www.ft.com/con tent/71ed9f88-9f5b-11ea-b65d-489c67b0d85d.

69. "Biological Weapons in the Former Soviet Union: An Interview with Dr. Kenneth Alibek," *Nonproliferation Review* (Spring/Summer 1999), pp. 1–10.

70. Clark Whelton, "Say Your Prayers and Take Your Chances: Remembering the 1957 Asian Flu Pandemic," *City Journal*, March 13, 2020, https://www.city-journal.org/1957-asian-flu-pandemic.

71. Henderson et al., "Public Health and Medical Responses," pp. 270, 272.

72. Justin McCarthy, "Americans Differ Greatly in Readiness to Return to Normal," Gallup, April 30, 2020, https://news.gallup.com/poll/309578/americans-differ-greatly-readiness-return-normal.aspx.

73. R. J. Reinhart, "Roundup of Gallup COVID-19 Coverage," October 19, 2020, https://news.gallup.com /opinion/gallup/308126/roundup-gallup-covid-coverage.aspx.

74. Michele Gelfand et al., "Cultural and Institutional Factors Predicting the Infection Rate and Mortality Likelihood of the COVID-19 Pandemic," PsyArXiv, April 1, 2020, https://doi.org/10.31234/osf.io /m7f8a.

75. Charles Murray, *Coming Apart: The State of White America, 1960–2010* (New York: Crown Forum, 2012).

76. Office of Personnel Management, "Historical Federal Workforce Tables," https://www.opm.gov/policy -data-oversight/data-analysis-documentation/federal-employment-reports/historical-tables/executive -branch-civilian-employment-since-1940/.

77. U.S. Bureau of Labor Statistics, "All Employees, Government [USGOVT]," retrieved from FRED: Federal Reserve Bank of St. Louis, https://fred.stlouisfed.org/series/USGOVT.

78. U.S. Bureau of Labor Statistics, "All Employees, Government."

79. Federal Reserve Bank of St. Louis and U.S. Office of Management and Budget, "Gross Federal Debt as Percent of Gross Domestic Product [GFDGPA188S]," retrieved from FRED: Federal Reserve Bank of St. Louis, https://fred.stlouisfed.org/series/GFDGPA188S.

80. "Budget Projections: Debt Will Exceed the Size of the Economy This Year," Committee for a Responsible Federal Budget, April 13, 2020, http://www.crfb.org/blogs/budget-projections-debt-will-exceed-size -economy-year.

81. Oshinsky, *Polio: An American Story*, p. 8.

82. Oshinsky, *Polio: An American Story*, p. 53.

83. Oshinsky, *Polio: An American Story*, p. 162.

84. Oshinsky, *Polio: An American Story*, p. 204.

85. Oshinsky, *Polio: An American Story*, p. 218.

86. Oshinsky, *Polio: An American Story*, p. 219.

87. Oshinsky, *Polio: An American Story*, p. 268.

88. Richard Krause, "The Swine Flu Episode and the Fog of Epidemics," *Emerging Infectious Diseases* 12, no. 1 (January 2006), pp. 40–43, https://doi.org/10.3201/eid1201.051132.

89. Homeland Security Council, *National Strategy for Pandemic Influenza* (November 2005), https:// www.cdc.gov/flu/pandemic-resources/pdf/pandemic-influenza-strategy-2005.pdf.

90. David C. Morrison, "Pandemics and National Security," *Great Decisions* (2006), pp. 93–102, https://www.jstor.org/stable/43682459.

91. James Fallows, "The 3 Weeks That Changed Everything," *Atlantic,* June 29, 2020, https://www.the atlantic.com/politics/archive/2020/06/how-white-house-coronavirus-response-went-wrong/613591/.

92. Anna Mummert et al., "A Perspective on Multiple Waves of Influenza Pandemics," *PLOS One,* April 23, 2013, https://doi.org/10.1371/journal.pone.0060343.

93. Petersen et al., "Comparing SARS-CoV-2 with SARS-CoV and Influenza." See also "2009 H1N1 Pandemic (H1N1pdm09 Virus)," CDC, https://www.cdc.gov/flu/pandemic-resources/2009-h1n1-pandemic.html.

94. Executive Office of the President of the United States, "Playbook for Early Response to High-Consequence Emerging Infectious Disease Threats and Biological Incidents," n.d., https://assets.documentcloud.org/documents/6819268/Pandemic-Playbook.pdf.

95. A. Moya et al., "The Population Genetics and Evolutionary Epidemiology of RNA Viruses," *Nature Reviews* 2 (2004), pp. 279–88.

96. Randy Shilts, *And the Band Played On: Politics, People and the AIDS Epidemic* (London: Souvenir Press, 2011).

97. Shilts, *And the Band Played On,* pp. 68f.

98. Shilts, *And the Band Played On,* pp. 73f.

99. Shilts, *And the Band Played On,* p. 165.

100. Shilts, *And the Band Played On,* p. 229.

101. Shilts, *And the Band Played On,* pp. 242f.

102. "How HIV/AIDS Changed the World," *Economist,* June 25, 2020, https://www.economist.com/books-and-arts/2020/06/25/how-hiv/aids-changed-the-world.

103. Natasha Geiling, "The Confusing and At-Times Counterproductive 1980s Response to the AIDS Epidemic," *Smithsonian,* December 4, 2013, https://www.smithsonianmag.com/history/the-confusing-and-at-times-counterproductive-1980s-response-to-the-aids-epidemic-180948611/.

104. Shilts, *And the Band Played On,* p. 129.

105. Shilts, *And the Band Played On,* pp. 319f., 450ff.

106. Shilts, *And the Band Played On,* p. 593.

107. Laurie Garrett, "Ebola's Lessons: How the WHO Mishandled the Crisis," *Foreign Affairs* 94, no. 5 (September/October 2015), pp. 84f.

108. Peter Piot, *No Time to Lose: A Life in Pursuit of Deadly Viruses* (New York and London: W. W. Norton, 2012), pp. 183f.

109. Piot, *No Time to Lose,* pp. 100, 191.

110. Piot, *No Time to Lose,* pp. 108f., 167.

111. See, e.g., Romualdo Pastor-Satorras and Alessandro Vespignani, "Immunization of Complex Networks," Abdus Salam International Centre for Theoretical Physics, February 1, 2008.

112. David M. Auerbach et al., "Cluster of Cases of the Acquired Immune Deficiency Syndrome. Patients Linked by Sexual Contact," *American Journal of Medicine* 76, no. 3 (1984), pp. 487–92, https://doi.org/10.1016/0002-9343(84)90668-5. Dugas was later wrongly identified as "patient zero," the first AIDS case in the United States. In fact, the authors of the 1984 paper had originally designated him "Patient O" for "Out-of-California."

113. Filio Marineli et al., "Mary Mallon (1869–1938) and the History of Typhoid Fever," *Annals of Gastroenterology* 26, no. 2 (2013), pp. 132–34, https://www.ncbi.nlm.nih.gov/pmc/articles/PMC3959940/.

114. "Trends in Sexual Behavior and the HIV Pandemic," *American Journal of Public Health* 82, no. 11 (1992), p. 1459.

115. See, in general, Jonathan Engel, *The Epidemic: A Global History of AIDS* (Washington, D.C.: Smithsonian Books, 2006).

116. "How HIV/AIDS Changed the World," *Economist.*

117. Calder Walton, "Intelligence and Coronavirus: Rethinking US National Security: An Applied History Analysis," unpublished paper, Harvard University (May 2020).

118. UNAIDS, *How AIDS Changed Everything: MDG 6: 15 Years, 15 Lessons of Hope from the AIDS Response* (New York: United Nations, 2016), https://www.unaids.org/en/resources/documents/2015/MDG6_15years-15lessonsfromtheAIDSresponse.

119. Marshall H. Becker and Jill G. Joseph, "AIDS and Behavioral Change to Reduce Risk: A Review," *American Journal of Public Health* 78, no. 4 (1988), pp. 394–410.

120. Joel A. Feinleib and Robert T. Michael, "Reported Changes in Sexual Behavior in Response to AIDS in the United States," *Preventive Medicine* 27, no. 3 (May 1998), pp. 400–411, https://doi.org/10.1006/pmed.1998.0270.

121. Muazzam Nasrullah et al., "Factors Associated with Condom Use Among Sexually Active U.S. Adults, National Survey of Family Growth, 2006–2010 and 2011–2013," *Journal of Sexual Medicine* 14, no. 4 (April 2017), pp. 541–50, https://doi.org10.1016/j.jsxm.2017.02.015. See also Wenjia Zhu, Samuel A. Bazzi, and Angel R. Bazzi, "Behavioral Changes Following HIV Seroconversion During the Historical Expansion of HIV Treatment in the United States," *AIDS* 33, no. 1 (January 2, 2019), pp. 113–21,

https://journals.lww.com/aidsonline/fulltext/2019/01020/behavioral_changes_following_hiv_sero conversion.12.aspx.

122. Gus Cairns, "Behaviour Change Interventions in HIV Prevention: Is There Still a Place for Them?," NAM AIDS Map, April 12, 2017, https://www.aidsmap.com/news/apr-2017/behaviour-change-interventions -hiv-prevention-there-still-place-them.

123. UNAIDS, *How AIDS Changed Everything*, p. 33.

124. Tony Barnett and Justin Parkhurst, "HIV/AIDS: Sex, Abstinence, and Behaviour Change," *Lancet,* September 2005, https://doi.org/10.1016/S1473-3099(05)70219-X; Emily Oster, "HIV and Sexual Behavior Change: Why Not Africa?," *Journal of Health Economics* 31, no. 1 (January 2012), pp. 35–49, https://www.sciencedirect.com/science/article/abs/pii/S016762961100172X.

125. Brooke E. Wells and Jean M. Twenge, "Changes in Young People's Sexual Behavior and Attitudes, 1943–1999: A Cross-Temporal Meta-Analysis," *Review of General Psychology* 9, no. 3 (September 2005), pp. 249–61.

126. Nicholas H. Wolfinger, "Nine Decades of Promiscuity," Institute for Family Studies, February 6, 2018, https://ifstudies.org/blog/nine-decades-of-promiscuity.

127. Steven Reinberg, "Only About One-Third of Americans Use Condoms: CDC," WebMD, August 10, 2017, https://www.webmd.com/sex/news/20170810/only-about-one-third-of-americans-use-condoms -cdc#1; Rachael Rettner, "US Men's Condom Use Is on the Rise," *LiveScience,* August 10, 2017, https://www.livescience.com/60095-condom-use-men.html.

128. Peter Ueda, Catherine H. Mercer, and Cyrus Ghaznavi, "Trends in Frequency of Sexual Activity and Number of Sexual Partners Among Adults Aged 18 to 44 Years in the US, 2000–2018," *JAMA Network Open* 3, no. 6 (2020), https://doi.org/10.1001/jamanetworkopen.2020.3833.

129. National Survey of Sexual Attitudes and Lifestyles, Natsal, http://www.natsal.ac.uk/home.aspx.

130. Kaye Wellings et al., "Changes in, and Factors Associated with, Frequency of Sex in Britain: Evidence from Three National Surveys of Sexual Attitudes and Lifestyles (Natsal)," *BMJ* 365, no. l1525 (2019), pp. 1–9, https://doi.org/10.1136/bmj.l1525.

131. Ueda, Mercer, and Ghaznavi, "Trends in Frequency of Sexual Activity," eTable 6.

132. CDC, "HIV in the United States and Dependent Areas," https://www.cdc.gov/hiv/statistics/overview /ataglance.html.

133. CDC, "2018 STD Surveillance Report," https://www.cdc.gov/nchhstp/newsroom/2019/2018-STD -surveillance-report.html.

134. James Gorman, "Are Face Masks the New Condoms?," *New York Times,* April 18, 2020, https://www .nytimes.com/2020/04/18/health/coronavirus-mask-condom.html.

135. For Rees's "Long Now" interview on the subject in 2010, see FORA.tv, "Biotech Disaster by 2020? Martin Rees Weighs the Risks," September 14, 2010, YouTube video, 3:50, https://www.youtube.com/watch?v =zq-OBNft2OM.

136. Details of the bet can be found at Bet 9, Long Bets Project, http://longbets.org/9/.

137. Steven Pinker, *Enlightenment Now: The Case for Reason, Science, Humanism, and Progress* (New York: Viking, 2018), pp. 142, 301, 307.

138. Laurie Garrett, "The Next Pandemic," *Foreign Affairs,* July/August 2005, https://www.foreignaffairs .com/articles/2005-07-01/next-pandemic.

139. Dan Balz, "America Was Unprepared for a Major Crisis. Again," *Washington Post,* April 4, 2020, https://www.washingtonpost.com/graphics/2020/politics/america-was-unprepared-for-a-major-crisis -again/.

140. Michael Osterholm, "Preparing for the Next Pandemic," *Foreign Affairs,* July/August 2005, https://www.foreignaffairs.com/articles/2005-07-01/preparing-next-pandemic.

141. Larry Brilliant, "My Wish: Help Me Stop Pandemics," February 2006, TED video, 25:38, https://www .ted.com/talks/larry_brilliant_my_wish_help_me_stop_pandemics.

142. Ian Goldin and Mike Mariathasan, *The Butterfly Defect: How Globalization Creates Systemic Risks and What to Do About It* (Princeton, NJ: Princeton University Press, 2014), chap. 6.

143. Bill Gates, "The Next Outbreak: We're Not Ready," March 2015, TED video, 8:25, https://www.ted .com/talks/bill_gates_the_next_outbreak_we_re_not_ready.

144. Robert G. Webster, *Flu Hunter: Unlocking the Secrets of a Virus* (Otago, New Zealand: University of Otago Press, 2018).

145. Ed Yong, "The Next Plague Is Coming. Is America Ready?," *Atlantic,* July/August 2018, https://www .theatlantic.com/magazine/archive/2018/07/when-the-next-plague-hits/561734/.

146. Thoughty2, "This Is the New Killer Virus That Will End Humanity," November 15, 2019, YouTube video, 15:35, https://www.youtube.com/watch?v=-Jhz0pVSKtI&app=desktop.

147. Lawrence Wright, *The End of October* (New York: Random House, 2020). This book was presumably completed in 2019.

148. Peter Frankopan, "We Live in the Age of the Pandemic. This Is What We Need to Do About It," *Prospect,* December 8, 2019, https://www.prospectmagazine.co.uk/magazine/pandemic-likelihood-preparedness -uk-who-global.

149. A. S. Fauci, "Infectious Diseases: Considerations for the 21st Century," IDSA lecture, *Clinical Infectious Diseases* 32 (2001), pp. 675–78. On the difficulties with TB vaccines, see Morven E. M. Wilkie and

Helen McShane, "TB Vaccine Development: Where Are We and Why Is It So Difficult?," *Thorax* 70 (2015), pp. 299–301, https://doi.org/10.1136/thoraxjnl-2014-205202.

150. David M. Morens et al., "The Challenge of Emerging and Re-emerging Infectious Diseases," *Nature* 430 (July 8, 2004), pp. 242–49; Robin A. Weiss, "The Leeuwenhoek Lecture, 2001: Animal Origins of Human Infectious Diseases," *Philosophical Transactions of the Royal Society Biological Sciences* 356 (2001), pp. 957–77. See also Dorothy H. Crawford, *Deadly Companions: How Microbes Shaped Our History* (Oxford: Oxford University Press, 2007), pp. 214f.

151. K. E. Jones et al., "Global Trends in Emerging Infectious Diseases," *Nature* 451 (February 2008), pp. 990–94.

152. Vittoria Colizza, Alain Barrat, Marc Barthélemy, and Alessandro Vespignani, "The Role of the Airline Transportation Network in the Prediction and Predictability of Global Epidemics," *PNAS* 103, no. 7 (2006), pp. 2015–20. See also Globalization 101, "Health and Globalization," SUNY Levin Institute, http://www.globalization101.org.

153. Stephen S. Morse, "Emerging Viruses: Defining the Rules for Viral Traffic," *Perspectives in Biology and Medicine* 34, no. 3 (1991), pp. 387–409; Joshua Lederberg, "Infectious Diseases as an Evolutionary Paradigm," *Emerging Infectious Diseases* 3, no. 4 (December 1997), pp. 417–23. See also Mark Honigsbaum, *The Pandemic Century: A History of Global Contagion from the Spanish Flu to Covid-19* (London: Penguin, 2020), pp. 165f.

154. D. Campbell-Lendrum, "Global Climate Change: Implications for International Public Health Policy," *Bulletin of the World Health Organization* 85, no. 3 (2007), pp. 235–37. See also World Health Organization, *Climate Change and Human Health: Risks and Responses, Summary* (Geneva: WHO, 2003).

155. Kristian G. Andersen et al., "The Proximal Origin of SARS-CoV-2," *Nature Medicine* 26 (March 17, 2020), pp. 450–52, https://www.nature.com/articles/s41591-020-0820-9.

156. Petersen et al., "Comparing SARS-CoV-2 with SARS-CoV and Influenza."

157. Barabási, *Network Science*, chap. 10.

158. J. O. Lloyd-Smith et al., "Superspreading and the Effect of Individual Variation on Disease Emergence," *Nature* 438 (2005), pp. 355–59, https://www.nature.com/articles/nature04153.

159. See, in general, Thomas Abraham, *Twenty-First Century Plague: The Story of SARS* (Baltimore: John Hopkins University Press, 2007).

160. Abraham, *Twenty-First Century Plague*, p. 87.

161. Abraham, *Twenty-First Century Plague*, pp. 101–4.

162. Richard D. Smith, "Responding to Global Infectious Disease Outbreaks: Lessons from SARS on the Role of Risk Perception, Communication and Management," *Social Science and Medicine* 63 (2006), pp. 3113–23.

163. V. Rossi and John Walker, "Assessing the Economic Impact and Costs of Flu Pandemics Originating in Asia," Oxford Economic Forecasting Group (2005), pp. 1–23.

164. "COVID-19 Science Update for March 27th: Super-Spreaders and the Need for New Prediction Models," *Quillette*, March 27, 2020, https://quillette.com/2020/03/27/covid-19-science-update-for-march-27-super-spreaders-and-the-need-for-new-prediction-models/.

165. Petersen et al., "Comparing SARS-CoV-2 with SARS-CoV and Influenza," table 1.

166. David Quammen, *Ebola: The Natural and Human History* (London: Bodley Head, 2014), loc. 702–15, Kindle; Richard Preston, *The Hot Zone* (New York: Random House, 1994), p. 68.

167. Garrett, "Ebola's Lessons," pp. 80–107.

168. Honigsbaum, *Pandemic Century*, pp. 202f.

169. Garrett, "Ebola's Lessons," pp. 94f.

170. Garrett, "Ebola's Lessons," p. 97.

171. Zeynep Tufekci, "Ebola: The Real Reason Everyone Should Panic," *Medium*, October 23, 2014, https://medium.com/message/ebola-the-real-reason-everyone-should-panic-889f32740e3e.

172. John Poole, "'Shadow' and 'D-12' Sing an Infectious Song About Ebola," *Morning Edition*, NPR, August 19, 2014, https://www.npr.org/sections/goatsandsoda/2014/08/19/341412011/shadow-and-d-12-sing-an-infectious-song-about-ebola.

Chapter 8: The Fractal Geometry of Disaster

1. Airline Accident Fatalities per Year, 1946–2017, Aviation Safety Network, https://aviation-safety.net/graphics/infographics/Airliner-Accident-Fatalities-Per-Year-1946-2017.jpg.

2. Airliner Accidents per 1 Million Flights, 1977–2017, Aviation Safety Network, https://aviation-safety.net/graphics/infographics/Fatal-Accidents-Per-Mln-Flights-1977-2017.jpg.

3. Sebastian Junger, *The Perfect Storm* (New York: W. W. Norton, 1997).

4. "Meteorologists Say 'Perfect Storm' Not So Perfect," *Science Daily*, June 29, 2000, https://www.sciencedaily.com/releases/2000/06/000628101549.htm.

5. James Reason, *Human Error* (Cambridge: Cambridge University Press, 1990), p. 175.

6. Jens Rasmussen, "The Definition of Human Error and a Taxonomy for Technical Systems Design," in *New Technology and Human Error*, ed. J. Rasmussen, K. Duncan, and J. Leplat (London: Wiley, 1987), pp. 23–30.

7. James B. Battles, "Disaster Prevention: Lessons Learned from the *Titanic*," *Baylor University Medical Center Proceedings* 14, no. 2 (April 2001), pp. 150–53.

8. Roy Mengot, "*Titanic* and the Iceberg," Titanic Research and Modeling Association, https://web .archive.org/web/20130920234448/http://titanic-model.com/db/db-02/rm-db-2.html.

9. "Did Anyone Really Think the *Titanic* Was Unsinkable?," *Britannica,* https://www.britannica.com /story/did-anyone-really-think-the-titanic-was-unsinkable.

10. History.com, "The *Titanic*: Sinking & Facts," November 9, 2009, updated March 10, 2020, https:// www.history.com/topics/early-20th-century-us/titanic.

11. Battles, "Disaster Prevention," p. 151.

12. Andrew Wilson, *Shadow of the* Titanic: *The Extraordinary Stories of Those Who Survived* (New York: Atria, 2012), p. 7. See also Frances Wilson, *How to Survive the* Titanic, *or The Sinking of J. Bruce Ismay* (London: Bloomsbury, 2012).

13. Atlanticus, "The Unlearned Lesson of the *Titanic*," *Atlantic* (August 1913), https://www.theatlantic .com/magazine/archive/1913/08/the-unlearned-lesson-of-the-titanic/308866/.

14. Mikael Elinder and Oscar Erixson, "Every Man for Himself! Gender, Norms and Survival in Maritime Disasters," IFN Working Paper No. 913 (April 2, 2012), Research Institute of Industrial Economics (Stockholm).

15. Bob Vosseller, "Remembering the *Hindenburg* Is Important for All," *Jersey Shore Online,* May 6, 2017, https://www.jerseyshoreonline.com/ocean-county/remembering-hindenburg-passion-important/.

16. National Geographic Channel, *Seconds from Disaster: The* Hindenburg (2005), dir. by Yavar Abbas, YouTube video, 1:06:29, https://www.youtube.com/watch?v=mCQ0uk3AWQ8&t=2811s.

17. Joanna Walters, "The *Hindenburg* Disaster, 80 Years On: A 'Perfect Storm of Circumstances,'" *Guardian,* May 7, 2017, https://www.theguardian.com/us-news/2017/may/07/hindenburg-disaster-80th -anniversary.

18. Karl E. Weick, "The Vulnerable System: An Analysis of the Tenerife Air Disaster," *Journal of Management* 16, no. 3 (1990), p. 573.

19. Diane Tedeschi, "Crash in the Canary Islands," *Air & Space Magazine,* June 2019, https://www.air spacemag.com/history-of-flight/reviews-crash-in-canary-islands-180972227/.

20. John David Ebert, "The Plane Crash at Tenerife: What It Unconceals," in *The Age of Catastrophe: Disaster and Humanity in Modern Times* (Jefferson, NC, and London: McFarland & Co., 2012), loc. 60, 598–612, Kindle.

21. Weick, "Vulnerable System," p. 573.

22. Tedeschi, "Crash in the Canary Islands."

23. Weick, "Vulnerable System," p. 587.

24. Terence Hunt, "NASA Suggested Reagan Hail *Challenger* Mission in State of Union," Associated Press, March 12, 1986, https://apnews.com/00a395472559b3afcd22de473da2e65f.

25. Margaret Lazarus Dean, "The Oral History of the Space Shuttle *Challenger* Disaster," *Popular Mechanics,* January 28, 2019, https://www.popularmechanics.com/space/a18616/an-oral-history-of-the-space -shuttle-challenger-disaster/.

26. John Schwartz and Matthew L. Ward, "NASA's Curse? 'Groupthink' Is 30 Years Old and Still Going Strong," *New York Times,* March 9, 2003, https://www.nytimes.com/2003/03/09/weekinreview/the -nation-nasa-s-curse-groupthink-is-30-years-old-and-still-going-strong.html.

27. Richard A. Clarke and R. P. Eddy, *Warnings: Finding Cassandras to Stop Catastrophes* (New York: Harper-Collins, 2018), pp. 11–13.

28. Wade Robison, Roger Boisjoly, David Hoeker, and Stefan Young, "Representation and Misrepresentation: Tufte and the Morton Thiokol Engineers on the *Challenger*," *Science and Engineering Ethics* 8, no. 1 (2002), p. 72.

29. Roger Boisjoly, "Ethical Decisions—Morton Thiokol and the Space Shuttle Disaster," *ASME Proceedings,* December 13–18, 1987, p. 4.

30. See also Diane Vaughan, *The* Challenger *Launch Decision* (Chicago: University of Chicago Press, 1996), pp. 155, 343.

31. Joe Atkinson, "Engineer Who Opposed *Challenger* Launch Offers Personal Look at Tragedy," *Researcher News* (Langley Research Center, Hampton, VA), October 2012, https://www.nasa.gov/centers/langley /news/researchernews/rn_Colloquium1012.html.

32. Lazarus Dean, "Oral History of the Space Shuttle *Challenger* Disaster."

33. Richard Feynman, *"What Do You Care What Other People Think?": Further Adventures of a Curious Character* (New York: W. W. Norton, 1988).

34. Feynman, *"What Do You Care,"* pp. 138ff.

35. Feynman, *"What Do You Care,"* pp. 179f.

36. Feynman, *"What Do You Care,"* pp. 181–84.

37. Richard Feynman, "Personal Observations on the Reliability of the Shuttle," appendix F to the Rogers Commission report, https://science.ksc.nasa.gov/shuttle/missions/51-l/docs/rogers-commission /Appendix-F.txt.

38. Feynman, *"What Do You Care,"* p. 212.

39. Feynman, *"What Do You Care,"* pp. 213–17.
40. Allan J. McDonald and James R. Hansen, *Truth, Lies, and O-Rings: Inside the Space Shuttle* Challenger *Disaster* (Gainesville: University Press of Florida, 2009), pp. 91f.
41. McDonald and Hansen, *Truth, Lies, and O-Rings*, pp. 102–10.
42. WJXT, "Challenger: *A Rush to Launch*," posted by Jason Payne, January 28, 2016, YouTube video, 50:21, https://www.youtube.com/watch?v=2FehGJQlOf0.
43. McDonald and Hansen, *Truth, Lies, and O-Rings*, p. 107.
44. Serhii Plokhy, *Chernobyl: History of a Tragedy* (London: Penguin, 2018), p. 347.
45. "The Real Chernobyl," dir. by Stephanie DeGroote, Sky News (2019).
46. Plokhy, *Chernobyl*, pp. 46–49, 321–22, 347.
47. World Nuclear Association, "Chernobyl Accident 1986," https://www.world-nuclear.org/information -library/safety-and-security/safety-of-plants/chernobyl-accident.aspx.
48. Plokhy, *Chernobyl*, pp. 321–22.
49. World Nuclear Association, "Chernobyl Accident 1986."
50. Plokhy, *Chernobyl*, pp. 46–49.
51. Plokhy, *Chernobyl*, p. 347.
52. World Nuclear Association, "RBMK Reactors—Appendix to Nuclear Power Reactors," https://www .world-nuclear.org/information-library/nuclear-fuel-cycle/nuclear-power-reactors/appendices /rbmk-reactors.aspx.
53. United Nations Scientific Committee on the Effects of Atomic Radiation, *UNSCEAR Report to the General Assembly: Sources and Effects of Ionizing Radiation* (New York: United Nations, 2018), pp. 5, 15–17.
54. International Atomic Energy Agency, "Chernobyl's Legacy: Health, Environmental and Socio-Economic Impacts," in *The Chernobyl Forum, 2003–2005*, 2nd rev. version (Vienna, 2006), p. 8, http://www.iaea .org/Publications/Booklets/Chernobyl/chernobyl.pdf. See also UN Chernobyl Forum Expert Group "Health," *Health Effects of the Chernobyl Accident and Special Health Care Programmes* (Geneva: World Health Organization, 2006).
55. J. Little, "The Chernobyl Accident, Congenital Anomalies and Other Reproductive Outcomes," *Paediatric and Perinatal Epidemiology* 7, no. 2 (April 1993), pp. 121–51, https://doi.org/10.1111/j.1365-3016 .1993.tb00388.x.
56. Story Hinckley, "Chernobyl Will Be Unhabitable for at Least 3,000 Years, Say Nuclear Experts," *Christian Science Monitor*, April 24, 2016, https://www.csmonitor.com/World/Global-News/2016/0424 /Chernobyl-will-be-unhabitable-for-at-least-3-000-years-say-nuclear-experts.
57. Yu A. Izrael et al., "The Atlas of Caesium-137 Contamination of Europe After the Chernobyl Accident," Joint Study Project of the CEC/CIS Collaborative Programme on the Consequences of the Chernobyl Accident (n.d.), https://inis.iaea.org/collection/NCLCollectionStore/_Public/31/056/31056824.pdf.
58. "The Real Chernobyl."
59. United States Nuclear Regulatory Commission, "Backgrounder on the Three Mile Island Accident" (June 2018), https://www.nrc.gov/reading-rm/doc-collections/fact-sheets/3mile-isle.html.
60. Three Mile Island Special Inquiry Group, *Human Factors Evaluation of Control Room Design and Operator Performance at Three Mile Island-2*, NUREG/CR-1270, vol. I (Washington, D.C.: United States Nuclear Regulatory Commission, January 1980), pp. v–vi, https://www.osti.gov/servlets/purl/5603680.
61. Erin Blakemore, "How the Three Mile Island Accident Was Made Even Worse by a Chaotic Response," History.com, March 27, 2019, https://www.history.com/news/three-mile-island-evacuation-orders -controversy.
62. Federal Emergency Management Agency, *Evacuation Planning in the TMI Accident* (Washington, D.C.: FEMA, January 1980), pp. 167–70, https://apps.dtic.mil/dtic/tr/fulltext/u2/a080104.pdf.
63. "A Presidential Tour to Calm Fears," *Washington Post*, April 10, 1979, https://www.washingtonpost .com/wp-srv/national/longterm/tmi/stories/ch10.htm.
64. Charles B. Perrow, "The President's Commission and the Normal Accident," in *Accident at Three Mile Island: The Human Dimensions*, ed. D. Sils, C. Wolf, and V. Shelanski (Boulder, CO: Westview Press, 1982), pp. 173–84.
65. Tayler Lonsdale, "Complexity Kills: What Regulators Should Learn from the Grenfell Tower Fire," July 31, 2017, https://medium.com/@tayler_lonsdale/complexity-kills-what-regulators-should-learn-from-the -grenfell-tower-fire-21ec3cdfde47.
66. See Mary Douglas and Aaron Wildavsky, *Risk and Culture: An Essay on the Selection of Technical and Environmental Dangers* (Berkeley: University of California Press, 1982); Ulrich Beck, *Risikogesellschaft: Auf dem Wege in eine andere Moderne* (Frankfurt am Main: Suhrkamp, 1982).

Chapter 9: The Plagues

1. Bulletin of the Atomic Scientists Science and Security Board, "Closer Than Ever: It Is 100 Seconds to Midnight," ed. John Mecklin, https://thebulletin.org/doomsday-clock/current-time/.
2. "Greta Thunberg's Remarks at the Davos Economic Forum," *New York Times*, January 23, 2020, https:// www.nytimes.com/2020/01/21/climate/greta-thunberg-davos-transcript.html.

3. M. Bauwens et al., "Impact of Coronavirus Outbreak on NO_2 Pollution Assessed Using TROPOMI and OMI Observations," *Geophysical Research Letters* 47, no. 11 (May 6, 2020), pp. 1–9, https://doi.org/10.1029/2020GL087978.

4. Ben Goldfarb, "Lockdowns Could Be the 'Biggest Conservation Action' in a Century," *Atlantic,* July 6, 2020, https://www.theatlantic.com/science/archive/2020/07/pandemic-roadkill/613852/.

5. "Facts + Statistics: Mortality Risk," Insurance Information Institute, https://www.iii.org/fact-statistic/facts-statistics-mortality-risk; Kenneth D. Kochanek et al., "Deaths: Final Data for 2017," *National Vital Statistics Reports* 68, no. 9 (June 24, 2019), pp. 1–77, https://www.cdc.gov/nchs/data/nvsr/nvsr68/nvsr68_09-508.pdf.

6. CDC Wonder, "About Underlying Cause of Death, 1999–2018," https://wonder.cdc.gov/ucd-icd10.html.

7. COVID-19 Dashboard, Center for Systems Science and Engineering (CSSE), Johns Hopkins University, https://gisanddata.maps.arcgis.com/apps/opsdashboard/index.html#/bda7594740fd40299423467b48e9ecf6.

8. "United States Coronavirus Cases," Worldometers, https://www.worldometers.info/coronavirus/country/us/.

9. "COVID-19 Projections: United States of America," Institute for Health Metrics and Evaluation (IHME), August 6, 2020, https://covid19.healthdata.org/united-states-of-america; "United States COVID-19 Simulator," Massachusetts General Hospital (MGH) Institute for Technology Assessment, August 10, 2020, https://analytics-tools.shinyapps.io/covid19simulator06/.

10. Andrew Clark et al., "Global, Regional, and National Estimates of the Population at Increased Risk of Severe COVID-19 Due to Underlying Health Conditions in 2020: A Modelling Study," *Lancet Global Health* 8, no. 8 (June 15, 2020), pp. E1003–E1017, https://doi.org/10.1016/S2214-109X(20)30264-3.

11. Josh Rogin, "State Department Cables Warned of Safety Issues at Wuhan Lab Studying Bat Coronaviruses," *Washington Post,* April 14, 2020, https://www.washingtonpost.com/opinions/2020/04/14/state-department-cables-warned-safety-issues-wuhan-lab-studying-bat-coronaviruses/; Adam Sage, "Coronavirus: China Bars Safety Experts from Wuhan Lab," *Times* (London), April 22, 2020, https://www.thetimes.co.uk/edition/news/coronavirus-china-bars-safety-experts-from-wuhan-lab-brbm9rwtm.

12. Wu Fan et al., "A New Coronavirus Associated with Human Respiratory Disease in China," *Nature* 579 (February 3, 2020), pp. 265–69, https://doi.org/10.1038/s41586-020-2008-3.

13. Kristian G. Andersen et al., "The Proximal Origin of SARS-CoV-2," *Nature Medicine* 26 (March 17, 2020), pp. 450–52, www.nature.com/articles/s41591-020-0820-9; Li Xiaojun et al., "Emergence of SARS-CoV-2 Through Recombination and Strong Purifying Selection," *Science Advances* 6, no. 27 (July 1, 2020), pp. 1–11, https://doi.org/10.1126/sciadv.abb9153.

14. The following two paragraphs are based on Julia Belluz, "Did China Downplay the Coronavirus Outbreak Early On?," *Vox,* January 27, 2020, https://www.vox.com/2020/1/27/21082354/coronavirus-outbreak-wuhan-china-early-on-lancet; Dali L. Yang, "China's Early Warning System Didn't Work on COVID-19. Here's the Story," *Washington Post,* February 24, 2020, https://www.washingtonpost.com/politics/2020/02/24/chinas-early-warning-system-didnt-work-covid-19-heres-story/; Zhuang Pinghui, "Chinese Laboratory That First Shared Coronavirus Genome with World Ordered to Close for 'Rectification,' Hindering Its COVID-19 Research," *South China Morning Post,* February 28, 2020, https://www.scmp.com/news/china/society/article/3052966/chinese-laboratory-first-shared-coronavirus-genome-world-ordered; Sue-Lin Wong and Yuan Yang, "China Tech Groups Censored Information About Coronavirus," March 3, 2020, https://www.ft.com/content/35d7c414-5d53-11ea-8033-fa40a0d65a98; Sharri Markson, "Coronavirus NSW: Dossier Lays Out Case Against China Bat Virus Program," *Daily Telegraph,* May 4, 2020, https://www.dailytelegraph.com.au/coronavirus/bombshell-dossier-lays-out-case-against-chinese-bat-virus-program/news-story/55add857058731c9c71c0e96ad17da60.

15. Nicholas A. Christakis, *Apollo's Arrow: The Profound and Enduring Impact of Coronavirus on the Way We Live* (New York: Little, Brown Spark, 2020), p. 5.

16. "China Delayed Releasing Coronavirus Info, Frustrating WHO," Associated Press, June 2, 2020, https://apnews.com/3c061794970661042b18d5aeaaed9fae.

17. Elaine Okanyene Nsoesie et al., "Analysis of Hospital Traffic and Search Engine Data in Wuhan China Indicates Early Disease Activity in the Fall of 2019," Harvard Medical School Scholarly Articles (2020), pp. 1–10, https://dash.harvard.edu/handle/1/42669767. For critiques of this paper, see Christopher Giles, Benjamin Strick, and Song Wanyuan, "Coronavirus: Fact-Checking Claims It Might Have Started in August 2019," BBC News, June 15, 2020, https://www.bbc.com/news/world-asia-china-53005768, and Zhao Yusha and Leng Shumei, "Doctors Reject 'Error-Filled' Harvard Paper," *Global Times,* June 10, 2020, https://www.globaltimes.cn/content/1191172.shtml.

18. Lanhee J. Chen, "Lost in Beijing: The Story of the WHO," *Wall Street Journal,* April 8, 2020, https://www.wsj.com/articles/lost-in-beijing-the-story-of-the-who-11586365090; Dan Blumenthal and Nicholas Eberstadt, "China Unquarantined," *National Review,* June 22, 2020, https://www.nationalreview.com/magazine/2020/06/22/our-disastrous-engagement-of-china/#slide-1.

19. Katsuji Nakazawa, "China's Inaction for 3 Days in January at Root of Pandemic," *Nikkei Asian Review,* March 19, 2020, https://asia.nikkei.com/Editor-s-Picks/China-up-close/China-s-inaction-for-3-days-in-January-at-root-of-pandemic.

20. Wu Jin et al., "How the Virus Got Out," *New York Times,* March 22, 2020, https://www.nytimes.com /interactive/2020/03/22/world/coronavirus-spread.html.

21. Li Ruiyun et al., "Substantial Undocumented Infection Facilitates the Rapid Dissemination of Novel Coronavirus (SARS-CoV-2)," *Science* 368, no. 6490 (May 1, 2020), pp. 489–93, https://doi.org/10.1126 /science.abb3221. See also Wang Chaolong et al., "Evolving Epidemiology and Impact of Non-Pharmaceutical Interventions on the Outbreak of Coronavirus Disease 2019 in Wuhan, China," MedRxiv, March 6, 2020, pp. 1–30, https://doi.org/10.1101/2020.03.03.20030593.

22. Steven Sanche et al., "High Contagiousness and Spread of Severe Acute Respiratory Syndrome Coronavirus 2," *Emerging Infectious Diseases* 26, no. 7 (July 2020), pp. 1470–77, https://doi.org /10.3201/eid2607.200282.

23. Zheng Ruizhi et al., "Spatial Transmission of COVID-19 Via Public and Private Transportation in China," *Travel Medicine and Infectious Disease* 34 (March–April 2020), https://doi.org/10.1016/j .tmaid.2020.101626.

24. Benjamin F. Maier and Dirk Brockmann, "Effective Containment Explains Sub-Exponential Growth in Confirmed Cases of Recent COVID-19 Outbreak in Mainland China," MedRxiv, February 20, 2020, pp. 1–9, https://doi.org/10.1101/2020.02.18.20024414.

25. Maier and Brockmann, "Effective Containment Explains Sub-Exponential Growth"; Tian Huaiyu et al., "An Investigation of Transmission Control Measures During the First 50 Days of the COVID-19 Epidemic in China," *Science* 368, no. 6491 (May 8, 2020), pp. 638–42, https://doi.org/10.1126/science .abb6105.

26. Peter Hessler, "How China Controlled the Coronavirus," *New Yorker,* August 10, 2020, https://www .newyorker.com/magazine/2020/08/17/how-china-controlled-the-coronavirus.

27. "Readyscore Map," Prevent Epidemics, https://preventepidemics.org/map.

28. "2019 Global Health Security Index," https://www.ghsindex.org/.

29. Sawyer Crosby et al., "All Bets Are Off for Measuring Pandemic Preparedness," Think Global Health, June 30, 2020, https://www.thinkglobalhealth.org/article/all-bets-are-measuring-pandemic-preparedness.

30. "Coronavirus Health Safety Countries Ranking," Deep Knowledge Group, April 2, 2020, https://www .dkv.global/covid-19-health-safety.

31. Christakis, *Apollo's Arrow,* pp. 13–16.

32. Hamada S. Badr et al., "Association Between Mobility Patterns and COVID-19 Transmission in the USA: A Mathematical Modelling Study," *Lancet Infectious Diseases,* July 1, 2020, pp. 1–8, https://doi.org /10.1016/S1473-3099(20)30553-3. See also Stan Oklobdzija, "Visualization of NYT COVID-19 Data," University of California, San Diego, August 14, 2020, http://acsweb.ucsd.edu/~soklobdz/covid_map .html.

33. Hassani M. Behroozh and Yutong (Yuri) Song, "COVID-19 Application," ShinyApps, https://behroozh .shinyapps.io/COVID19/.

34. Denise Lu, "The True Coronavirus Toll in the U.S. Has Already Surpassed 200,000," *New York Times,* August 13, 2020, https://www.nytimes.com/interactive/2020/08/12/us/covid-deaths-us.html.

35. National Center for Health Statistics, "Excess Deaths Associated with COVID-19," https://www.cdc .gov/nchs/nvss/vsrr/covid19/excess_deaths.htm.

36. Charles Tallack, "Understanding Excess Mortality: Comparing COVID-19's Impact in the UK to Other European Countries," Health Foundation, June 30, 2020, https://www.health.org.uk/news-and-comment /charts-and-infographics/comparing-covid-19-impact-in-the-uk-to-european-countries.

37. "Coronavirus Tracked: The Latest Figures as Countries Fight COVID-19 Resurgence," *Financial Times,* August 14, 2020, https://www.ft.com/content/a2901ce8-5eb7-4633-b89c-cbdf5b386938.

38. Era Iyer, "Some Are Winning—Some Are Not: Which States and Territories Do Best in Beating COVID-19?," End Coronavirus, https://www.endcoronavirus.org/states?itemId=wja54gdfp032z0770l s4y81fw8cq66.

39. Tomas Pueyo, "Coronavirus: Why You Must Act Now," *Medium,* March 10, 2020, https://medium .com/@tomaspueyo/coronavirus-act-today-or-people-will-die-f4d3d9cd99ca.

40. Jacob B. Aguilar et al., "A Model Describing COVID-19 Community Transmission Taking into Account Asymptomatic Carriers and Risk Mitigation," MedRxiv, August 11, 2020, pp. 1–32, https://doi.org /10.1101/2020.03.18.20037994; Sanche et al., "High Contagiousness."

41. Eskild Petersen et al., "Comparing SARS-CoV-2 with SARS-CoV and Influenza Pandemics," *Lancet Infectious Diseases* 20, no. 9 (September 2020), pp. E238–E244, https://doi.org/10.1016/S1473-3099(20) 30484-9.

42. See, e.g., Arnaud Fontanet et al., "Cluster of COVID-19 in Northern France: A Retrospective Closed Cohort Study," MedRxiv, April 23, 2020, pp. 1–22, https://doi.org/10.1101/2020.04.18.20071134.

43. "COVID-19 Pandemic Planning Scenarios," CDC, July 10, 2020, https://www.cdc.gov/coronavirus /2019-ncov/hcp/planning-scenarios.html.

44. Kim Jeong-min et al., "Identification of Coronavirus Isolated from a Patient in Korea with COVID-19," *Osong Public Health and Research Perspectives* 11, no. 1 (February 2020), pp. 3–7, https://doi.org/10.24171 /j.phrp.2020.11.1.02; Joshua L. Santarpia et al., "Aerosol and Surface Transmission Potential of SARS-CoV-2," MedRxiv, June 3, 2020, pp. 1–19, https://www.medrxiv.org/content/10.1101/2020.03.23 .20039446v2.

45. Valentyn Stadnytskyi et al., "The Airborne Lifetime of Small Speech Droplets and Their Potential Importance in SARS-CoV-2 Transmission," *PNAS* 117, no. 22 (June 2, 2020), pp. 11875–77, https://doi .org/10.1073/pnas.2006874117; Lydia Bourouiba, "Turbulent Gas Clouds and Respiratory Pathogen Emissions: Potential Implications for Reducing Transmission of COVID-19," *Journal of the American Medical Association* (henceforth *JAMA*) 323, no. 18 (March 26, 2020), pp. 1837–38, https://doi.org /10.1001/jama.2020.4756.

46. Jonathan Kay, "COVID-19 Superspreader Events in 28 Countries: Critical Patterns and Lessons," *Quillette*, April 23, 2020, https://quillette.com/2020/04/23/covid-19-superspreader-events-in-28-countries -critical-patterns-and-lessons/; Lidia Morawska and Donald K. Milton, "It Is Time to Address Airborne Transmission of COVID-19," *Clinical Infectious Diseases,* July 6, 2020, pp. 1–9, https://doi.org/10.1093 /cid/ciaa939.

47. Kimberly A. Prather, Chia C. Wang, and Robert T. Schooley, "Reducing Transmission of SARS-CoV-2," *Science* 368, no. 6498, June 26, 2020, pp. 1422–24, https://doi.org/10.1126/science.abc6197; Richard O. J. H. Stutt et al., "A Modelling Framework to Assess the Likely Effectiveness of Facemasks in Combination with 'Lock-Down' in Managing the COVID-19 Pandemic," *Proceedings of the Royal Society* 476, no. 2238 (June 10, 2020), pp. 1–21, https://doi.org/10.1098/rspa.2020.0376. For the unconvincing case against masks, see Graham P. Martin, Esmée Hanna, and Robert Dingwall, "Face Masks for the Public During COVID-19: An Appeal for Caution in Policy," SocArXiv, April 25, 2020, pp. 1–7, https:// doi.org/10.31235/osf.io/uyzxe.

48. Qian Hua et al., "Indoor Transmission of SARS-CoV-2," MedRxiv, April 7, 2020, pp. 1–22, https://doi .org/10.1101/2020.04.04.20053058.

49. Jordan Peccia et al., "SARS-CoV-2 RNA Concentrations in Primary Municipal Sewage Sludge as a Leading Indicator of COVID-19 Outbreak Dynamics," MedRxiv, June 12, 2020, pp. 1–12, https://doi.org /10.1101/2020.05.19.20105999; Li Yun-yun, Wang Ji-xiang, and Chen Xi, "Can a Toilet Promote Virus Transmission? From a Fluid Dynamics Perspective," *Physics of Fluids* 32, no. 6 (June 16, 2020), pp. 1–15, https://doi.org/10.1063/5.0013318.

50. Multiple papers pursued this probably wrong hypothesis: see Wang Jingyuan et al., "High Temperature and High Humidity Reduce the Transmission of COVID-19," May 22, 2020, pp. 1–33, available at SSRN, http://dx.doi.org/10.2139/ssrn.3551767; Ma Yueling et al., "Effects of Temperature Variation and Humidity on the Mortality of COVID-19 in Wuhan," MedRxiv, March 18, 2020, pp. 1–13, https:// doi.org/10.1101/2020.03.15.20036426; Qi Hongchao et al., "COVID-19 Transmission in Mainland China Is Associated with Temperature and Humidity: A Time-Series Analysis," MedRxiv, March 30, 2020, pp. 1–19, https://doi.org/10.1101/2020.03.30.20044099; Mohammad M. Sajadi et al., "Temperature, Humidity and Latitude Analysis to Predict Potential Spread and Seasonality for COVID-19," April 6, 2020, pp. 1–18, available at SSRN, http://dx.doi.org/10.2139/ssrn.3550308; Kyle Meng, "Research: Working Papers," http://www.kylemeng.com/research; Qasim Bukhari and Yusuf Jameel, "Will Coronavirus Pandemic Diminish by Summer?," April 18, 2020, pp. 1–15, available at SSRN, http:// dx.doi.org/10.2139/ssrn.3556998; Mohammad M. Sajadi et al., "Temperature, Humidity and Latitude Analysis to Estimate Potential Spread and Seasonality of Coronavirus Disease 2019 (COVID-19)," *JAMA Network Open* 3, no. 6 (June 11, 2020), pp. 1–11, https://doi.org/10.1001/jamanetworkopen.2020.11834.

51. Cristina Menni et al., "Real-Time Tracking of Self-Reported Symptoms to Predict Potential COVID-19," *Nature Medicine* 26 (May 11, 2020), pp. 1037–40, https://doi.org/10.1038/s41591-020-0916-2; Tyler Wagner et al., "Augmented Curation of Medical Notes from a Massive EHR System Reveals Symptoms of Impending COVID-19 Diagnosis," MedRxiv, June 11, 2020, pp. 1–13, https://doi.org/10.1101/2020.04 .19.20067660.

52. Henrik Salje et al., "Estimating the Burden of SARS-CoV-2 in France," *Science* 369, no. 6500 (July 10, 2020), pp. 208–11, https://doi.org/10.1126/science.abc3517.

53. Liu Xiaoqing et al., "COVID-19 Does Not Lead to a 'Typical' Acute Respiratory Distress Syndrome," *American Journal of Respiratory and Critical Care Medicine* 201, no. 10 (May 15, 2020), pp. 1299–1300, https://doi.org/10.1164/rccm.202003-0817LE.

54. Derek Thompson, "COVID-19 Cases Are Rising, So Why Are Deaths Flatlining?," *Atlantic,* July 9, 2020, https://www.theatlantic.com/ideas/archive/2020/07/why-covid-death-rate-down/613945/.

55. Maximilian Ackermann et al., "Pulmonary Vascular Endothelialitis, Thrombosis, and Angiogenesis in COVID-19," *New England Journal of Medicine* (henceforth *NEJM*) 383 (July 9, 2020), pp. 120–28, https://doi.org/10.1056/NEJMoa2015432.

56. Jennifer Beam Dowd et al., "Demographic Science Aids in Understanding the Spread and Fatality Rates of COVID-19," *PNAS* 117, no. 18 (May 5, 2020), pp. 9696–98, https://doi.org/10.1073/pnas.2004911117.

57. Jason Douglas and Daniel Michaels, "New Data Reveal Just How Deadly COVID-19 Is for the Elderly," *Wall Street Journal,* June 27, 2020, https://www.wsj.com/articles/new-data-reveal-just-how-deadly -covid-19-is-for-the-elderly-11593250200.

58. Graziano Onder, Giovanni Rezza, and Silvio Brusaferro, "Case-Fatality Rate and Characteristics of Patients Dying in Relation to COVID-19 in Italy," *JAMA* 323, no. 18 (March 23, 2020), pp. 1775–76, https://doi.org/10.1001/jama.2020.4683; Giacomo Grasselli et al., "Baseline Characteristics and Outcomes of 1591 Patients Infected with SARS-CoV-2 Admitted to ICUs of the Lombardy Region, Italy," *JAMA* 323, no. 16 (April 6, 2020), pp. 1574–81, https://doi.org/10.1001/jama.2020.5394.

59. Annemarie B. Docherty et al., "Features of 16,749 Hospitalised UK Patients with COVID-19 Using the ISARIC WHO Clinical Characterisation Protocol," MedRxiv, April 28, 2020, pp. 1–21, https://doi.org/10.1101/2020.04.23.20076042; Elizabeth Williamson et al., "OpenSAFELY: Factors Associated with COVID-19-Related Hospital Death in the Linked Electronic Health Records of 17 Million Adult NHS Patients," MedRxiv, May 7, 2020, pp. 1–22, https://doi.org/10.1101/2020.05.06.20092999. See also Tom Whipple and Kat Lay, "Diabetes Sufferers Account for Quarter of Hospital Coronavirus Deaths," *Times* (London), May 15, 2020, https://www.thetimes.co.uk/article/diabetes-sufferers-account-for-quarter-of-hospital-coronavirus-deaths-lpf2rnkpf.

60. Petersen et al., "Comparing SARS-CoV-2 with SARS-CoV and Influenza"; Christopher M. Petrilli et al., "Factors Associated with Hospitalization and Critical Illness Among 4,103 Patients with COVID-19 Disease in New York City," MedRxiv, April 11, 2020, pp. 1–25, https://doi.org/10.1101/2020.04.08.20057794. See also Paul Overberg and Jon Kamp, "U.S. Deaths Are Up Sharply, Though COVID-19's Precise Toll Is Murky," *Wall Street Journal,* May 15, 2020, https://www.wsj.com/articles/covid-19s-exact-toll-is-murky-though-u-s-deaths-are-up-sharply-11589555652.

61. Dilip DaSilva, "Introducing the Proximity Solution: A Strategy to Win the COVID-19 War," *Medium,* April 14, 2020, https://medium.com/@dilip.dasilva/introducing-the-proximity-solution-a-strategy-to-win-the-covid-19-war-70d5d109a9fa.

62. "When COVID-19 Deaths Are Analysed by Age, America Is an Outlier," *Economist,* June 24, 2020, https://www.economist.com/graphic-detail/2020/06/24/when-covid-19-deaths-are-analysed-by-age-america-is-an-outlier; "Adult Obesity Facts," CDC, https://www.cdc.gov/obesity/data/adult.html.

63. Paolo Perini et al., "Acute Limb Ischaemia in Young, Non-Atherosclerotic Patients with COVID-19," *Lancet* 395, no. 10236 (May 5, 2020), p. 1546, https://doi.org/10.1016/S0140-6736(20)31051-5; Alexander E. Merkler et al., "Risk of Ischemic Stroke in Patients with Coronavirus Disease 2019 (COVID-19) vs Patients with Influenza," *JAMA Neurology,* July 2, 2020, https://doi.org/10.1001/jamaneurol.2020.2730; Ariana Eujung Cha, "Young and Middle-Aged People, Barely Sick with COVID-19, Are Dying of Strokes," *Washington Post,* April 25, 2020, https://www.washingtonpost.com/health/2020/04/24/strokes-coronavirus-young-patients/; Ariana Eujung Cha, "'Frostbite' Toes and Other Peculiar Rashes May Be Signs of Hidden Coronavirus Infection, Especially in the Young," *Washington Post,* April 29, 2020, https://www.washingtonpost.com/health/2020/04/29/coronavirus-rashes-toes/.

64. Chris Smith, "Coronavirus Can Harm Your Body Even If You're Asymptomatic," *Boy Genius Report (BGR) Media,* June 17, 2020, https://bgr.com/2020/06/17/coronavirus-asymptomatic-spread-virus-can-harm-lungs-immune-system/.

65. Angelo Carfì et al., "Persistent Symptoms in Patients After Acute COVID-19," *JAMA* 324, no. 6 (July 9, 2020), pp. 603–5, https://doi.org/10.1001/jama.2020.12603.

66. Silvia Garazzino et al., "Multicentre Italian Study of SARS-CoV-2 Infection in Children and Adolescents, Preliminary Data as at 10 April 2020," *EuroSurveillance* 25, no. 18 (May 7, 2020), https://doi.org/10.2807/1560-7917.ES.2020.25.18.2000600; Julie Toubiana et al., "Kawasaki-Like Multisystem Inflammatory Syndrome in Children During the COVID-19 Pandemic in Paris, France: Prospective Observational Study," *BMJ* 369 (June 3, 2020), pp. 1–7, https://doi.org/10.1136/bmj.m2094.

67. Florian Götzinger et al., "COVID-19 in Children and Adolescents in Europe: A Multinational, Multicentre Cohort Study," *Lancet Child and Adolescent Health,* June 25, 2020, pp. 1–9, https://doi.org/10.1016/S2352-4642(20)30177-2.

68. John Eligon et al., "Black Americans Face Alarming Rates of Coronavirus Infection in Some States," *New York Times,* April 14, 2020, https://www.nytimes.com/2020/04/07/us/coronavirus-race.html; Overberg and Kamp, "U.S. Deaths Are Up Sharply."

69. Elizabeth J. Williamson et al., "Factors Associated with COVID-19-Related Death Using OpenSAFELY," *Nature,* July 8, 2020, pp. 1–17, https://doi.org/10.1038/s41586-020-2521-4. See also William Wallis, "How Somalis in East London Were Hit by the Pandemic," *Financial Times,* June 21, 2020, https://www.ft.com/content/aaa2c3cd-eea6-4cfa-a918-9eb7d1c230f4.

70. Neeraj Bhala et al., "Sharpening the Global Focus on Ethnicity and Race in the Time of COVID-19," *Lancet* 395, no. 10238 (May 8, 2020), pp. P1673–P1676, https://doi.org/10.1016/S0140-6736(20)31102-8. See also "The COVID-19 Racial Data Tracker," Atlantic COVID Tracking Project, https://covidtracking.com/race.

71. David A. Martinez et al., "SARS-CoV-2 Positivity Rate for Latinos in the Baltimore–Washington, D.C. Area," *JAMA* 324, no. 4 (June 18, 2020), pp. 392–95, https://doi.org/10.1001/jama.2020.11374; Samantha Artiga and Matthew Rae, "The COVID-19 Outbreak and Food Production Workers: Who Is At Risk?," *Kaiser Family Foundation News,* June 3, 2020, https://www.kff.org/coronavirus-covid-19/issue-brief/the-covid-19-outbreak-and-food-production-workers-who-is-at-risk/; Jonathan M. Wortham et al., "Characteristics of Persons Who Died with COVID-19—United States, February 12–May 18, 2020," *CDC Morbidity and Mortality Weekly Report (MMWR)* 69, no. 28 (July 17, 2020), pp. 923–29, http://dx.doi.org/10.15585/mmwr.mm6928e1. On Native Americans, see James Bikales, "Native American Tribal Nations Take Tougher Line on COVID-19 as States Reopen," *The Hill,* June 21, 2020, https://thehill.com/homenews/state-watch/503770-native-american-tribal-nations-take-tougher-line-on-covid-19-as-states, but also Ryan M. Close and Myles J. Stone, "Contact Tracing for Native Americans

in Rural Arizona," *NEJM* 383, no. 3 (July 16, 2020), pp. E15–E16, https://doi.org/10.1056/NEJMc20 23540.

72. Nasar Meer et al. "The Social Determinants of Covid-19 and BAME Disproportionality," Justice in Global Health Emergencies and Humanitarian Crises, May 5, 2020, https://www.ghe.law.ed.ac.uk /the-social-determinants-of-covid-19-and-bame-disproportionality-repost-by-nasar-meer-and -colleagues/. See also Wallis, "Somalis in East London," and Hugo Zeberg and Svante Pääbo, "The Major Genetic Risk Factor for Severe COVID-19 Is Inherited from Neandertals," BioRxiv, July 3, 2020, https://www.biorxiv.org/content/10.1101/2020.07.03.186296v1.

73. Gideon Meyerowitz-Katz, "Here's Why Herd Immunity Won't Save Us from the COVID-19 Pandemic," *Science Alert,* March 30, 2020, https://www.sciencealert.com/why-herd-immunity-will-not-save-us -from-the-covid-19-pandemic; Haley E. Randolph and Luis B. Barreiro, "Herd Immunity: Understand- ing COVID-19," *Immunity* 52, no. 5 (May 19, 2020), pp. 737–41, https://doi.org/10.1016/j.immuni.2020 .04.012.

74. Liu Tao et al., "Prevalence of IgG Antibodies to SARS-CoV-2 in Wuhan—Implications for the Ability to Produce Long-Lasting Protective Antibodies Against SARS-CoV-2," MedRxiv, June 16, 2020, pp. 1–30, https://doi.org/10.1101/2020.06.13.20130252; Henry M. Staines et al., "Dynamics of IgG Seroconver- sion and Pathophysiology of COVID-19 Infections," MedRxiv, June 9, 2020, pp. 1–21, https://doi.org /10.1101/2020.06.07.20124636; Long Quan-Xin et al., "Clinical and Immunological Assessment of Asymptomatic SARS-CoV-2 Infections," *Nature Medicine* 26 (June 18, 2020), pp. 1200–1204, https://doi .org/10.1038/s41591-020-0965-6; F. Javier Ibarrondo et al., "Rapid Decay of Anti-SARS-CoV-2 Anti- bodies in Persons with Mild COVID-19," *NEJM,* July 21, 2020, pp. 1–2, https://doi.org/10.1056 /NEJMc2025179.

75. Bao Linlin et al., "Reinfection Could Not Occur in SARS-CoV-2 Infected Rhesus Macaques," BioRxiv, March 14, 2020, pp. 1–20, https://doi.org/10.1101/2020.03.13.990226; Deng Wei et al., "Primary Ex- posure to SARS-CoV-2 Protects Against Reinfection in Rhesus Macaques," *Science* 369, no. 6505 (Au- gust 14, 2020), pp. 818–23, https://doi.org/10.1126/science.abc5343; "News Room: Press Release," Korean Centers for Disease Control, https://www.cdc.go.kr/board/board.es?mid=a30402000000& bid=0030; Roman Woelfel et al., "Clinical Presentation and Virological Assessment of Hospitalized Cases of Coronavirus Disease 2019 in a Travel-Associated Transmission Cluster," MedRxiv, March 8, 2020, pp. 1–16, https://doi.org/10.1101/2020.03.05.20030502; Ania Wajnberg et al., "Humoral Im- mune Response and Prolonged PCR Sensitivity in a Cohort of 1343 SARS-CoV-2 Patients in the New York City Region," MedRxiv, May 5, 2020, pp. 1–17, https://doi.org/10.1101/2020.04.30.20085613. However, see Apoorva Mandavilli, "First Documented Coronavirus Reinfection Reported in Hong Kong," *New York Times,* August 24, 2020, https://www.nytimes.com/2020/08/24/health/coronavirus -reinfection.html.

76. Paul K. Hegarty et al., "BCG Vaccination May Be Protective Against COVID-19," March 2020, pp. 1–8, Research Gate, https://doi.org/10.13140/RG.2.2.35948.10880; Martha K. Berg et al., "Mandated Ba- cillus Calmette-Guérin (BCG) Vaccination Predicts Flattened Curves for the Spread of COVID-19," MedRxiv, June 12, 2020, pp. 1–15, https://doi.org/10.1101/2020.04.05.20054163; Akiko Iwasaki and Nathan D. Grubaugh, "Why Does Japan Have So Few Cases of COVID-19?," *European Molecular Biol- ogy Organization (EMBO) Molecular Medicine* 12, no. 5 (May 8, 2020), pp. 1–3, https://doi.org/10.15252 /emmm.202012481; Luis E. Escobar, Alvaro Molina-Cruz, and Carolina Barillas-Mury, "BCG Vaccine Protection from Severe Coronavirus Disease 2019 (COVID-19)," *PNAS,* June 9, 2020, pp. 1–7, https:// doi.org/10.1073/pnas.2008410117.

77. Zhao Jiao et al., "Relationship Between the ABO Blood Group and the COVID-19 Susceptibility," MedRxiv, March 27, 2020, pp. 1–18, https://doi.org/10.1101/2020.03.11.20031096; David Ellinghaus et al., "Genomewide Association Study of Severe COVID-19 with Respiratory Failure," *NEJM,* June 17, 2020, pp. 1–13, https://doi.org/10.1056/NEJMoa2020283; Gabi Zietsman, "One Blood Type Seems to Be More Resistant Against COVID-19," *Health24 Infectious Diseases,* June 15, 2020, https://www .health24.com/Medical/Infectious-diseases/Coronavirus/one-blood-type-seems-to-be-more -resistant-against-covid-19-20200613-2.

78. Takuya Sekine et al., "Robust T Cell Immunity in Convalescent Individuals with Asymptomatic or Mild COVID-19," BioRxiv, June 29, 2020, pp. 1–35, https://doi.org/10.1101/2020.06.29.174888; Li Junwei et al., "Mapping the T Cell Response to COVID-19," *Nature Signal Transduction and Targeted Therapy* 5, no. 112 (July 2, 2020), pp. 1–2, https://doi.org/10.1038/s41392-020-00228-1; Alessandro Sette and Shane Crotty, "Pre-Existing Immunity to SARS-CoV-2: The Knowns and Unknowns," *Nature Reviews Immunology* 20 (July 7, 2020), pp. 457–58, https://doi.org/10.1038/s41577-020-0389-z; Floriane Gal- laise et al., "Intrafamilial Exposure to SARS-CoV-2 Induces Cellular Immune Response Without Sero- conversion," MedRxiv, June 22, 2020, pp. 1–15, https://doi.org/10.1101/2020.06.21.20132449; Paul W. Franks and Joacim Rocklöv, "Coronavirus: Could It Be Burning Out After 20% of a Population Is Infected?," *The Conversation,* June 29, 2020, https://theconversation.com/coronavirus-could-it-be-burning -out-after-20-of-a-population-is-infected-141584; Julian Braun et al., "Presence of SARS-CoV-2 Reac- tive T Cells in COVID-19 Patients and Healthy Donors," MedRxiv, April 22, 2020, pp. 1–12, https://doi .org/10.1101/2020.04.17.20061440; Kevin W. Ng et al., "Pre-Existing and *De Novo* Humoral Immunity

to SARS-CoV-2 in Humans," BioRxiv, July 23, 2020, pp. 1–38, https://doi.org/10.1101/2020.05.14 .095414; Nikolai Eroshenko et al., "Implications of Antibody-Dependent Enhancement of Infection for SARS-CoV-2 Countermeasures," *Nature Biotechnology* 38 (June 5, 2020), pp. 789–91, https://doi.org /10.1038/s41587-020-0577-1.

79. UnHerd, "Karl Friston: Up to 80% Not Even Susceptible to COVID-19," June 4, 2020, YouTube video, 34:14, https://youtu.be/dUOFeVIrOPg; Laura Spinney, "COVID-19 Expert Karl Friston: 'Germany May Have More Immunological Dark Matter,'" *Guardian,* May 31, 2020, https://www.theguardian.com /world/2020/may/31/covid-19-expert-karl-friston-germany-may-have-more-immunological-dark -matter.

80. Jia Yong et al., "Analysis of the Mutation Dynamics of SARS-CoV-2 Reveals the Spread History and Emergence of RBD Mutant with Lower ACE2 Binding Affinity," BioRxiv, April 11, 2020, pp. 1–17, https://doi.org/10.1101/2020.04.09.034942; B. Korber et al., "Spike Mutation Pipeline Reveals the Emergence of a More Transmissible Form of SARS-CoV-2," BioRxiv, April 30, 2020, pp. 1–33, https:// doi.org/10.1101/2020.04.29.069054. See also Stephen Chen, "Coronavirus's Ability to Mutate Has Been Vastly Underestimated, and Mutations Affect Deadliness of Strains, Chinese Study Finds," *South China Morning Post,* April 20, 2020, https://www.scmp.com/news/china/science/article/3080771 /coronavirus-mutations-affect-deadliness-strains-chinese-study.

81. Joshua Geleris et al., "Observational Study of Hydroxychloroquine in Hospitalized Patients with Covid-19," *NEJM,* June 18, 2020, https://www.nejm.org/doi/full/10.1056/nejmoa2012410; Alexandre B. Cavalcanti et al., "Hydroxychloroquine With or Without Azithromycin in Mild-to-Moderate Covid-19," *NEJM,* July 23, 2020, https://www.nejm.org/doi/full/10.1056/NEJMoa2019014; David R. Boulware et al., "A Randomized Trial of Hydroxychloroquine as Postexposure Prophylaxis for Covid-19," *NEJM,* July 23, 2020, https://www.nejm.org/doi/full/10.1056/NEJMoa2016638.

82. "COVID-19 Vaccine Tracker," Faster Cures, Milken Institute, August 14, 2020, https://www.covid -19vaccinetracker.org/. See, in general, Tung Thanh Le et al., "The COVID-19 Vaccine Development Landscape," *Nature Reviews Drug Discovery* 19 (April 9, 2020), pp. 305–6, https://doi.org/10.1038 /d41573-020-00073-5.

83. Stuart A. Thompson, "How Long Will a Vaccine Really Take?," *New York Times,* April 30, 2020, https:// www.nytimes.com/interactive/2020/04/30/opinion/coronavirus-covid-vaccine.html.

84. Nicholas Kumleben, R. Bhopal, T. Czypionka, L. Gruer, R. Kock, Justin Stebbing, and F. L. Stigler, "Test, Test, Test for COVID-19 Antibodies: The Importance of Sensitivity, Specificity and Predictive Powers," *Public Health* 185 (August 2020), pp. 88–90, https://doi.org/10.1016/j.puhe.2020.06.006.

85. Albert-László Barabási, *Network Science* (Cambridge: Cambridge University Press, 2016), chap. 10.

86. I owe this point to Cecilia Mascolo of Cambridge University.

87. Matthew J. Ferrari et al., "Network Frailty and the Geometry of Herd Immunity," *Proceedings of the Royal Society B: Biological Sciences* 273, no. 1602 (November 7, 2006), pp. 2743–48, https://doi.org /10.1098/rspb.2006.3636. See also M. Gabriela Gomes et al., "Individual Variation in Susceptibility or Exposure to SARS-CoV-2 Lowers the Herd Immunity Threshold," MedRxiv, May 21, 2020, pp. 1–10, https://doi.org/10.1101/2020.04.27.20081893.

88. Tom Britton, Frank Ball, and Pieter Trapman, "The Disease-Induced Herd Immunity Level for COVID-19 Is Substantially Lower than the Classical Herd Immunity Level," *Quantitative Biology: Populations and Evolution,* May 8, 2020, pp. 1–15, https://arxiv.org/abs/2005.03085. See also Ricardo Aguas et al., "Herd Immunity Thresholds for SARS-CoV-2 Estimated from Unfolding Epidemics," MedRxiv, July 24, 2020, https://doi.org/10.1101/2020.07.23.20160762.

89. Charles Musselwhite, Erel Avineri, and Yusak Susilo, "Editorial JTH 16—The Coronavirus Disease COVID-19 and Its Implications for Transport and Health," *Journal of Transport & Health* 16 (March 2020), https://doi.org/10.1016/j.jth.2020.100853.

90. Michael Laris, "Scientists Know Ways to Help Stop Viruses from Spreading on Airplanes. They're Too Late for This Pandemic," *Washington Post,* April 29, 2020, https://www.washingtonpost.com/local /trafficandcommuting/scientists-think-they-know-ways-to-combat-viruses-on-airplanes-theyre-too -late-for-this-pandemic/2020/04/20/83279318-76ab-11ea-87da-77a8136c1a6d_story.html.

91. U.S. Department of Commerce, ITA, National Travel and Tourism Office.

92. "Historical Flight Status," FlightStats by Cerium, https://www.flightstats.com/v2/historical-flight /subscribe.

93. For my debate on this subject with Daniel Bell, see Daniel A. Bell, "Did the Chinese Government Deliberately Export COVID-19 to the Rest of the World?," Danielabell.com, April 21, 2020, https:// danielabell.com/2020/04/21/did-the-chinese-government-deliberately-export-covid-19-to-the -rest-of-the-world/; Niall Ferguson, "Six Questions for Xi Jinping: An Update," Niallferguson.com, April 21, 2020, http://www.niallferguson.com/blog/six-questions-for-xi-jinping-an-update; Niall Ferguson, "Six Questions for Xi Jinping: Another Update," Niallferguson.com, May 26, 2020, http://www .niallferguson.com/blog/six-questions-for-xi-jinping-another-update.

94. Matteo Chinazzi et al., "The Effect of Travel Restrictions on the Spread of the 2019 Novel Coronavirus (2019-nCoV) Outbreak," MedRxiv, February 11, 2020, pp. 1–12, https://doi.org/10.1101/2020.02.09 .20021261.

95. Steve Eder et al., "430,000 People Have Traveled from China to U.S. Since Coronavirus Surfaced," *New York Times,* April 4, 2020, https://www.nytimes.com/2020/04/04/us/coronavirus-china-travel -restrictions.html.

96. Phillip Connor, "More than Nine-in-Ten People Worldwide Live in Countries with Travel Restrictions amid COVID-19," Fact Tank, Pew Research Center, April 1, 2020, https://www.pewresearch.org/fact -tank/2020/04/01/more-than-nine-in-ten-people-worldwide-live-in-countries-with-travel -restrictions-amid-covid-19/; Anthony Faiola, "The Virus That Shut Down the World," *Washington Post,* June 26, 2020, https://www.washingtonpost.com/graphics/2020/world/coronavirus-pandemic -globalization/?itid=hp_hp-banner-main_virus-shutdown-630pm.

97. "Relative Risk of Importing a Case of 2019-nCoV," Google Data Studio, August 17, 2020, https:// datastudio.google.com/u/0/reporting/3ffd36c3-0272-4510-a140-39e288a9f15c/page/U5lCB. See also Matteo Chinazzi et al., "Estimating the Risk of Sustained Community Transmission of COVID-19 Outside Mainland China," March 11, 2020, pp. 1–11, https://www.mobs-lab.org/uploads /6/7/8/7/6787877/estimating_the_risk_of_sustained_community_transmission_of_covid-19_outside _china.pdf.

98. Javier Salas and Mariano Zafra, "An Analysis of Three COVID-19 Outbreaks: How They Happened and How They Can Be Avoided," *El País English: Science & Tech,* June 17, 2020, https://english.elpais.com /spanish_news/2020-06-17/an-analysis-of-three-covid-19-outbreaks-how-they-happened-and-how -they-can-be-avoided.html; Liu Xiaopeng and Zhang Sisen, "COVID-19: Face Masks and Human-to- Human Transmission," *Influenza and Other Respiratory Viruses* 14, no. 4 (March 29, 2020), pp. 472–73, https://doi.org/10.1111/irv.12740.

99. Lara Goscé and Anders Johansson, "Analysing the Link Between Public Transport Use and Airborne Transmission: Mobility and Contagion in the London Underground," *Environmental Health* 17, no. 84 (December 4, 2018), pp. 1–11, https://doi.org/10.1186/s12940-018-0427-5; Jeffrey E. Harris, "The Subways Seeded the Massive Coronavirus Epidemic in New York City," NBER Working Paper No. 27021 (August 2020), https://doi.org/10.3386/w27021; Stephen M. Kissler et al., "Reductions in Commut- ing Mobility Predict Geographic Differences in SARS-CoV-2 Prevalence in New York City," Harvard School of Public Health Scholarly Articles (2020), pp. 1–15, http://nrs.harvard.edu/urn-3:HUL.In stRepos:42665370.

100. Bi Qifang et al., "Epidemiology and Transmission of COVID-19 in 391 Cases and 1286 of Their Close Contacts in Shenzhen, China: A Retrospective Cohort Study," *Lancet Infectious Diseases* 20, no. 8 (Au- gust 1, 2020), pp. P911–P919, https://doi.org/10.1016/S1473-3099(20)30287-5.

101. Christian Bayer and Moritz Kuhn, "Intergenerational Ties and Case Fatality Rates: A Cross-Country Analysis," *VoxEU & CEPR,* March 20, 2020: https://voxeu.org/article/intergenerational-ties-and-case -fatality-rates.

102. Liu Jingtao, Huang Jiaquan, and Xiang Dandan, "Large SARS-CoV-2 Outbreak Caused by Asymptom- atic Traveler, China," *Emerging Infectious Diseases* 26, no. 9 (June 30, 2020), https://doi.org/10.3201 /eid2609.201798.

103. Terry C. Jones et al., "An Analysis of SARS-CoV-2 Viral Load by Patient Age," MedRxiv, June 9, 2020, pp. 1–19, https://doi.org/10.1101/2020.06.08.20125484. See also Gretchen Vogel and Jennifer Couzin- Frankel, "Should Schools Reopen? Kids' Role in Pandemic Still a Mystery," *Science,* May 4, 2020, https://doi.org/10.1126/science.abc6227.

104. Didier Jourdan, Nicola Gray, and Michael Marmot, "Re-Opening Schools: What Knowledge Can We Rely Upon?," UNESCO Chair Global Health and Education, May 4, 2020, https://unescochair-ghe.org /2020/05/04/re-opening-schools-what-knowledge-can-we-rely-upon/.

105. "Amid Surge in Israeli Virus Cases, Schools in Outbreak Areas to Be Shuttered," *Times of Israel,* May 30, 2020, https://www.timesofisrael.com/amid-spike-in-virus-cases-schools-in-outbreak-areas-set-to -shutter/. For other school outbreaks, see Q. J. Leclerc et al., "What Settings Have Been Linked to SARS- CoV-2 Transmission Clusters?," *Wellcome Open Research* 5, no. 83 (2020), https://wellcomeopen research.org/articles/5-83.

106. Faris Mokhtar, "How Singapore Flipped from Virus Hero to Cautionary Tale," Bloomberg, April 21, 2020, https://www.bloomberg.com/news/articles/2020-04-21/how-singapore-flipped-from-virus -hero-to-cautionary-tale.

107. Tomas Pueyo, "Coronavirus: The Basic Dance Steps Everybody Can Follow," *Medium,* April 23, 2020, https://medium.com/@tomaspueyo/coronavirus-the-basic-dance-steps-everybody-can-follow -b3d216daa343. See also Julie Scagell, "Study Finds Spikes in Coronavirus Cases Linked to In-Person Restaurant Dining," *Yahoo! Life,* July 4, 2020, https://www.yahoo.com/lifestyle/study-finds-spikes -coronavirus-cases-161559634.html.

108. Yuki Furuse et al., "Clusters of Coronavirus Disease in Communities, Japan, January–April 2020," *Emerging Infectious Diseases* 26, no. 9 (June 10, 2020), https://doi.org/10.3201/eid2609.202272.

109. Shin Young Park et al., "Coronavirus Disease Outbreak in Call Center, South Korea," *Emerging Infec- tious Diseases* 26, no. 8 (April 23, 2020), https://doi.org/10.3201/eid2608.201274.

110. Leclerc et al., "What Settings Have Been Linked to SARS-CoV-2 Transmission Clusters?" See also Kay, "COVID-19 Superspreader Events."

111. David Pegg, Robert Booth, and David Conn, "Revealed: The Secret Report That Gave Ministers Warning of Care Home Coronavirus Crisis," *Guardian,* May 7, 2020, https://www.theguardian.com/world /2020/may/07/revealed-the-secret-report-that-gave-ministers-warning-of-care-home-coronavirus -crisis; Richard Coker, "'Harvesting' Is a Terrible Word—but It's What Has Happened in Britain's Care Homes," *Guardian,* May 8, 2020, https://www.theguardian.com/commentisfree/2020/may/08/care -home-residents-harvested-left-to-die-uk-government-herd-immunity; Robert Booth, "Coronavirus: Real Care Home Death Toll Double Official Figure, Study Says," *Guardian,* May 13, 2020, https://www .theguardian.com/world/2020/may/13/coronavirus-real-care-home-death-toll-double-official -figure-study-says. Cf. Tom McTague, "How the Pandemic Revealed Britain's National Illness," *Atlantic,* August 20, 2020, https://www.theatlantic.com/international/archive/2020/08/why-britain-failed -coronavirus-pandemic/615166/.

112. Gregg Girvan, "Nursing Homes and Assisted Living Facilities Account for 45% of COVID-19 Deaths," Foundation for Research on Equal Opportunity, May 7, 2020, https://freopp.org/the-covid-19-nursing -home-crisis-by-the-numbers-3a47433c3f70. See also Jessica Silver-Greenberg and Amy Julia Harris, "'They Just Dumped Him Like Trash': Nursing Homes Evict Vulnerable Residents," *New York Times,* July 23, 2020, https://www.nytimes.com/2020/06/21/business/nursing-homes-evictions-discharges -coronavirus.html, and Karen Yourish et al., "One-Third of All U.S. Coronavirus Deaths Are Nursing Home Residents or Workers," *New York Times,* May 11, 2020, https://www.nytimes.com/interactive /2020/05/09/us/coronavirus-cases-nursing-homes-us.html.

113. Joaquin Sapien and Joe Sexton, "'Fire Through Dry Grass': Andrew Cuomo Saw COVID-19's Threat to Nursing Homes. Then He Risked Adding to It," *ProPublica,* June 16, 2020, https://www.propublica .org/article/fire-through-dry-grass-andrew-cuomo-saw-covid-19-threat-to-nursing-homes-then -he-risked-adding-to-it.

114. Figures up to mid-June. Adelina Comas-Herrera, "Mortality Associated with COVID-19 Outbreaks in Care Homes: Early International Evidence," International Long Term Care Policy Network, June 26, 2020, https://ltccovid.org/wp-content/uploads/2020/06/Mortality-associated-with-COVID-among -people-who-use-long-term-care-26-June-1.pdf.

115. F. A. Hayek, *The Constitution of Liberty: The Definitive Edition,* ed. Ronald Hamowy, vol. 17 of *The Collected Works of F. A. Hayek* (Abingdon, UK: Routledge, 2011 [1960]), p. 421.

116. Jamie Lloyd-Smith (@jlloydsmith), "Couldn't resist such nice data and dusted off my old code," Twitter, May 20, 2020, 12:11 a.m., https://twitter.com/jlloydsmith/status/1262989192948146176; Kai Kupferschmidt, "Why Do Some COVID-19 Patients Infect Many Others, Whereas Most Don't Spread the Virus at All?," *Science,* May 19, 2020, https://www.sciencemag.org/news/2020/05/why-do-some -covid-19-patients-infect-many-others-whereas-most-don-t-spread-virus-all.

117. Akira Endo et al., "Estimating the Overdispersion in COVID-19 Transmission Using Outbreak Sizes Outside China," *Wellcome Open Research* 5, no. 67 (July 10, 2020), https://doi.org/10.12688/well comeopenres.15842.1.

118. Dillon Adam et al., "Clustering and Superspreading Potential of Severe Acute Respiratory Syndrome Coronavirus 2 (SARS-CoV-2) Infections in Hong Kong," May 21, 2020, pp. 1–27, Research Square, https://doi.org/10.21203/rs.3.rs-29548/v1.

119. Michael Worobey et al., "The Emergence of SARS-CoV-2 in Europe and the U.S.," BioRxiv, May 23, 2020, pp. 1–26, https://doi.org/10.1101/2020.05.21.109322; Carl Zimmer, "Coronavirus Epidemics Began Later Than Believed, Study Concludes," *New York Times,* May 27, 2020, https://www.nytimes .com/2020/05/27/health/coronavirus-spread-united-states.html.

120. Merle M. Böhmer et al., "Investigation of a COVID-19 Outbreak in Germany Resulting from a Single Travel-Associated Primary Case: A Case Series," *Lancet Infectious Diseases* 20, no. 8 (August 1, 2020), pp. P920–P928, https://doi.org/10.1016/S1473-3099(20)30314-5.

121. Haroon Siddique, "'Super-Spreader' Brought Coronavirus from Singapore to Sussex via France," *Guardian,* February 10, 2020, https://www.theguardian.com/world/2020/feb/10/super-spreader-brought -coronavirus-from-singapore-to-sussex-via-france.

122. Marco Hernandez, Simon Scarr, and Manas Sharma, "The Korean Clusters: How Coronavirus Cases Exploded in South Korean Churches and Hospitals," Reuters, March 20, 2020, https://graphics.reuters .com/CHINA-HEALTH-SOUTHKOREA-CLUSTERS/0100B5G33SB/index.html.

123. Eric Reguly, "Italy Investigates a Hospital That Failed to Catch a Coronavirus Super-Spreader as Infection Cases Rise," *Globe and Mail* (Toronto), March 11, 2020, https://www.theglobeandmail.com/world /article-italy-investigates-hospital-that-failed-to-catch-a-coronavirus-super/.

124. Carey Goldberg, "Single Conference Linked to Most Mass. Coronavirus Cases Looks Like a 'Super-spreading Event,'" WBUR News, March 12, 2020, https://www.wbur.org/commonhealth/2020/03/12 /coronavirus-outbreak-biogen-conference-superspreading; Drew Karedes, "Hotel at Center of Biogen Meeting Linked to COVID-19 Outbreak in Boston Closed Indefinitely," Boston 25 News, March 12, 2020, https://www.boston25news.com/news/hotel-center-biogen-meeting-linked-covid-19-outbreak -boston-closed-indefinitely/B3UTQ553RBF2BLK4A7AK4T77UI/.

125. Jonathan Saltzman, "Biogen Conference Likely Led to 20,000 COVID-19 Cases in Boston Area, Researchers Say," *Boston Globe,* August 25, 2020, https://www.bostonglobe.com/2020/08/25/business

/biogen-conference-likely-led-20000-covid-19-cases-boston-area-researchers-say/. See also Jacob Lemieux et al., "Phylogenetic Analysis of SARS-CoV-2 in the Boston Area Highlights the Role of Recurrent Importation and Superspreading Events," MedRxiv, August 25, 2020, https://www.medrxiv.org /content/10.1101/2020.08.23.20178236v1.

126. Lea Hamner et al., "High SARS-CoV-2 Attack Rate Following Exposure at a Choir Practice—Skagit County, Washington, March 2020," *CDC Morbidity and Mortality Weekly Report (MMWR)* 69, no. 19 (May 12, 2020), pp. 606–10, http://dx.doi.org/10.15585/mmwr.mm6919e6.

127. Per Block et al., "Social Network-Based Distancing Strategies to Flatten the COVID-19 Curve in a Post-Lockdown World," May 27, 2020, pp. 1–28, ArXiv, https://arxiv.org/abs/2004.07052; Jose Parra-Moyano and Raquel Rosés, "The Network and the Curve: The Relevance of Staying at Home," *Medium,* March 16, 2020, https://medium.com/@raquelroses2/the-network-and-the-curve-the-relevance-of-staying-at-home -a65bb73f3893.

128. Theresa Kuchler, Dominic Russel, and Johannes Stroebel, "The Geographic Spread of COVID-19 Correlates with the Structure of Social Networks as Measured by Facebook," NBER Working Paper No. 26990 (August 2020), pp. 1–22, http://www.nber.org/papers/w26990.

129. Jaron Lanier and E. Glen Weyl, "How Civic Technology Can Help Stop a Pandemic," *Foreign Affairs,* March 20, 2020, https://www.foreignaffairs.com/articles/asia/2020-03-20/how-civic-technology-can -help-stop-pandemic; Lee Yimou, "Taiwan's New 'Electronic Fence' for Quarantines Leads Waves of Virus Monitoring," *Reuters: Technology News,* March 20, 2020, https://www.reuters.com/article /us-health-coronavirus-taiwan-surveillanc/taiwans-new-electronic-fence-for-quarantines-leads -wave-of-virus-monitoring-idUSKBN2170SK; Tomas Pueyo, "Coronavirus: Learning How to Dance," *Medium,* April 20, 2020, https://medium.com/@tomaspueyo/coronavirus-learning-how-to-dance -b8420170203e.

130. Chen-Hua Chen et al., "Taipei Lockdown: Three Containment Models to Flatten the Curve," *Tianxia (CommonWealth),* April 7, 2020, https://web.cw.com.tw/covid19-taipei-lockdown-en/index.html.

131. Dennis Normile, "Coronavirus Cases Have Dropped Sharply in South Korea. What's the Secret to Its Success?," *Science,* March 17, 2020, https://www.sciencemag.org/news/2020/03/coronavirus-cases -have-dropped-sharply-south-korea-whats-secret-its-success. See also Max Fisher and Choe Sang-Hun, "How South Korea Flattened the Curve," *New York Times,* April 10, 2020, https://www.nytimes.com /2020/03/23/world/asia/coronavirus-south-korea-flatten-curve.html, and Juhwan Oh et al., "National Response to COVID-19 in the Republic of Korea and Lessons Learned for Other Countries," *Health Systems & Reform* 6, no. 1 (April 29, 2020), pp. 1–10, https://www.tandfonline.com/doi/full/10.1080 /23288604.2020.1753464.

132. Zeynep Tufekci, "How Hong Kong Did It," *Atlantic,* May 12, 2020, https://www.theatlantic.com/tech nology/archive/2020/05/how-hong-kong-beating-coronavirus/611524/.

133. Aravind Sesagiri Raamkumar et al., "Measuring the Outreach Efforts of Public Health Authorities and the Public Response on Facebook During the COVID-19 Pandemic in Early 2020: A Cross-Country Comparison," *Journal of Medical Internet Research* 22, no. 5 (2020), pp. 1–12, https://www.jmir.org/2020/5 /e19334/pdf. For a survey of Asian contact-tracing apps, see Huang Yasheng, Sun Meicen, and Sui Yuze, "How Digital Contact Tracing Slowed COVID-19 in East Asia," *Harvard Business Review,* April 15, 2020, https://hbr.org/2020/04/how-digital-contact-tracing-slowed-covid-19-in-east-asia.

134. John Authers, "Stocks Rally Suggests Turning Point in Coronavirus Fight," *Bloomberg Opinion,* April 6, 2020, https://www.bloomberg.com/opinion/articles/2020-04-07/stocks-rally-suggests-turning-point -in-coronavirus-fight.

135. Michael Worobey et al., "The Emergence of SARS-CoV-2 in Europe and North America," *Science,* September 10, 2020, https://science.sciencemag.org/content/early/2020/09/11/science.abc8169.

136. Stephen Grey and Andrew MacAskill, "Special Report: Johnson Listened to His Scientists About Coronavirus—but They Were Slow to Sound the Alarm," Reuters, April 7, 2020, https://www.reuters .com/article/us-health-coronavirus-britain-path-speci/special-report-johnson-listened-to-his -scientists-about-coronavirus-but-they-were-slow-to-sound-the-alarm-idUSKBN21P1VF.

137. James Forsyth, "Boris Johnson Knows the Risk He Is Taking with His Coronavirus Strategy," *Spectator,* March 14, 2020, https://www.spectator.co.uk/article/Boris-Johnson-knows-the-risk-he-is-taking-with -his-coronavirus-strategy.

138. Neil Ferguson et al., "Report 9: Impact of Non-Pharmaceutical Interventions (NPIs) to Reduce COVID-19 Mortality and Healthcare Demand," Imperial College COVID-19 Response Team, March 16, 2020, https://spiral.imperial.ac.uk:8443/handle/10044/1/77482. See also, for similar estimates in a leaked Public Health England briefing, Denis Campbell, "UK Coronavirus Crisis 'to Last Until Spring 2021 and Could See 7.9m Hospitalised,'" *Guardian,* March 15, 2020, https://www.theguardian.com/world/2020 /mar/15/uk-coronavirus-crisis-to-last-until-spring-2021-and-could-see-79m-hospitalised.

139. Sarah Knapton, "Two Thirds of Coronavirus Victims May Have Died This Year Anyway, Government Adviser Says," *Daily Telegraph,* March 25, 2020, https://www.telegraph.co.uk/news/2020/03/25/two -thirds-patients-die-coronavirus-would-have-died-year-anyway/.

140. Sue Denim, "Code Review of Ferguson's Model," Lockdown Sceptics, May 10, 2020, https://lockdown sceptics.org/code-review-of-fergusons-model/; David Richards and Konstantin Boudnik, "Neil Fergu-

son's Imperial Model Could Be the Most Devastating Software Mistake of All Time," *Daily Telegraph,* May 16, 2020, https://www.telegraph.co.uk/technology/2020/05/16/neil-fergusons-imperial-model-could-devastating-software-mistake/.

141. Alistair Haimes, "Ignoring the COVID Evidence," *The Critic,* July–August 2020, https://thecritic.co.uk/issues/july-august-2020/ignoring-the-covid-evidence/; McTague, "How the Pandemic Revealed Britain's National Illness."

142. For a complete compilation, see Democratic Coalition, "Trump Lied, Americans Died," May 8, 2020, YouTube video, 6:20, https://www.youtube.com/watch?time_continue=8&v=dzAQnD0Oz14. See also Christakis, *Apollo's Arrow,* pp. 153, 156f.

143. Bob Woodward, *Rage* (New York: Simon & Schuster, 2020).

144. James Fallows, "The 3 Weeks That Changed Everything," *Atlantic,* June 29, 2020, https://www.the atlantic.com/politics/archive/2020/06/how-white-house-coronavirus-response-went-wrong/613591/.

145. Michael D. Shear et al., "Inside Trump's Failure: The Rush to Abandon Leadership Role on the Virus," *New York Times,* July 18, 2020, https://www.nytimes.com/2020/07/18/us/politics/trump-coronavirus-response-failure-leadership.html; David Crow and Hannah Kuchler, "US Coronavirus Surge: 'It's a Failure of National Leadership,'" *Financial Times,* July 17, 2020, https://www.ft.com/content/787125ba-5707-4718-858b-1e912fee0a38.

146. Zeynep Tufekci, "It Wasn't Just Trump Who Got It Wrong," *Atlantic,* March 24, 2020, https://www.the atlantic.com/technology/archive/2020/03/what-really-doomed-americas-coronavirus-response/608596/.

147. "President Trump Job Approval," *Real Clear Politics,* https://www.realclearpolitics.com/epolls/other/president_trump_job_approval-6179.html.

148. Pandemic and All-Hazards Preparedness and Advancing Innovation Act of 2019, S.1379, 116th Cong. (2019), https://www.congress.gov/bill/116th-congress/senate-bill/1379.

149. "A National Blueprint for Biodefense: Leadership and Major Reform Needed to Optimize Efforts," Bipartisan Report of the Blue Ribbon Study Panel on Biodefense, October 2015, https://biodefensecommission.org/reports/a-national-blueprint-for-biodefense/.

150. "News," Bipartisan Commission on Defense, https://biodefensecommission.org/news/.

151. White House, *National Biodefense Strategy* (Washington, D.C.: Government Printing Office, 2018), https://www.whitehouse.gov/wp-content/uploads/2018/09/National-Biodefense-Strategy.pdf.

152. Judge Glock, "Why Two Decades of Pandemic Planning Failed," *Medium,* April 9, 2020, https://medium.com/@judgeglock/why-two-decades-of-pandemic-planning-failed-a20608d05800.

153. "Evolution of Biodefense Policy with Dr. Robert Kadlec," Robert Strauss Center, October 18, 2018, https://www.youtube.com/watch?list=UUPLAYER_RobertStraussCenter&v=6U4e4029SpE.

154. Niall Ferguson, *The Great Degeneration: How Institutions Decay and Economies Die* (New York: Penguin Press, 2013).

155. Josh Margolin and James Gordon Meek, "Intelligence Report Warned of Coronavirus Crisis as Early as November: Sources," ABC News, April 8, 2020, https://abcnews.go.com/Politics/intelligence-report-warned-coronavirus-crisis-early-november-sources/story?id=70031273; Fallows, "3 Weeks That Changed Everything."

156. Michael D. Shear, Sheri Fink, and Noah Welland, "Inside the Trump Administration, Debate Raged over What to Tell Public," *New York Times,* March 9, 2020, https://www.nytimes.com/2020/03/07/us/politics/trump-coronavirus.html; Jonathan Swan and Margaret Talev, "Navarro Memos Warning of Mass Coronavirus Death Circulated in January," *Axios,* April 7, 2020, https://www.axios.com/exclusive-navarro-deaths-coronavirus-memos-january-da3f08fb-dce1-4f69-89b5-ea048f8382a9.html; Philip A. Wallach and Justus Myers, "The Federal Government's Coronavirus Response—Public Health Timeline," Brookings, March 31, 2020, https://www.brookings.edu/research/the-federal-governments-coronavirus-actions-and-failures-timeline-and-themes/.

157. Paul Kane, "Early On, Cheney and Cotton Warned About the Coronavirus. They Still Face Pushback in the GOP," *Washington Post,* April 4, 2020, https://www.washingtonpost.com/powerpost/early-on-cheney-and-cotton-warned-about-the-coronavirus-they-still-face-push-back-in-the-gop/2020/04/04/d6676200-75df-11ea-87da-77a8136c1a6d_story.html.

158. Robert Costa and Philip Rucker, "Woodward Book: Trump Says He Knew Coronavirus Was 'Deadly,'" *Washington Post,* September 9, 2020, https://www.washingtonpost.com/politics/bob-woodward-rage-book-trump/2020/09/09/0368fe3c-efd2-11ea-b4bc-3a2098fc73d4_story.html.

159. Greg Miller, Josh Dawsey, and Aaron C. Davis, "One Final Viral Infusion: Trump's Move to Block Travel from Europe Triggered Chaos and a Surge of Passengers from the Outbreak's Center," *Washington Post,* May 23, 2020, https://www.washingtonpost.com/world/national-security/one-final-viral-infusion-trumps-move-to-block-travel-from-europe-triggered-chaos-and-a-surge-of-passengers-from-the-outbreaks-center/2020/05/23/64836a00-962b-11ea-82b4-c8db161ff6e5_story.html.

160. Fallows, "3 Weeks That Changed Everything."

161. Anne Applebaum, "The Coronavirus Called America's Bluff," *Atlantic,* March 15, 2020, https://www.theatlantic.com/ideas/archive/2020/03/coronavirus-showed-america-wasnt-task/608023/; Jon Cohen,

"The United States Badly Bungled Coronavirus Testing—but Things May Soon Improve," *Science,* February 28, 2020, https://www.sciencemag.org/news/2020/02/united-states-badly-bungled-coronavirus-testing-things-may-soon-improve.

162. Robinson Meyer and Alexis C. Madrigal, "Exclusive: The Strongest Evidence Yet That America Is Botching Coronavirus Testing," *Atlantic,* March 6, 2020, https://www.theatlantic.com/health/archive/2020/03/how-many-americans-have-been-tested-coronavirus/607597/; Christopher Weaver, Betsy McKay, and Brianna Abbott, "America Needed Coronavirus Tests. The Government Failed," *Wall Street Journal,* March 19, 2020, https://www.wsj.com/articles/how-washington-failed-to-build-a-robust-coronavirus-testing-system-11584552147; Lazaro Gamio, Cai Weiyi, and Adeel Hassan, "Where the U.S. Stands Now on Coronavirus Testing," *New York Times,* March 27, 2020, https://www.nytimes.com/interactive/2020/03/26/us/coronavirus-testing-states.html.

163. Joel Eastwood, Paul Overberg, and Rob Barry, "Why We Don't Know How Many Americans Are Infected with Coronavirus—and Might Never Know," *Wall Street Journal,* April 4, 2020, https://www.wsj.com/articles/why-we-dont-know-how-many-americans-are-infected-with-coronavirusand-might-never-know-11586005200.

164. Veronique de Rugy, "The Monumental Failure of the CDC," American Institute for Economic Research, April 11, 2020, https://www.aier.org/article/the-monumental-failure-of-the-cdc/; Bret Stephens, "COVID-19 and the Big Government Problem," *New York Times,* April 10, 2020, https://www.nytimes.com/2020/04/10/opinion/coronavirus-FDA.html.

165. Eric Lipton et al., "The C.D.C. Waited 'Its Entire Existence for This Moment.' What Went Wrong?," *New York Times,* June 3, 2020, https://www.nytimes.com/2020/06/03/us/cdc-coronavirus.html.

166. Sheri Fink, "Worst-Case Estimates for U.S. Coronavirus Deaths," *New York Times,* March 13, 2020, https://www.nytimes.com/2020/03/13/us/coronavirus-deaths-estimate.html. See also Lydia Ramsey Pflanzer, "One Slide in a Leaked Presentation for U.S. Hospitals Reveals That They're Preparing for Millions of Hospitalizations as the Outbreak Unfolds," *Business Insider,* March 6, 2020, https://www.businessinsider.com/presentation-us-hospitals-preparing-for-millions-of-hospitalizations-2020-3.

167. Li Ruoran et al., "The Demand for Inpatient and ICU Beds for COVID-19 in the U.S.: Lessons from Chinese Cities," Harvard Library Office for Scholarly Communication (March 2020), pp. 1–17, https://dash.harvard.edu/bitstream/handle/1/42599304/Inpatient%20ICU%20beds%20needs%20for%20COVID-19%20medRxiv.pdf?sequence=1&isAllowed=y; Margot Sanger-Katz, Sarah Kliff, and Alicia Parlapiano, "These Places Could Run Out of Hospital Beds as Coronavirus Spreads," *New York Times,* March 17, 2020, https://www.nytimes.com/interactive/2020/03/17/upshot/hospital-bed-shortages-coronavirus.html.

168. Demographia, *Demographia World Urban Areas: 16th Annual Edition* (June 2020), pp. 1–94, http://demographia.com/db-worldua.pdf.

169. "TSA Travel Checkpoint Numbers for 2020 and 2019," U.S. Transportation Security Administration, https://www.tsa.gov/coronavirus/passenger-throughput.

170. Tony Romm, Elizabeth Dwoskin, and Craig Timberg, "U.S. Government, Tech Industry Discussing Ways to Use Smartphone Location Data to Combat Coronavirus," *Washington Post,* March 17, 2020, https://www.washingtonpost.com/technology/2020/03/17/white-house-location-data-coronavirus/.

171. Fred Sainz, "Apple and Google Partner on COVID-19 Contact Tracing Technology," April 10, 2020, https://www.apple.com/newsroom/2020/04/apple-and-google-partner-on-covid-19-contact-tracing-technology/.

172. Patrick McGree, "Apple and Google Announce New Contact-Tracing Tool," *Financial Times,* September 1, 2020, https://www.ft.com/content/0ed38c49-fafe-4e7b-bd57-44c705ba52f7.

173. Derek Watkins et al., "How the Virus Won," *New York Times,* June 25, 2020, https://www.nytimes.com/interactive/2020/us/coronavirus-spread.html; Benedict Carey and James Glanz, "Travel from New York City Seeded Wave of U.S. Outbreaks," *New York Times,* July 16, 2020, https://www.nytimes.com/2020/05/07/us/new-york-city-coronavirus-outbreak.html.

174. Google, "COVID-19 Community Mobility Reports," https://www.google.com/covid19/mobility/; SafeGraph, "Shelter in Place Index: The Impact of Coronavirus on Human Movement," https://www.safegraph.com/dashboard/covid19-shelter-in-place.

175. Wang Shuo, "U.S. Ventilator Data Tells Me Wuhan Really Took a Bullet for China," *Caixin Global,* March 29, 2020, https://www.caixinglobal.com/2020-03-29/as-us-sits-on-ample-ventilator-supply-china-wages-must-win-battle-to-contain-covid-19-in-hubei-101535747.html; Sharon Begley, "With Ventilators Running Out, Doctors Say the Machines Are Overused for COVID-19," *STAT News,* April 8, 2020, https://www.statnews.com/2020/04/08/doctors-say-ventilators-overused-for-covid-19/.

176. Joe Sexton and Joaquin Sapien, "Two Coasts. One Virus. How New York Suffered Nearly 10 Times the Number of Deaths as California," *ProPublica,* May 16, 2020, https://www.propublica.org/article/two-coasts-one-virus-how-new-york-suffered-nearly-10-times-the-number-of-deaths-as-california. See also Britta L. Jewell and Nicholas P. Jewell, "The Huge Cost of Waiting to Contain the Pandemic," *New York Times,* April 14, 2020, https://www.nytimes.com/2020/05/20/us/coronavirus-distancing-deaths.html.

177. Badr et al., "Association Between Mobility Patterns." See also Unacast, "Social Distancing Scoreboard," https://www.unacast.com/covid19/social-distancing-scoreboard.

178. Ding Wenzhi et al., "Social Distancing and Social Capital: Why U.S. Counties Respond Differently to COVID-19," NBER Working Paper No. 27393 (June 2020), pp. 1–33, https://www.nber.org/papers/w27393.

179. Christopher DeMuth, "Can the Administrative State Be Tamed?," *Journal of Legal Analysis* 8, no. 1 (Spring 2016), pp. 121–90.

180. Philip Zelikow, "To Regain Policy Competence: The Software of American Public Problem-Solving," *Texas National Security Review* 2, no. 4 (August 2019), pp. 110–27, http://dx.doi.org/10.26153/tsw/6665.

181. Francis Fukuyama, *Political Order and Political Decay: From the Industrial Revolution to the Globalisation of Democracy* (London: Profile Books, 2014), p. 469.

182. Marc Andreessen, "It's Time to Build," Andreessen Horowitz, April 18, 2020, https://a16z.com/2020/04/18/its-time-to-build/; Ezra Klein, "Why We Can't Build," *Vox,* April 22, 2020, https://www.vox.com/2020/4/22/21228469/marc-andreessen-build-government-coronavirus; Steven M. Teles, "Kludgeocracy: The American Way of Policy," New America Foundation, December 2012, pp. 1–11, https://static.newamerica.org/attachments/4209-kludgeocracy-the-american-way-of-policy/Teles_Steven_Kludgeocracy_NAF_Dec2012.d8a805aa40e34bca9e2fecb018a3dcb0.pdf.

183. For just one of many examples: Jeff Horwitz and Deepa Seetharaman, "Facebook Executives Shut Down Efforts to Make the Site Less Divisive," *Wall Street Journal,* May 26, 2020, https://www.wsj.com/articles/facebook-knows-it-encourages-division-top-executives-nixed-solutions-11590507499.

184. "Coronavirus: How a Misleading Map Went Global," BBC News, February 19, 2020.

185. Lena H. Sun, "CDC to Cut by 80 Percent Efforts to Prevent Global Disease Outbreak," *Washington Post,* February 1, 2018, https://www.washingtonpost.com/news/to-your-health/wp/2018/02/01/cdc-to-cut-by-80-percent-efforts-to-prevent-global-disease-outbreak/; Glenn Kessler, "No, Trump Didn't Shut Down 37 of 47 Global Anti-Pandemic Programs," *Washington Post,* March 4, 2020, https://www.washingtonpost.com/politics/2020/03/04/no-trump-didnt-shut-down-37-47-global-anti-pandemic-programs/.

186. Leonardo Bursztyn et al., "Misinformation During a Pandemic," Becker Friedman Institute for Economics Working Paper No. 2020-044 (June 2020), pp. 1–118, https://bfi.uchicago.edu/wp-content/uploads/BFI_WP_202044.pdf.

187. Andrey Simonov et al., "The Persuasive Effect of Fox News: Non-Compliance with Social Distancing During the COVID-19 Pandemic," NBER Working Paper No. 27237 (July 2020), pp. 1–70, http://www.nber.org/papers/w27237.

188. Lijian Zhao (@zlj517), "CDC was caught on the spot," Twitter, March 12, 2020, 8:37 a.m., https://twitter.com/zlj517/status/1238111898828066823.

189. Steven Lee Myers, "China Spins Tale That the U.S. Army Started the Coronavirus Epidemic," *New York Times,* March 13, 2020, https://www.nytimes.com/2020/03/13/world/asia/coronavirus-china-conspiracy-theory.html.

190. Edward Wong, Matthew Rosenberg, and Julian E. Barnes, "Chinese Agents Helped Spread Messages That Sowed Virus Panic in U.S., Officials Say," *New York Times,* April 22, 2020, https://www.nytimes.com/2020/04/22/us/politics/coronavirus-china-disinformation.html.

191. Virginia Alvino Young, "Nearly Half of the Twitter Accounts Discussing 'Reopening America' May Be Bots," Carnegie Mellon University School of Computer Science, May 20, 2020, https://www.cs.cmu.edu/news/nearly-half-twitter-accounts-discussing-reopening-america-may-be-bots.

192. "Analysis of June 2020 Twitter Takedowns Linked to China, Russia and Turkey," Stanford Internet Observatory Cyber Policy Center blog, June 11, 2020, https://cyber.fsi.stanford.edu/io/news/june-2020-twitter-takedown#china.

193. Dominic Kennedy, "British Academics Sharing Coronavirus Conspiracy Theories Online," *Times* (London), April 11, 2020, https://www.thetimes.co.uk/article/british-academics-sharing-coronavirus-conspiracy-theories-online-v8nn99zmv.

194. Ben Norton (@BenjaminNorton), "@TheGrayzoneNews we published the exposé many people have asked for," Twitter, July 9, 2020, 11:15 a.m., https://twitter.com/BenjaminNorton/status/1281275778316095491; Jeremy Loffredo and Michele Greenstein, "Why the Bill Gates Global Health Empire Promises More Empire and Less Public Health," *The Gray Zone,* July 8, 2020, https://thegrayzone.com/2020/07/08/bill-gates-global-health-policy/.

195. Kevin Roose, "Get Ready for a Vaccine Information War," *New York Times,* June 3, 2020, https://www.nytimes.com/2020/05/13/technology/coronavirus-vaccine-disinformation.html.

196. Karen Kornbluh, Ellen P. Goodman, and Eli Weiner, "Safeguarding Democracy Against Disinformation," German Marshall Fund of the United States, March 24, 2020, http://www.gmfus.org/publications/safeguarding-democracy-against-disinformation.

197. Neil F. Johnson et al., "The Online Competition Between Pro- and Anti-Vaccination Views," *Nature* 582 (May 13, 2020), pp. 230–33, https://www.nature.com/articles/s41586-020-2281-1; Ari Sen and Brandy Zadrozny, "QAnon Groups Have Millions of Members on Facebook, Documents Show," NBC News, August 10, 2020, https://www.nbcnews.com/tech/tech-news/qanon-groups-have-millions-members-facebook-documents-show-n1236317.

198. "Conspiracies of Corona," Pulsar Platform, https://www.pulsarplatform.com/resources/the-conspiracies-of-corona/.

199. Horwitz and Seetharaman, "Facebook Executives Shut Down Efforts."
200. Kathleen Hall Jamieson and Dolores Albarracín, "The Relation Between Media Consumption and Misinformation at the Outset of the SARS-CoV-2 Pandemic in the U.S.," *Harvard Kennedy School Misinformation Review* 1 (April 20, 2020), pp. 1–22, https://misinforeview.hks.harvard.edu/article/the-relation-between-media-consumption-and-misinformation-at-the-outset-of-the-sars-cov-2-pandemic-in-the-us/.
201. "On Coronavirus and Conspiracies," *Public Policy and the Past* (blog), April 17, 2020, http://publicpolicypast.blogspot.com/2020/04/on-coronavirus-and-conspiracies.html. But see also Stephen Cushion et al., "Coronavirus: Fake News Less of a Problem Than Confusing Government Messages—New Study," *The Conversation,* June 12, 2020, https://theconversation.com/coronavirus-fake-news-less-of-a-problem-than-confusing-government-messages-new-study-140383.
202. Andrew Romano, "New Yahoo News/YouGov Poll Shows Coronavirus Conspiracy Theories Leading on the Right May Hamper Vaccine Efforts," *Yahoo! News,* May 22, 2020, https://news.yahoo.com/new-yahoo-news-you-gov-poll-shows-coronavirus-conspiracy-theories-spreading-on-the-right-may-hamper-vaccine-efforts-152843610.html.
203. Katarina Rebello et al., "Covid-19 News and Information from State-Backed Outlets Targeting French, German and Spanish-Speaking Social Media Users: Understanding Chinese, Iranian, Russian and Turkish Outlets," Computational Propaganda Project (COMPROP), Oxford Internet Institute, University of Oxford, https://kq.freepressunlimited.org/evidence/covid-19-news-and-information-from-state-backed-outlets-targeting-french-german-and-spanish-speaking-social-media-users-understanding-chinese-iranian-russian-and-turkish-outlets/.
204. Rex Chapman (@RexChapman), "This angry Florida woman argued today against the mask mandate," Twitter, June 24, 2020, 4:01 p.m., https://twitter.com/RexChapman/status/1275912010555932672.
205. Will Sommer, "Trump's New Favorite COVID Doctor Believes in Alien DNA, Demon Sperm, and Hydroxychloroquine," *Daily Beast,* July 28, 2020, https://www.thedailybeast.com/stella-immanuel-trumps-new-covid-doctor-believes-in-alien-dna-demon-sperm-and-hydroxychloroquine.

Chapter 10: The Economic Consequences of the Plague

1. John Maynard Keynes, *The Economic Consequences of the Peace* (New York: Harcourt, Brace, and Howe: 1920).
2. Keynes, *Economic Consequences of the Peace,* p. 268.
3. Olivier Accominotti and David Chambers, "If You're So Smart: John Maynard Keynes and Currency Speculation in the Interwar Years," *Journal of Economic History* 76, no. 23 (2016), pp. 342–86, https://doi.org/10.1017/S0022050716000589.
4. International Monetary Fund, "A Crisis Like No Other, an Uncertain Recovery," World Economic Outlook Update, June 2020, https://www.imf.org/en/Publications/WEO/Issues/2020/06/24/WEOUpdate June2020; "A Long and Difficult Ascent" (October 2020), https://www.imf.org/en/Publications/WEO/Issues/2020/06/24/WEOUpdateJune2020.
5. Chris Giles, "BoE Warns UK Set to Enter Worst Recession for 300 Years," *Financial Times,* May 7, 2020, https://www.ft.com/content/734e604b-93d9-43a6-a6ec-19e8b22dad3c.
6. Summers first used this line at an event at Harvard's Kennedy School of Government in November 2019.
7. Andrew Edgecliffe-Johnson, "U.S. Supply Chains and Ports Under Strain from Coronavirus," *Financial Times,* March 2, 2020, https://www.ft.com/content/5b5b8990-5a98-11ea-a528-dd0f971febbc.
8. Yuan Yang et al., "Hidden Infections Challenge China's Claim Coronavirus Is Under Control," *Financial Times,* March 26, 2020, https://www.ft.com/content/4aa35288-3979-44f7-b204-b881f473fca0.
9. Mike Bird, John Emont, and Shan Li, "China Is Open for Business, but the Postcoronavirus Reboot Looks Slow and Rocky," *Wall Street Journal,* March 26, 2020, https://www.wsj.com/articles/china-is-open-for-business-but-the-post-coronavirus-reboot-looks-slow-and-rocky-11585232600; Keith Bradsher, "China's Factories Are Back. Its Consumers Aren't," *New York Times,* April 28, 2020, https://www.nytimes.com/2020/04/28/business/china-coronavirus-economy.html.
10. John Liu et al., "China Abandons Hard Growth Target, Shifts Stimulus Focus to Jobs," Bloomberg, May 22, 2020, https://www.bloomberg.com/news/articles/2020-05-22/china-to-abandon-numerical-growth-target-amid-virus-uncertainty.
11. Frank Tang, "Coronavirus: China's Central Bank, Finance Ministry at Odds over Funding for Economic Recovery," *South China Morning Post,* May 6, 2020, https://www.scmp.com/economy/china-economy/article/3083193/coronavirus-chinas-central-bank-finance-ministry-odds-over; Frank Tang, "China's Top Bank Regulator Sees Surge of Bad Loans Straining Financial System in 2020, 2021," *South China Morning Post,* August 13, 2020, https://www.scmp.com/economy/china-economy/article/3097229/chinas-top-bank-regulator-sees-surge-bad-loans-straining.
12. Anthony Faiola, "The Virus That Shut Down the World," *Washington Post,* June 26, 2020, https://www.washingtonpost.com/graphics/2020/world/coronavirus-pandemic-globalization/?itid=hp_hp-banner-main_virus-shutdown-630pm.

13. Clara Ferreira Marques, "The Coronavirus Is a Human Credit Crunch," Bloomberg, March 4, 2020, https://www.bloomberg.com/opinion/articles/2020-03-04/coronavirus-is-a-human-version-of-the-credit-crunch.

14. "The State of the Restaurant Industry," OpenTable by Booking.com, https://www.opentable.com/state-of-industry.

15. SafeGraph, "The Impact of Coronavirus (COVID-19) on Foot Traffic," August 18, 2020, https://www.safegraph.com/dashboard/covid19-commerce-patterns.

16. Justin Baer, "The Day Coronavirus Nearly Broke the Financial Markets," *Wall Street Journal,* May 20, 2020, https://www.wsj.com/articles/the-day-coronavirus-nearly-broke-the-financial-markets-11589982288.

17. John Plender, "The Seeds of the Next Debt Crisis," *Financial Times,* March 3, 2020, https://www.ft.com/content/27cf0690-5c9d-11ea-b0ab-339c2307bcd4.

18. Eva Szalay, "Dollar Surge Stirs Talk of Multilateral Move to Weaken It," *Financial Times,* March 24, 2020, https://www.ft.com/content/931ddba6-6dd2-11ea-9bca-bf503995cd6f.

19. Andreas Schrimpf, Hyun Song Shin, and Vladyslav Sushko, "Leverage and Margin Spirals in Fixed Income Markets During the COVID-19 Crisis," *Bank of International Settlements Bulletin* 2 (April 2, 2020), https://www.bis.org/publ/bisbull02.htm.

20. Gavyn Davies, "A Strategy for the Dysfunctional U.S. Treasuries Market," *Financial Times,* March 22, 2020, https://www.ft.com/content/8df468f2-6a4e-11ea-800d-da70cff6e4d3.

21. Nick Timiraos and John Hilsenrath, "The Federal Reserve Is Changing What It Means to Be a Central Bank," *Wall Street Journal,* April 27, 2020, https://www.wsj.com/articles/fate-and-history-the-fed-tosses-the-rules-to-fight-coronavirus-downturn-11587999986.

22. Lev Menand, "Unappropriated Dollars: The Fed's Ad Hoc Lending Facilities and the Rules That Govern Them," European Corporate Governance Institute (ECGI)–Law Working Paper No. 518/2020 (May 22, 2020), http://dx.doi.org/10.2139/ssrn.3602740.

23. Joshua Jamerson, Andrew Duehren, and Natalie Andrews, "Senate Approves Nearly $2 Trillion in Coronavirus Relief," *Wall Street Journal,* March 26, 2020, https://www.wsj.com/articles/trump-administration-senate-democrats-said-to-reach-stimulus-bill-deal-11585113371.

24. "Budget Projections: Debt Will Exceed the Size of the Economy This Year," Committee for a Responsible Federal Budget blog, April 13, 2020, http://www.crfb.org/blogs/budget-projections-debt-will-exceed-size-economy-year.

25. Jeffrey M. Jones, "President Trump's Job Approval Rating Up to 49%," Gallup, March 24, 2020, https://news.gallup.com/poll/298313/president-trump-job-approval-rating.aspx.

26. Francis Wilkinson, "Gavin Newsom Declares California a 'Nation-State,'" Bloomberg, April 9, 2020, https://www.bloomberg.com/opinion/articles/2020-04-09/california-declares-independence-from-trump-s-coronavirus-plans; Scott Clement and Dan Balz, "Many Governors Win Bipartisan Support for Handling of Pandemic, but Some Republicans Face Blowback over Reopening Efforts," *Washington Post,* May 12, 2020, https://www.washingtonpost.com/politics/many-governors-win-bipartisan-support-for-handling-of-pandemic-but-some-republicans-face-blowback-over-reopening-efforts/2020/05/11/8e98500e-93d2-11ea-9f5e-56d8239bf9ad_story.html; "April 14–19 *Washington Post*–U. Md. Poll," *Washington Post,* May 5, 2020, https://www.washingtonpost.com/context/april-14-19-washington-post-u-md-poll/4521bb45-b844-4dbd-b72d-0a298cf7539a; "NBC News/*Wall Street Journal* Survey Study #200203," Hart Research Associates/Public Opinion Strategies, April 13–15, 2020, https://www.documentcloud.org/documents/6842659-200203-NBCWSJ-April-Poll-4-19-20-Release.html.

27. "Most Americans Say Trump Was Too Slow in Initial Response to Coronavirus Threat," Pew Research Center, April 16, 2020, https://www.people-press.org/2020/04/16/most-americans-say-trump-was-too-slow-in-initial-response-to-coronavirus-threat/.

28. "Coronavirus: Outbreak Concern," Civiqs, https://civiqs.com/results/coronavirus_concern?uncertainty.

29. Mat Krahn, "We all have Schrodinger's Virus now," Facebook, March 30, 2020, https://www.facebook.com/mat.krahn/posts/3076953808995462.

30. Patrick G. T. Walker et al., "The Global Impact of COVID-19 and Strategies for Mitigation and Suppression," Imperial College COVID-19 Response Team Report 12 (March 26, 2020), https://doi.org/10.25561/77735.

31. Nicholas Kristof and Stuart A. Thompson, "Trump Wants to 'Reopen America.' Here's What Happens If We Do," *New York Times,* March 25, 2020, https://www.nytimes.com/interactive/2020/03/25/opinion/coronavirus-trump-reopen-america.html.

32. Maria Chikina and Wesley Pegden, "A Call to Honesty in Pandemic Modeling," *Medium,* March 29, 2020, https://medium.com/@wpegden/a-call-to-honesty-in-pandemic-modeling-5c156686a64b.

33. Seth Flaxman et al., "Estimating the Number of Infections and the Impact of Non-Pharmaceutical Interventions on COVID-19 in 11 European Countries," Imperial College COVID-19 Response Team Report 13 (March 30, 2020), https://doi.org/10.25561/77731.

34. Walker et al., "The Global Impact of COVID-19."

35. Felicia Sonmez, "Texas Lt. Gov. Dan Patrick Comes Under Fire for Saying Seniors Should 'Take a Chance' on Their Own Lives for Sake of Grandchildren During Coronavirus Crisis," *Washington Post,* March 24, 2020, https://www.washingtonpost.com/politics/texas-lt-gov-dan-patrick-comes-under

-fire-for-saying-seniors-should-take-a-chance-on-their-own-lives-for-sake-of-grandchildren-during
-coronavirus-crisis/2020/03/24/e6f64858-6de6-11ea-b148-e4ce3fbd85b5_story.html.

36. Andrew Cuomo (@NYGovCuomo), "My mother is not expendable. Your mother is not expendable,"
    Twitter, March 24, 2020, 9:43 a.m., https://twitter.com/NYGovCuomo/status/1242477029083295746.
37. Thomas J. Kniesner and W. Kip Viscusi, "The Value of a Statistical Life," Vanderbilt Law Research Paper
    No. 19-15 (May 16, 2019), available at SSRN, http://dx.doi.org/10.2139/ssrn.3379967.
38. Greg Ip, "Economics vs. Epidemiology: Quantifying the Trade-Off," Wall Street Journal, April 15, 2020,
    https://www.wsj.com/articles/economics-vs-epidemiology-quantifying-the-trade-off-11586982855.
39. Andrew Scott, "How Aging Societies Should Respond to Pandemics," Project Syndicate, April 22, 2020,
    https://www.project-syndicate.org/commentary/how-aging-societies-should-respond-to-pandemics
    -by-andrew-scott-2020-04.
40. I am grateful to the late Edward Lazear for his guidance on this issue. For the alternative view that
    "from an economic perspective, our response was commensurate to the threat posed by the virus," see
    Nicholas A. Christakis, Apollo's Arrow: The Profound and Enduring Impact of Coronavirus on the Way
    We Live (New York: Little, Brown Spark, 2020), pp. 304f.
41. Christos A. Makridis and Jonathan Hartley, "The Cost of COVID-19: A Rough Estimate of the 2020 U.S.
    GDP Impact," Mercatus Center Special Edition Policy Brief, March 23, 2020, available at SSRN, http://
    dx.doi.org/10.2139/ssrn.3559139.
42. Jay Boice, "Experts Say the Coronavirus Outlook Has Worsened, but the Trajectory Is Still Unclear,"
    FiveThirtyEight, March 26, 2020, https://fivethirtyeight.com/features/experts-say-the-coronavirus
    -outlook-has-worsened-but-the-trajectory-is-still-unclear/.
43. Roman Marchant et al., "Learning as We Go: An Examination of the Statistical Accuracy of COVID-19
    Daily Death Count Predictions," May 26, 2020, https://arxiv.org/abs/2004.04734. For a critique of the
    models, see Andrea Saltelli et al., "Five Ways to Ensure That Models Serve Society: A Manifesto," Na-
    ture 582 (June 24, 2020), pp. 482–84, https://doi.org/10.1038/d41586-020-01812-9.
44. Eskild Petersen et al., "Comparing SARS-CoV-2 with SARS-CoV and Influenza Pandemics," Lancet In-
    fectious Diseases 20, no. 9 (September 2020), pp. E238–E244, https://doi.org/10.1016/S1473-3099(20)
    30484-9.
45. "EuroMOMO Bulletin," European Mortality Monitoring Project, http://www.euromomo.eu/; "Weekly
    Death Statistics: Dramatic Rise in Deaths in Early Spring," Eurostat, July 21, 2020, https://ec.europa
    .eu/eurostat/statistics-explained/index.php?title=Weekly_death_statistics&stable#Dramatic_rise
    _in_deaths_in_early_spring.
46. "Tracking COVID-19 Excess Deaths Across Countries," Economist, July 15, 2020, https://www.econo
    mist.com/graphic-detail/2020/04/16/tracking-covid-19-excess-deaths-across-countries; Jin Wu et al.,
    "Missing Deaths: Tracking the True Toll of the Coronavirus Outbreak," New York Times, July 31, 2020,
    https://www.nytimes.com/interactive/2020/04/21/world/coronavirus-missing-deaths.html; "Coro-
    navirus Tracked: The Latest Figures as Countries Fight COVID-19 Resurgence," Financial Times, Au-
    gust 18, 2020, https://www.ft.com/content/a26fbf7e-48f8-11ea-aeb3-955839e06441.
47. On the vexed question of attribution of death to COVID-19 and other causes of excess mortality, see
    John Lee, "The Way 'COVID Deaths' Are Being Counted Is a National Scandal," Spectator, May 30,
    2020, https://www.spectator.co.uk/article/the-way-covid-deaths-are-being-counted-is-a-national
    -scandal, and David Spiegelhalter, "COVID and 'Excess Deaths' in the Week Ending April 10th," Medium,
    April 24, 2020, https://medium.com/wintoncentre/covid-and-excess-deaths-in-the-week-ending-april
    -10th-20ca7d355ec4.
48. Sarah Caul et al., "Deaths Registered Weekly in England and Wales, Provisional: Week Ending 27
    March 2020," UK Office for National Statistics, April 7, 2020, https://www.ons.gov.uk/peoplepopula
    tionandcommunity/birthsdeathsandmarriages/deaths/bulletins/deathsregisteredweeklyinengland
    andwalesprovisional/weekending27march2020#deaths-registered-by-week.
49. Chris Giles, "UK Coronavirus Deaths More Than Double Official Figure, According to FT Study," Finan-
    cial Times, April 21, 2020, https://www.ft.com/content/67e6a4ee-3d05-43bc-ba03-e239799fa6ab.
50. "COVID-19 Daily Deaths," NHS England, https://www.england.nhs.uk/statistics/statistical-work-areas
    /covid-19-daily-deaths/.
51. Lewis Goodall (@lewis_goodall), "Looking through @ONS data on European deaths, it is v clear
    how poor the performance in England," Twitter, July 30, 2020, 11:15 a.m., https://twitter.com/lewis
    _goodall/status/1288886067039535104.
52. John Burn-Murdoch and Chris Giles, "UK Suffers Second-Highest Death Rate from Coronavirus," Fi-
    nancial Times, May 28, 2020, https://www.ft.com/content/6b4c784e-c259-4ca4-9a82-648ffde71bf0.
53. Harry Kennard (@HarryKennard), "ONS have updated their weekly mortality figures up to April 10th
    for England and Wales," Twitter, April 21, 2020, 2:59 a.m., https://twitter.com/HarryKennard/status
    /1252522319903436800.
54. "Coronavirus Tracked," Financial Times.
55. Burn-Murdoch and Giles, "UK Suffers Second-Highest Death Rate."
56. "Pneumonia and Influenza Surveillance from the National Center for Health Statistics Mortality Sur-
    veillance System," CDC FluView Interactive, https://gis.cdc.gov/grasp/fluview/mortality.html; "CO-
    VIDView Weekly Summary," COVIDView, CDC, https://www.cdc.gov/coronavirus/2019-ncov/covid

-data/covidview/index.html?CDC_AA_refVal=https%3A%2F%2Fwww.cdc.gov%2Fcoronavirus %2F2019-ncov%2Fcovid-data%2Fcovidview.html. See also Paul Overberg and Jon Kamp, "U.S. Deaths Are Up Sharply, Though COVID-19's Precise Toll Is Murky," *Wall Street Journal,* May 15, 2020, https:// www.wsj.com/articles/covid-19s-exact-toll-is-murky-though-u-s-deaths-are-up-sharply -11589555652.

57. Jeremy Samuel Faust and Carlos del Rio, "Assessment of Deaths from COVID-19 and from Seasonal Influenza," *JAMA Internal Medicine* 180, no. 8 (May 14, 2020), pp. 1045–46, https://doi.org/10.1001 /jamainternmed.2020.2306.

58. Robin Martin, "COVID vs. U.S. Daily Average Cause of Death," *Flourish,* April 21, 2020, https://public .flourish.studio/visualisation/1712761/.

59. Steven H. Woolf et al., "Excess Deaths from COVID-19 and Other Causes, March–April 2020," *JAMA* 324, no. 5 (July 1, 2020), pp. 510–13, https://doi.org/10.1001/jama.2020.11787.

60. Claudio Cancelli and Luca Foresti, "The Real Death Toll for COVID-19 Is at Least 4 Times the Official Numbers," *Corriere della Sera,* March 26, 2020, https://www.corriere.it/politica/20_marzo_26/the -real-death-toll-for-covid-19-is-at-least-4-times-the-official-numbers-b5af0edc-6eeb-11ea-925b -a0c3cdbe1130.shtml.

61. Centro Nacional de Epidemiología (ISCIII), "Vigilancia de los excesos de mortalidad por todas las causas," April 19, 2020, https://www.isciii.es/QueHacemos/Servicios/VigilanciaSaludPublicaRENAVE /EnfermedadesTransmisibles/MoMo/Documents/informesMoMo2020/MoMo_Situacion%20a %2019%20de%20abril_CNE.pdf.

62. Josh Katz and Margot Sanger-Katz, "Deaths in New York City Are More Than Double the Usual Total," *New York Times,* April 10, 2020, https://www.nytimes.com/interactive/2020/04/10/upshot/coronavirus -deaths-new-york-city.html.

63. Josh Kovensky, "How Many People Have Died in NYC During the COVID Pandemic?," *Talking Points Memo Muckraker,* April 14, 2020, https://talkingpointsmemo.com/muckraker/how-many-people-have -died-in-nyc-during-the-covid-pandemic. See also "Coronavirus Tracked," *Financial Times,* and Jin Wu et al., "Missing Deaths."

64. "COVID-19 Data and Tools," California State Government, https://public.tableau.com/views/COVID -19CasesDashboard_15931020425010/Cases. On the problems of Southern California, see James Temple, "There's Not One Reason California's COVID-19 Cases Are Soaring—There Are Many," *MIT Technology Review,* June 30, 2020, https://www.technologyreview.com/2020/06/30/1004696/theres -not-one-reason-californias-covid-19-cases-are-soaring-there-are-many/.

65. "Excess Deaths Associated with COVID-19," CDC National Center for Health Statistics, August 12, 2020, https://www.cdc.gov/nchs/nvss/vsrr/covid19/excess_deaths.htm.

66. "Estudio ENE-COVID19: Primera ronda: Estudio nacional de sero-epidemiología de la infección por SARS-CoV-2 en España: Informe preliminar," Gobierno de España Ministerio de Ciencia e Innovación /Ministerio de Sanidad, May 13, 2020, https://www.ciencia.gob.es/stfls/MICINN/Ministerio/FICHE ROS/ENECOVID_Informe_preliminar_cierre_primera_ronda_13Mayo2020.pdf; Travis P. Baggett et al., "COVID-19 Outbreak at a Large Homeless Shelter in Boston: Implications for Universal Testing," MedRxiv, April 15, 2020, https://doi.org/10.1101/2020.04.12.20059618; Bill Chappell and Paige Pfleger, "73% of Inmates at an Ohio Prison Test Positive for Coronavirus," *Coronavirus Live Updates,* NPR, April 20, 2020, https://www.npr.org/sections/coronavirus-live-updates/2020/04/20/838943211 /73-of-inmates-at-an-ohio-prison-test-positive-for-coronavirus.

67. Joseph Goldstein, "68% Have Antibodies in This Clinic. Can a Neighborhood Beat a Next Wave?," *New York Times,* July 10, 2020, https://www.nytimes.com/2020/07/09/nyregion/nyc-coronavirus-antibodies .html.

68. Eran Bendavid et al., "COVID-19 Antibody Seroprevalence in Santa Clara County, California," MedRxiv, April 30, 2020, https://doi.org/10.1101/2020.04.14.20062463.

69. "COVID-19 in Iceland—Statistics from 15 June 2020," Ministry of Health of Iceland, https://www .covid.is/data; "Estudio ENE-COVID19: Primera ronda."

70. Daniel Howdon, Jason Oke, and Carl Heneghan, "Estimating the Infection Fatality Ratio in England," Centre for Evidence-Based Medicine, August 21, 2020, https://www.cebm.net/covid-19/estimating -the-infection-fatality-ratio-in-england/.

71. John P. A. Ioannidis, "The Infection Fatality Rate of COVID-19 Inferred from Seroprevalence Data," MedRxiv, July 14, 2020, https://doi.org/10.1101/2020.05.13.20101253; "COVID-19 Pandemic Planning Scenarios," CDC, July 10, 2020, https://www.cdc.gov/coronavirus/2019-ncov/hcp/planning-scenarios .html; Lucy C. Okell et al., "Have Deaths in Europe Plateaued Due to Herd Immunity?," *Lancet* 395, no. 10241 (June 11, 2020), pp. E110–E111, https://doi.org/10.1016/S0140-6736(20)31357-X; Smriti Mallapaty, "How Deadly Is the Coronavirus? Scientists Are Close to an Answer," *Nature* 582 (June 16, 2020), pp. 467–68, https://doi.org/10.1038/d41586-020-01738-2.

72. Gideon Meyerowitz-Katz and Lea Merone, "A Systematic Review and Meta-Analysis of Published Research Data on COVID-19 Infection-Fatality Rates," MedRxiv, July 7, 2020, https://doi.org/10.1011 /2020.05.03.20089854; Brianna Abbott and Jason Douglas, "How Deadly Is COVID-19? Researchers Are Getting Closer to an Answer," *Wall Street Journal,* July 21, 2020, https://www.wsj.com/articles /how-deadly-is-covid-19-researchers-are-getting-closer-to-an-answer-11595323801.

73. Javier Perez-Saez et al., "Serology-Informed Estimates of SARS-CoV-2 Infection Fatality Risk in Geneva, Switzerland," OSF Preprints, June 15, 2020, https://doi.org/10.31219/osf.io/wdbpe.

74. John Burn-Murdoch, "Some Fresh Analysis of the Factors That Do—and Do Not—Appear to Influence the Pace of Countries' COVID-19 Outbreaks," April 13, 2020, https://threadreaderapp.com/thread /1249821596199596034.html. See also Okell et al., "Have Deaths in Europe Plateaued?"

75. T. J. Rodgers, "Do Lockdowns Save Many Lives? In Most Places, the Data Say No," *Wall Street Journal,* April 26, 2020, https://www.wsj.com/articles/do-lockdowns-save-many-lives-is-most-places-the-data -say-no-11587930911. See also the research by Marko Kolanavic and J.P. Morgan.

76. "Coronavirus Government Response Tracker," Oxford University Blavatnik School of Government, August 6, 2020, https://www.bsg.ox.ac.uk/research/research-projects/oxford-covid-19-government -response-tracker; Thomas Hale et al., "Variation in Government Responses to COVID-19," Blavatnik School of Government (BSG) Working Paper Series BSG-WP-2020/032, Version 6.0 (May 27, 2020), https://www.bsg.ox.ac.uk/sites/default/files/2020-05/BSG-WP-2020-032-v6.0.pdf.

77. Elaine He, "The Results of Europe's Lockdown Experiment Are In," Bloomberg, May 19, 2020, https:// www.bloomberg.com/graphics/2020-opinion-coronavirus-europe-lockdown-excess-deaths-recession. See also James Scruton et al., "GDP First Quarterly Estimate, UK: January to March 2020," UK Office for National Statistics, May 13, 2020, https://www.ons.gov.uk/economy/grossdomesticproductgdp /bulletins/gdpfirstquarterlyestimateuk/januarytomarch2020; JohannesBorgen (@jeuasommenulle), "This is v. interesting - basically oxford econ did a huge database of world lockdown measures and ONS regressed it against known GDP prints," Twitter, May 13, 2020, 2:11 a.m., https://twitter.com /jeuasommenulle/status/1260482683936915456.

78. Okell et al., "Have Deaths in Europe Plateaued?"

79. Joseph A. Lewnard and Nathan C. Lo, "Scientific and Ethical Basis for Social-Distancing Interventions Against COVID-19," *Lancet Infectious Diseases* 20, no. 6 (June 1, 2020), pp. P631–P633, https://doi.org /10.1016/S1473-3099(20)30190-0.

80. Lai Shengjie et al., "Effect of Non-Pharmaceutical Interventions for Containing the COVID-19 Outbreak in China," MedRxiv, March 13, 2020, https://doi.org/10.1011/2020.03.03.20029843; Zhang Juanjuan et al., "Changes in Contact Patterns Explain the Dynamics of the COVID-19 Outbreak in China," *Science* 368, no. 6498 (June 26, 2020), pp. 1481–86, https://doi.org/10.1126/science.abb8001.

81. Solomon Hsiang et al., "The Effect of Large-Scale Anti-Contagion Policies on the COVID-19 Pandemic," *Nature* 584 (June 8, 2020), pp. 262–67, https://doi.org/10.1038/s41586-020-2404-8.

82. Amnon Shashua and Shai Shalev-Shwartz, "The Day After COVID-19 Lockdown: Need to Focus on the Vulnerable," *Medium,* April 27, 2020, https://medium.com/@amnon.shashua/the-day-after-covid-19 -lockdown-need-to-focus-on-the-vulnerable-42c0a360a27; Alexander Chudik, M. Hashem Pesaran, and Alessandro Rebucci, "Mandated and Targeted Social Isolation Policies Flatten the COVID-19 Curve and Can Help Mitigate the Associated Employment Losses," *VoxEU & CEPR,* May 2, 2020, https:// voxeu.org/article/mandated-targeted-social-isolation-can-flatten-covid-19-curve-and-mitigate -employment-losses; Alexander Chudik, M. Hashem Pesaran, and Alessandro Rebucci, "Voluntary and Mandatory Social Distancing: Evidence on COVID-19 Exposure Rates from Chinese Provinces and Selected Countries," Carey Business School Research Paper No. 20-03, Johns Hopkins University (April 15, 2020), available at SSRN, https://ssrn.com/abstract=3576703. See also M. Gabriela Gomes et al., "Individual Variation in Susceptibility or Exposure to SARS-CoV-2 Lowers the Herd Immunity Threshold," MedRxiv, May 21, 2020, https://doi.org/10.1101/2020.04.27.20081893.

83. Greg Ip, "New Thinking on Covid Lockdowns: They're Overly Blunt and Costly," *Wall Street Journal,* August 24, 2020, https://www.wsj.com/articles/covid-lockdowns-economy-pandemic-recession -business-shutdown-sweden-coronavirus-11598281419.

84. Flavia Rotondi, Boris Groendahl, and Stefan Nicola, "Europe's Reopening Road Map: How 11 Countries Are Beginning to Lift Lockdowns," *Fortune,* May 4, 2020, https://fortune.com/2020/05/04/reopen -economy-europe-italy-spain-france/.

85. Karin Modig and Marcus Ebeling, "Excess Mortality from COVID-19: Weekly Excess Death Rates by Age and Sex for Sweden," MedRxiv, May 15, 2020, https://doi.org/10.1101/2020.05.10.20096909.

86. "Mobilitätsindikatoren auf Basis von Mobilfunkdaten: Experimentelle Daten," Statistisches Bundesamt (Destatis), August 3, 2020, https://www.destatis.de/DE/Service/EXDAT/Datensaetze/mobilitaetsin dikatoren-mobilfunkdaten.html.

87. Alistair Haimes, "It's Hurting but It's Just Not Working," *The Critic,* April 24, 2020, https://thecritic .co.uk/its-hurting-but-its-just-not-working/; Fraser Nelson, "The Threat Has Passed, So Why Are Our Civil Liberties Still Suspended?," *Daily Telegraph,* June 18, 2020, https://www.telegraph.co.uk/politics /2020/06/18/threat-has-passed-civil-liberties-still-suspended/.

88. Justin McCarthy, "Americans Differ Greatly in Readiness to Return to Normal," Gallup, April 30, 2020, https://news.gallup.com/poll/309578/americans-differ-greatly-readiness-return-normal.aspx.

89. Apple Maps, "Mobility Trends Reports," https://www.apple.com/covid19/mobility. On the difference in behavior between Democrats and Republicans see, e.g., Marcus Painter and Tian Qiu, "Political Beliefs Affect Compliance with COVID-19 Social Distancing Orders," *VoxEU & CEPR,* May 11, 2020, https://voxeu.org/article/political-beliefs-and-compliance-social-distancing-orders.

90. Matthew Cleevely et al., "Stratified Periodic Testing: A Workable Testing Strategy for COVID-19," *VoxEU & CEPR,* May 6, 2020, https://voxeu.org/article/stratified-periodic-testing-covid-19; Edward Luce, "Inside Trump's Coronavirus Meltdown," *Financial Times,* May 13, 2020, https://www.ft.com/content/97dc7de6-940b-11ea-abcd-371e24b679ed; Abbott and Douglas, "How Deadly Is COVID-19?"

91. Luca Ferretti et al., "Quantifying SARS-CoV-2 Transmission Suggests Epidemic Control with Digital Contact Tracing," *Science* 368, no. 6491 (May 8, 2020), https://doi.org/10.1126/science.abb6936; Huang Yasheng, Sun Meicen, and Sui Yuze, "How Digital Contact Tracing Slowed COVID-19 in East Asia," *Harvard Business Review,* April 15, 2020, https://hbr.org/2020/04/how-digital-contact-tracing-slowed-covid-19-in-east-asia; Sharon Otterman, "N.Y.C. Hired 3,000 Workers for Contact Tracing. It's Off to a Slow Start," *New York Times,* June 21, 2020, https://www.nytimes.com/2020/06/21/nyregion/nyc-contact-tracing.html; I. Glenn Cohen, Lawrence O. Gostin, and Daniel J. Weitzner, "Digital Smartphone Tracking for COVID-19: Public Health and Civil Liberties in Tension," *JAMA* 323, no. 23 (May 27, 2020), pp. 2371–72, https://jamanetwork.com/journals/jama/fullarticle/2766675; Swathikan Chidambaram et al., "Observational Study of UK Mobile Health Apps for COVID-19," *Lancet Digital Health* 2 (June 24, 2020), pp. E388–E390, https://doi.org/10.1016/S2589-7500(20)30144-8.

92. Tomas Pueyo, "Coronavirus: The Hammer and the Dance," *Medium,* March 19, 2020, https://medium.com/@tomaspueyo/coronavirus-the-hammer-and-the-dance-be9337092b56.

93. Derek Watkins et al., "How the Virus Won," *New York Times,* June 25, 2020, https://www.nytimes.com/interactive/2020/us/coronavirus-spread.html.

94. John H. Cochrane, "Dumb Reopening Just Might Work," *The Grumpy Economist* (blog), May 4, 2020, https://johnhcochrane.blogspot.com/2020/05/dumb-reopening-might-just-work.html; John H. Cochrane, "An SIR Model with Behavior," *The Grumpy Economist* (blog), May 4, 2020, https://johnh cochrane.blogspot.com/2020/05/an-sir-model-with-behavior.html.

95. Austan Goolsbee and Chad Syverson, "Fear, Lockdown, and Diversion: Comparing Drivers of Pandemic Economic Decline 2020," NBER Working Paper No. 27432 (June 2020), https://doi.org/10.3386/w27432.

96. Chetan Ahya, "The Coronavirus Recession: Sharper but Shorter," *Morgan Stanley Ideas,* May 12, 2020, https://www.morganstanley.com/ideas/coronavirus-impact-on-global-growth; Gavyn Davies, "After Lockdowns, Economic Sunlight or a Long Hard Slog?," *Financial Times,* May 3, 2020, https://www.ft.com/content/f2b79b3a-8ae5-11ea-9dcb-fe6871f4145a.

97. Gita Gopinath, "The Great Lockdown: Worst Economic Downturn Since the Great Depression," *IMF-Blog,* April 14, 2020, https://blogs.imf.org/2020/04/14/the-great-lockdown-worst-economic-downturn-since-the-great-depression/; Gita Gopinath, "Reopening from the Great Lockdown: Uneven and Uncertain Recovery," *IMFBlog,* June 24, 2020, https://blogs.imf.org/2020/06/24/reopening-from-the-great-lockdown-uneven-and-uncertain-recovery/; James Politi, "Emerging Economies Forecast to Shrink for First Time in 60 Years," *Financial Times,* June 8, 2020, https://www.ft.com/content/47998ee3-b2d3-4066-a914-edbf60b797b5; "The World Economy on a Tightrope," OECD Economic Outlook (June 2020), https://www.oecd.org/economic-outlook/.

98. Scott R. Baker, Nicholas Bloom, Steven J. Davis, and Stephen J. Terry, "COVID-Induced Economic Uncertainty," NBER Working Paper No. 26983 (April 2020), https://www.nber.org/papers/w26983.

99. "Real-Time Data: The State of Hourly Work at U.S. Small Businesses," Homebase, https://joinhome base.com/data/covid-19; Laura Noonan, "'Where Is My Loan?,' Small Businesses Miss Out on U.S. Rescue Funds," *Financial Times,* April 20, 2020, https://www.ft.com/content/e6a06f94-5d2f-43a0-8aac-c7adddca0b0e; Neil Barofsky, "Why the Small-Business Bailout Went to the Big Guys," Bloomberg, April 30, 2020, https://www.bloomberg.com/opinion/articles/2020-04-30/why-small-business-bailout-went-to-shake-shack-and-ruth-s-chris.

100. Paul Krugman, "Notes on the Coronacoma (Wonkish)," *New York Times,* April 1, 2020, https://www.nytimes.com/2020/04/01/opinion/notes-on-the-coronacoma-wonkish.html; see also Noah Smith, "Paul Krugman Is Pretty Upbeat About the Economy," Bloomberg, May 27, 2020, https://www.bloom berg.com/opinion/articles/2020-05-27/paul-krugman-is-pretty-upbeat-about-coronavirus-economic-recovery.

101. Kenneth Rogoff, "Mapping the COVID-19 Recession," *Project Syndicate,* April 7, 2020, https://www.project-syndicate.org/commentary/mapping-covid19-global-recession-worst-in-150-years-by-kenneth-rogoff-2020-04.

102. "Fed Injection Postponing Economic Problems, Not Solving: Summers," Bloomberg, April 9, 2020, https://www.bloomberg.com/news/videos/2020-04-10/fed-injection-postponing-economic-problems-not-solving-summers-video.

103. John Cochrane, "Whack-a-Mole: The Long Run Virus," *The Grumpy Economist* (blog), April 4, 2020, https://johnhcochrane.blogspot.com/2020/04/whack-mole-long-run-virus.html.

104. Enda Curran and Hong Jinshan, "Chinese Factories Humming Doesn't Mean Anyone Is Buying," Bloomberg, May 30, 2020, https://www.bloomberg.com/news/articles/2020-05-30/chinese-factories-humming-doesn-t-mean-anyone-is-buying.

105. U.S. Bureau of Economic Analysis, "Personal Saving Rate [PSAVERT]," retrieved from FRED: Federal Reserve Bank of St. Louis, https://fred.stlouisfed.org/series/PSAVERT.

106. Greg Ip, "Signs of a V-Shaped Early-Stage Economic Recovery Emerge," *Wall Street Journal,* June 13, 2020, https://www.wsj.com/articles/signs-of-a-v-shaped-early-stage-economic-recovery-emerge-11592040600.

107. Jennifer Calfas, Brianna Abbott, and Andrew Restuccia, "Texas Pauses Reopening, as CDC Says Millions More May Have Had Coronavirus," *Wall Street Journal,* June 25, 2020, https://www.wsj.com/articles/coronavirus-latest-news-06-25-2020-11593070962; Greg Ip, "A Recovery That Started Out Like a V Is Changing Shape," *Wall Street Journal,* July 1, 2020, https://www.wsj.com/articles/a-reverse-square-root-recovery-11593602775.

108. "TSA Checkpoint Travel Numbers for 2020 and 2019," U.S. Transportation Security Administration, https://www.tsa.gov/coronavirus/passenger-throughput.

109. SafeGraph, "The Impact of Coronavirus (COVID-19) on Foot Traffic," August 17, 2020, https://www.safegraph.com/dashboard/covid19-commerce-patterns.

110. Apple Maps, "Mobility Trends Reports"; TomTom, "San Francisco Traffic," https://www.tomtom.com/en_gb/traffic-index/san-francisco-traffic/.

111. Raj Chetty et al., "Opportunity Insights Economic Tracker," https://tracktherecovery.org/; Emily Badger and Alicia Parlapiano, "The Rich Cut Their Spending. That Has Hurt All the Workers Who Count on It," *New York Times,* June 17, 2020, https://www.nytimes.com/2020/06/17/upshot/coronavirus-spending-rich-poor.html; Ip, "Recovery That Started Out Like a V."

112. "Impact of COVID-19 on Electricity Consumption and Particulate Pollution," Energy Policy Institute at the University of Chicago (EPIC), June 14, 2020, https://epic.uchicago.edu/area-of-focus/covid-19/.

113. Gavyn Davies, "Big Data Suggests a Difficult Recovery in U.S. Jobs Market," *Financial Times,* July 5, 2020, https://www.ft.com/content/607f24f5-71ed-452c-b68e-716145584e3d.

114. Alexandre Tanzi, "N.Y. Seen with 40% Drop in Tax Revenue, Steepest Fall in U.S.," Bloomberg, June 15, 2020, https://www.bloomberg.com/news/articles/2020-06-15/economists-forecast-at-least-30-tax-decline-for-10-u-s-states; David Harrison, "Recession Forces Spending Cuts on States, Cities Hit by Coronavirus," *Wall Street Journal,* July 8, 2020, https://www.wsj.com/articles/recession-forces-spending-cuts-on-states-cities-hit-by-coronavirus-11594200600.

115. Gavyn Davies, "Managing COVID Debt Mountains Is a Key Task for the Next Decade," *Financial Times,* June 7, 2020, https://www.ft.com/content/a371909e-a3fe-11ea-92e2-cbd9b7e28ee6; John Cochrane, "Perpetuities, Debt Crises, and Inflation," *The Grumpy Economist* (blog), June 8, 2020, https://johnhcochrane.blogspot.com/2020/06/perpetuities-debt-crises-and-inflation.html.

116. Timiraos and Hilsenrath, "Federal Reserve Is Changing What It Means."

117. Charles Goodhart and Manoj Pradhan, "Future Imperfect After Coronavirus," *VoxEU & CEPR,* March 27, 2020, https://voxeu.org/article/future-imperfect-after-coronavirus; Willem Buiter, "Paying for the COVID-19 Pandemic Will Be Painful," *Financial Times,* May 15, 2020, https://www.ft.com/content/d9041f04-9686-11ea-899a-f62a20d54625.

118. Ryan Banerjee, Aaron Mehrotra, and Fabrizio Zampolli, "Inflation at Risk from Covid-19," BIS Bulletin No. 28 (July 23, 2020), https://www.bis.org/publ/bisbull28.htm.

119. "News Release: CFS Divisia Monetary Data for the United States," Center for Financial Stability, July 22, 2020, http://www.centerforfinancialstability.org/amfm/Divisia_Jun20.pdf.

120. Faiola, "Virus That Shut Down the World."

121. Stephen Roach, "A Crash in the Dollar Is Coming," Bloomberg, June 8, 2020, https://www.bloomberg.com/opinion/articles/2020-06-08/a-crash-in-the-dollar-is-coming.

122. Katie Martin, Richard Henderson, and Eric Platt, "Markets: The 'Retail Bros' Betting on a Quick Recovery from the Pandemic," *Financial Times,* June 12, 2020, https://www.ft.com/content/dd6c7674-d0ed-4865-82ed-48ee169bc6cc; Richard Henderson, "Zero-Fee Trading Helps Citadel Securities Cash In on Retail Boom," *Financial Times,* June 21, 2020, https://www.ft.com/content/4a439398-88ab-442a-9927-e743a3ff609b.

123. "Coronavirus: Outbreak Concern," Civiqs. See Christos A. Makridis and Jonathan T. Rothwell, "The Real Cost of Political Polarization: Evidence from the COVID-19 Pandemic," June 29, 2020, available at SSRN, https://ssrn.com/abstract=3638373.

124. "President Trump Job Approval," RealClearPolitics, https://www.realclearpolitics.com/epolls/other/president_trump_job_approval-6179.html; "General Election: Trump vs. Biden," RealClearPolitics, https://www.realclearpolitics.com/epolls/2020/president/us/general_election_trump_vs_biden-6247.html; "Who Will Win the 2020 U.S. Presidential Election," PredictIt, https://www.predictit.org/markets/detail/3698/Who-will-win-the-2020-US-presidential-election.

125. Ian Bogost and Alexis C. Madrigal, "How Facebook Works for Trump," *Atlantic,* April 17, 2020, https://www.theatlantic.com/technology/archive/2020/04/how-facebooks-ad-technology-helps-trump-win/606403/.

126. Sheera Frenkel et al., "Facebook Employees Stage Virtual Walkout to Protest Trump Posts," *New York Times,* June 1, 2020, https://www.nytimes.com/2020/06/01/technology/facebook-employee-protest-trump.html; Mike Isaac, "Early Facebook Employees Disavow Zuckerberg's Stance on Trump Posts," *New York Times,* June 30, 2020, https://www.nytimes.com/2020/06/03/technology/facebook-trump-employees-letter.html; Kayla Gogarty and John Whitehouse, "Facebook Finally Removed Trump Campaign Ads with Inverted Red Triangle—an Infamous Nazi Symbol," Media Matters, June 18, 2020, https://www.mediamatters.org/facebook/facebook-let-trump-campaign-run-ads-inverted-red-triangle

-infamous-nazi-symbol; Megan Graham, "The Facebook Ad Boycotts Have Entered the Big Leagues. Now What?," CNBC News, June 29, 2020, https://www.cnbc.com/2020/06/27/the-facebook-ad-boycotts -have-entered-the-big-leagues-now-what.html.

127. Paul Bedard, "Poll: 20% of Democrats 'Think Biden Has Dementia,' 38% Among All Voters," *Washington Examiner,* June 29, 2020, https://www.washingtonexaminer.com/washington-secrets/poll-20-of -democrats-think-biden-has-dementia-38-among-all-voters.

128. Christakis, *Apollo's Arrow,* pp. 208–13.

129. George Packer, "We Are Living in a Failed State," *Atlantic,* June 2020, https://www.theatlantic.com /magazine/archive/2020/06/underlying-conditions/610261/.

130. "Remarks by President Trump, Vice President Pence, and Members of the Coronavirus Task Force in Press Briefing," March 18, 2020, https://www.whitehouse.gov/briefings-statements/remarks-president -trump-vice-president-pence-members-coronavirus-task-force-press-briefing-5/.

131. "Domestic Violence Has Increased During Coronavirus Lockdowns," *Economist,* April 22, 2020, https://www.economist.com/graphic-detail/2020/04/22/domestic-violence-has-increased-during -coronavirus-lockdowns?fsrc=scn/tw/te/bl/ed/dailychartdomesticviolencehasincreasedduringcoro naviruslockdownsgraphicdetail; Ryan Heath and Renuka Rayasam, "COVID's War on Women," *Politico,* April 29, 2020, https://www.politico.com/newsletters/politico-nightly-coronavirus-special-edition /2020/04/29/covids-war-on-women-489076; Amanda Taub and Jane Bradley, "As Domestic Abuse Rises, U.K. Failings Leave Victims in Peril," *New York Times,* July 2, 2020, https://www.nytimes.com /interactive/2020/07/02/world/europe/uk-coronavirus-domestic-abuse.html.

132. Giuliana Viglione, "How Many People Has the Coronavirus Killed?," *Nature* 585 (September 1, 2020), pp. 22–24, https://www.nature.com/articles/d41586-020-02497-w.

133. Shi Le et al., "Prevalence of and Risk Factors Associated with Mental Health Symptoms Among the General Population in China During the Coronavirus Disease 2019 Pandemic," *JAMA Network Open* 3, no. 7 (July 1, 2020), https://doi.org/10.1001/jamanetworkopen.2020.14053; Sun Yan et al., "Brief Report: Increased Addictive Internet and Substance Use Behavior During the COVID-19 Pandemic in China," *American Journal on Addictions* 29, no. 4 (June 4, 2020), pp. 268–70, https://doi.org/10.1111 /ajad.13066.

134. William Wan and Heather Long, "'Cries for Help': Drug Overdoses Are Soaring During the Coronavirus Pandemic," https://www.washingtonpost.com/health/2020/07/01/coronavirus-drug-overdose/.

135. Michael Holden, "COVID-19 Death Rate in Deprived Areas in England Double That of Better-Off Places: ONS," Reuters, May 1, 2020, https://www.reuters.com/article/us-health-coronavirus-britain-deprived -idUSKBN22D51O; Rishi K. Wadhera et al., "Variation in COVID-19 Hospitalizations and Deaths Across New York City Boroughs," *JAMA* 323, no. 21 (April 29, 2020), pp. 2192–95, https://doi.org/10.1001/jama .2020.7197.

136. Robert Armstrong, "Rising Markets and Inequality Grow from the Same Root," *Financial Times,* June 8, 2020, https://www.ft.com/content/a25bf8b6-a962-11ea-a766-7c300513fe47.

137. Megan Cassella, "Mounting Unemployment Crisis Fuels Racial Wealth Gap," *Politico,* June 5, 2020, https://www.politico.com/news/2020/06/04/unemployment-race-gap-301984.

138. Sean Illing, "Millennials Are Getting Screwed by the Economy. Again," *Vox,* April 21, 2020, https:// www.vox.com/policy-and-politics/2020/4/21/21221273/coronavirus-millennials-great-recession -annie-lowrey.

139. Sarah Chaney, "Women's Job Losses from Pandemic Aren't Good for Economic Recovery," *Wall Street Journal,* June 21, 2020, https://www.wsj.com/articles/womens-job-losses-from-pandemic-arent-good -for-economic-recovery-11592745164.

140. Tim Arango et al., "Fiery Clashes Erupt Between Police and Protesters over George Floyd Death," *New York Times,* June 10, 2020, https://www.nytimes.com/2020/05/30/us/minneapolis-floyd-protests .html.

141. Larry Buchanan, Quoctrung Bui, and Jugal K. Patel, "Black Lives Matter May Be the Largest Movement in U.S. History," *New York Times,* July 3, 2020, https://www.nytimes.com/interactive/2020/07/03/us /george-floyd-protests-crowd-size.html.

142. Dhaval M. Dave et al., "Black Lives Matter Protests, Social Distancing, and COVID-19," NBER Working Paper No. 27408 (June 2020), https://doi.org/10.3386/w27408.

143. Roudabeh Kishi and Sam Jones, "Demonstrations and Political Violence in America: New Data for Summer 2020," Armed Conflict Location & Event Data Project (ACLED), September 2020, https:// acleddata.com/2020/09/03/demonstrations-political-violence-in-america-new-data-for-summer -2020/.

144. Maggie Haberman, "Trump Threatens White House Protesters with 'Vicious Dogs' and 'Ominous Weapons,'" *New York Times,* May 30, 2020, https://www.nytimes.com/2020/05/30/us/politics/trump -threatens-protesters-dogs-weapons.html; Neil MacFarquhar, "Many Claim Extremists Are Sparking Protest Violence. But Which Extremists?," *New York Times,* June 22, 2020, https://www.nytimes.com /2020/05/31/us/george-floyd-protests-white-supremacists-antifa.html.

145. Jan Ransom and Annie Correal, "How the New York Protest Leaders Are Taking On the Establishment," *New York Times,* June 12, 2020, https://www.nytimes.com/2020/06/11/nyregion/nyc-george-floyd -protests.html.

146. Heather Mac Donald, "Darkness Falls: The Collapse of the Rule of Law Across the Country, Intensified by Antifa Radicals, Is Terrifying," *City Journal,* May 31, 2020, https://www.city-journal.org/terrifying-collapse-of-the-rule-of-law.

147. James Rainey, Dakota Smith, and Cindy Chang, "Growing the LAPD Was Gospel at City Hall. George Floyd Changed That," *Los Angeles Times,* June 5, 2020, https://www.latimes.com/california/story/2020-06-05/eric-garcetti-lapd-budget-cuts-10000-officers-protests.

148. Dave et al., "Black Lives Matter Protests, Social Distancing, and COVID-19."

149. Ashley Southall and Neil MacFarquhar, "Gun Violence Spikes in N.Y.C., Intensifying Debate over Policing," *New York Times,* July 17, 2020, https://www.nytimes.com/2020/06/23/nyregion/nyc-shootings-surge.html.

150. Omar Wasow, "Agenda Seeding: How 1960s Black Protests Moved Elites, Public Opinion and Voting," forthcoming submission to the *American Political Science Review* (2020), http://omarwasow.com/APSR_protests3_1.pdf.

151. Nexstar Media Wire, "Exclusive Poll Shows Support for George Floyd Protests, Disapproval of Trump's Response," KXAN News, June 3, 2020, https://www.kxan.com/news/exclusive-poll-shows-support-for-george-floyd-protests-disapproval-of-trumps-response/.

152. Nate Cohn and Kevin Quealy, "How Public Opinion Has Moved on Black Lives Matter," *New York Times,* June 10, 2020, https://www.nytimes.com/interactive/2020/06/10/upshot/black-lives-matter-attitudes.html; Amy Mitchell et al., "In Protest Response, Americans Say Donald Trump's Message Has Been Wrong, News Media Coverage Good," Pew Research Center, June 12, 2020, https://www.journalism.org/2020/06/12/in-protest-response-americans-say-donald-trumps-message-has-been-wrong-news-media-coverage-good/.

153. Mark Joyella, "Tucker Carlson Has Highest-Rated Program in Cable News History," *Forbes,* June 30, 2020, https://www.forbes.com/sites/markjoyella/2020/06/30/tucker-carlson-has-highest-rated-program-in-cable-news-history/#61b7e0056195.

154. Theresa Braine, "White Cops and Community Members Wash Black Faith Leaders' Feet at Protest," *New York Daily News,* June 9, 2020, https://www.nydailynews.com/news/national/ny-white-cops-community-wash-black-faith-leaders-feet-forgiveness-20200609-yl4gmoau4nclvgndlldgeqlj3y-story.html.

155. Maria Viti (@selfdeclaredref), "Bethesda," Twitter, June 2, 2020, 2:11 p.m., https://twitter.com/selfdeclaredref/status/1267911752462843904.

156. Shaggie (@Shaggie_Tweets), "A powerful show of unity and support," Twitter, May 31, 2020, 7:53 p.m., https://twitter.com/shaggie_tweets/status/1267273066461007872.

157. For a good commentary on "Third-Wave Antiracism," see John McWhorter, "Kneeling in the Church of Social Justice," *Reason,* June 29, 2020, https://reason.com/2020/06/29/kneeling-in-the-church-of-social-justice/.

158. Dominick Mastrangelo, "'Systemically, Racism Can Only Be White': Demonstrator Confronts Police in DC," *Washington Examiner,* June 25, 2020, https://www.washingtonexaminer.com/news/systemically-racism-can-only-be-white-demonstrator-confronts-police-in-dc.

159. Hannah Natanson et al., "Protesters Denounce Abraham Lincoln Statue in D.C., Urge Removal of Emancipation Memorial," *Washington Post,* June 26, 2020, https://www.washingtonpost.com/local/protesters-denounce-abraham-lincoln-statue-in-dc-urge-removal-of-emancipation-memorial/2020/06/25/02646910-b704-11ea-a510-55bf26485c93_story.html.

160. James Simpson, *Under the Hammer: Iconoclasm in the Anglo–American Tradition* (Oxford: Oxford University Press, 2010).

161. Hanna Lustig, "Teens on TikTok Are Exposing a Generational Rift Between Parents and Kids over How They Treat Black Lives Matter Protests," *Insider,* June 3, 2020, https://www.insider.com/tiktok-george-floyd-black-lives-matter-teens-parents-racist-views-2020-6.

162. Justin Wolfers (@JustinWolfers), "This Chicago economist has angered a lot of his fellow econs," Twitter, June 9, 2020, 2:05 p.m., https://twitter.com/JustinWolfers/status/1270446931668500480.

163. "Most Want to Prosecute Historic Statue Vandals," *Rasmussen Reports,* July 9, 2020, https://www.rasmussenreports.com/public_content/politics/current_events/racism/most_want_to_prosecute_historic_statue_vandals.

164. Federal Bureau of Investigation, "NICS Firearms Checks: Month/Year," https://www.fbi.gov/file-repository/nics_firearm_checks_-_month_year.pdf/view.

165. Nate Cohn and Kevin Quealy, "Nothing Divides Voters Like Owning a Gun," *New York Times,* October 5, 2017, https://www.nytimes.com/interactive/2017/10/05/upshot/gun-ownership-partisan-divide.html.

166. Julia P. Schleimer et al., "Firearm Purchasing and Firearm Violence in the First Months of the Coronavirus Pandemic in the United States," MedRxiv, July 4, 2020, https://doi.org/10.1011/2020.07.02.20145508.

167. Larry Diamond and Edward B. Foley, "The Terrifying Inadequacy of American Election Law," *Atlantic,* September 8, 2020, https://www.theatlantic.com/ideas/archive/2020/09/terrifying-inadequacy-american-election-law/616072/.

168. Dan Balz and Emily Guskin, "Biden Leads Trump in *Post*-ABC Poll as President's Coronavirus Rating Slips," *Washington Post,* May 30, 2020, https://www.washingtonpost.com/politics/biden-leads-trump-in-post-abc-poll-as-presidents-coronavirus-rating-slips/2020/05/29/37c0dac8-a1d1-11ea-9590

-1858a893bd59_story.html; "Two-Thirds of Americans Expect Presidential Election Will Be Disrupted by COVID-19," Pew Research Center, April 28, 2020, https://www.people-press.org/2020/04/28/two -thirds-of-americans-expect-presidential-election-will-be-disrupted-by-covid-19/.

169. Xu Shunqing and Li Yuanyuan, "Beware the Second Wave of COVID-19," *Lancet* 395, no. 10233 (April 25, 2020), pp. P1321–P1322, https://www.thelancet.com/journals/lancet/article/PIIS0140-6736(20) 30845-X/fulltext. See also Lena H. Sun, "CDC Director Warns Second Wave of Coronavirus Is Likely to Be Even More Devastating," *Washington Post,* April 21, 2020, https://www.washingtonpost.com /health/2020/04/21/coronavirus-secondwave-cdcdirector/.

170. Accominotti and Chambers, "If You're So Smart."

Chapter 11: The Three-Body Problem

1. Liu Cixin, *The Three-Body Problem,* trans. Ken Liu (New York: Tor Books, 2014).

2. Niall Ferguson, "Donald Trump's Trade War Is Now a Tech War," *Sunday Times,* February 3, 2019, http:// www.niallferguson.com/journalism/politics/donald-trumps-trade-war-is-now-a-tech-world-war.

3. Andrew Browne, "Foothills of a Cold War," Bloomberg, November 21, 2020, https://www.bloomberg .com/news/newsletters/2019-11-21/-foothills-of-a-cold-war.

4. Yao Yang, "Is a New Cold War Coming?" (interview), *Beijing Cultural Review,* April 28, 2020, available at Reading the China Dream, https://www.readingthechinadream.com/yao-yang-the-new-cold-war .html.

5. Orville Schell, "The Death of Engagement," *The Wire China,* June 7, 2020, https://www.thewirechina .com/2020/06/07/the-birth-life-and-death-of-engagement/.

6. John Garnaut, "Ideology in Xi Jinping's China," *Sinocism* newsletter, January 16, 2020, https://sinocism .com/p/engineers-of-the-soul-ideology-in.

7. Dan Blumenthal and Nicholas Eberstadt, "China Unquarantined," *National Review,* June 4, 2020, https://www.nationalreview.com/magazine/2020/06/22/our-disastrous-engagement-of-china /#slide-1.

8. Katsuji Nakazawa, "Xi Fears Japan-Led Manufacturing Exodus from China," *Nikkei Asian Review,* April 16, 2020, https://asia.nikkei.com/Editor-s-Picks/China-up-close/Xi-fears-Japan-led-manufacturing -exodus-from-China.

9. Dave Lawlor, "Josh Hawley Crafts the Case Against China," *Axios,* May 20, 2020, https://www.axios .com/josh-hawley-china-policy-f9e1fc01-2883-4db7-a721-fbb3f7aeacb8.html.

10. Steven Erlanger, "Global Backlash Builds Against China over Coronavirus," *New York Times,* May 3, 2020, https://www.nytimes.com/2020/05/03/world/europe/backlash-china-coronavirus.html.

11. Yu Yongding and Kevin P. Gallagher, "COVID-19 and the Thucydides Trap," Project Syndicate, April 24, 2020, https://www.project-syndicate.org/commentary/covid-thucydides-trap-by-yu-yongding-and -kevin-p-gallagher-2020-04.

12. Robert B. Zoellick, "The U.S. Doesn't Need a New Cold War," *Wall Street Journal,* May 18, 2020, https://www.wsj.com/articles/the-u-s-doesnt-need-a-new-cold-war-11589842987.

13. Niall Ferguson and Moritz Schularick, "Chimerical? Think Again," *Wall Street Journal,* February 5, 2007, https://www.wsj.com/articles/SB117063838651997830.

14. "China Opens $45 Trillion Financial Market as U.S. Closes," *People's Daily,* June 15, 2020, http:// en.people.cn/n3/2020/0615/c90000-9700486.html.

15. Kat Devlin, Laura Silver, and Christine Huang, "U.S. Views of China Increasingly Negative amid Coro- navirus Outbreak," Pew Research Center, April 21, 2020, https://www.pewresearch.org/global/2020 /04/21/u-s-views-of-china-increasingly-negative-amid-coronavirus-outbreak/; Craig Kafura, "Are Millennials China Doves or China Hawks?," Chicago Council on Foreign Affairs, April 7, 2020, https:// www.thechicagocouncil.org/blog/running-numbers/lcc/are-millennials-china-doves-or-china -hawks.

16. Laura Silver, Kat Devlin, and Christine Huang, "Americans Fault China for Its Role in the Spread of COVID-19," Pew Research Center, July 30, 2020, https://www.pewresearch.org/global/2020/07/30 /americans-fault-china-for-its-role-in-the-spread-of-covid-19/.

17. John Bolton, *The Room Where It Happened* (New York: Simon & Schuster, 2020), quoted in "John Bolton: The Scandal of Trump's China Policy," *Wall Street Journal,* June 17, 2020, https://www.wsj .com/articles/john-bolton-the-scandal-of-trumps-china-policy-11592419564.

18. "Chaguan," "Elites in Beijing See America in Decline, Hastened by Trump," *Economist,* June 11, 2020, https://www.economist.com/china/2020/06/11/elites-in-beijing-see-america-in-decline-hastened -by-trump.

19. Michèle A. Flournoy, "How to Prevent a War in Asia," *Foreign Affairs,* June 18, 2020, https://www .foreignaffairs.com/articles/united-states/2020-06-18/how-prevent-war-asia.

20. Christian Brose, *The Kill Chain: Defending America in the Future of High-Tech Warfare* (New York: Ha- chette, 2020).

21. Bernhard Zand, "Kishore Mahbubani: 'There Are Better Ways to Deal with Asia and China,'" *Der Spie- gel,* April 8, 2020, https://www.spiegel.de/international/world/political-scientist-kishore-mahbubani -on-the-asian-century-a-79680d54-17be-4dd2-bc8c-796101581f31.

22. Kishore Mahbubani, "Kishore Mahbubani on the Dawn of the Asian Century," *Economist,* April 20, 2020, https://www.economist.com/open-future/2020/04/20/by-invitation-kishore-mahbubani.

23. Martin Jacques, *When China Rules the World: The End of the Western World and the Birth of a New Global Order,* 2nd ed. (London: Penguin, 2012).

24. Daniel Bell, *The China Model: Political Meritocracy and the Limits of Democracy* (Princeton, NJ: Princeton University Press, 2016).

25. See, e.g., "Pro-People Policies, Dutiful Citizens Effective in China's COVID-19 Fight" (interview with Daniel Bell), *Global Times,* May 2, 2020, https://www.globaltimes.cn/content/1187304.shtml.

26. Edward Luce, "Inside Trump's Coronavirus Meltdown," *Financial Times,* May 13, 2020, https://www.ft.com/content/97dc7de6-940b-11ea-abcd-371e24b679ed.

27. John Micklethwait and Adrian Wooldridge, "The Virus Should Wake Up the West," Bloomberg, April 13, 2020, https://www.bloomberg.com/opinion/articles/2020-04-13/coronavirus-pandemic-is-wake-up-call-to-reinvent-the-state.

28. Lawrence Summers, "COVID-19 Looks Like a Hinge in History," *Financial Times,* May 14, 2020, https://www.ft.com/content/de643ae8-9527-11ea-899a-f62a20d54625.

29. Patrick Wintour, "Coronavirus: Who Will Be Winners and Losers in New World Order," *Guardian,* April 11, 2020, https://www.theguardian.com/world/2020/apr/11/coronavirus-who-will-be-winners-and-losers-in-new-world-order.

30. Anne Applebaum, "The Rest of the World Is Laughing at Trump," *Atlantic,* May 3, 2020, https://www.theatlantic.com/ideas/archive/2020/05/time-americans-are-doing-nothing/611056/.

31. Harold James, "Late Soviet America," Project Syndicate, July 1, 2020, https://www.project-syndicate.org/commentary/american-decline-under-trump-lessons-from-soviet-union-by-harold-james-2020-07.

32. Wade Davis, "The Unraveling of America," *Rolling Stone,* August 6, 2020, https://www.rollingstone.com/politics/political-commentary/covid-19-end-of-american-era-wade-davis-1038206/.

33. Gideon Rachman, "Coronavirus and the Threat to U.S. Supremacy," *Financial Times,* April 13, 2020, https://www.ft.com/content/2e8c8f76-7cbd-11ea-8fdb-7ec06edeef84; Joseph S. Nye Jr., "Coronavirus Will Not Change the Global Order," *Foreign Policy,* April 16, 2020, https://foreignpolicy.com/2020/04/16/coronavirus-pandemic-china-united-states-power-competition/.

34. Richard Haass, "The Pandemic Will Accelerate History Rather Than Reshape It," *Foreign Affairs,* April 7, 2020, https://www.foreignaffairs.com/articles/united-states/2020-04-07/pandemic-will-accelerate-history-rather-reshape-it.

35. Ray Dalio, *The Changing World Order: Why Nations Succeed and Fail* (New York: Avid Reader Press, 2021), https://www.principles.com/the-changing-world-order/.

36. Peter Turchin, "Dynamics of Political Instability in the United States, 1780–2010," *Journal of Peace Research* 49, no. 4 (July 2012). See also Peter Turchin, *Ages of Discord: A Structural-Demographic Analysis of American History* (Chaplin, CT: Beresta Books, 2016), esp. 241f.

37. David Mamet, "The Code and the Key," *National Review,* June 1, 2020, https://www.nationalreview.com/magazine/2020/06/01/the-code-and-the-key/.

38. Henry A. Kissinger, "The Coronavirus Pandemic Will Forever Alter the World Order," *Wall Street Journal,* April 3, 2020, https://www.wsj.com/articles/the-coronavirus-pandemic-will-forever-alter-the-world-order-11585953005.

39. Jon Meacham, *Destiny and Power: The American Odyssey of George Herbert Walker Bush* (New York: Random House, 2015), p. 60.

40. Niall Ferguson, *Colossus: The Rise and Fall of the American Empire* (New York: Penguin, 2004), pp. 148f., 339f.

41. Brendan Simms, *Unfinest Hour: Britain and the Destruction of Bosnia* (London: Allen Lane, 2001), p. 56.

42. For a vivid account, see George Packer, *Our Man: Richard Holbrooke and the End of the American Century* (New York: Alfred A. Knopf, 2019).

43. "Bosnia War Dead Figure Announced," BBC, June 21, 2007, quoting the Research and Documentation Center in Sarajevo, http://news.bbc.co.uk/2/hi/europe/6228152.stm.

44. Samantha Power, *"A Problem from Hell": America and the Age of Genocide* (London: HarperCollins, 2003), p. 381. See also William Shawcross, *Deliver Us from Evil: Warlords and Peacekeepers in a World of Endless Conflict* (New York: Simon & Schuster, 2000).

45. Richard A. Clarke, *Against All Enemies: Inside America's War on Terror—What Really Happened* (New York: Free Press, 2004), p. 232. See also pp. 28–32, pp. 227ff.

46. Ron Suskind, *The One Percent Doctrine* (New York: Simon & Schuster, 2008).

47. Ron Suskind, quoting a "senior adviser" to President Bush, in "Without a Doubt: Faith, Certainty and the Presidency of George W. Bush," *New York Times Magazine,* October 17, 2004, https://www.nytimes.com/2004/10/17/magazine/faith-certainty-and-the-presidency-of-george-w-bush.html.

48. Timothy Garton Ash, *Free World: America, Europe, and the Surprising Future of the West* (New York: Vintage, 2005), p. 102.

49. "Text of President Bush's Press Conference," *New York Times,* April 13, 2004.

50. Kathleen T. Rhem, "U.S. Not Interested in Iraqi Oil, Rumsfeld Tells Arab World," American Forces Press Service, February 26, 2003, https://archive.defense.gov/news/newsarticle.aspx?id=29374.

51. "Immediate Release: Casualty Status," U.S. Department of Defense, August 17, 2020, https://www.defense.gov/casualty.pdf.
52. "The Public Record of Violent Deaths Following the 2003 Invasion of Iraq," Iraq Body Count, accessed August 16, 2020, https://www.iraqbodycount.org/.
53. "Costs of War: Afghan Civilians," Watson Institute of International and Public Affairs, Brown University (January 2020): https://watson.brown.edu/costsofwar/costs/human/civilians/afghan.
54. Neta C. Crawford, "United States Budgetary Costs and Obligations of Post-9/11 Wars Through FY2020: $6.4 Trillion," Watson Institute, Brown University, November 13, 2019, https://watson.brown.edu/costsofwar/files/cow/imce/papers/2019/US%20Budgetary%20Costs%20of%20Wars%20November%202019.pdf.
55. Niall Ferguson, "Applying History in Real Time: A Tale of Two Crises," Impact of the Past lecture series, Institute of Advanced Study, Princeton, NJ, October 10, 2018.
56. "DoD News Briefing—Secretary Rumsfeld and Gen. Myers," U.S. Department of Defense Online Archive, February 12, 2002, https://archive.defense.gov/Transcripts/Transcript.aspx?TranscriptID=2636.
57. J. Luft and H. Ingham, "The Johari Window, a Graphic Model of Interpersonal Awareness," *Proceedings of the Western Training Laboratory in Group Development* (1955).
58. Donald Rumsfeld, *Known and Unknown: A Memoir* (New York: Sentinel, 2011), p. xvi. On the utility of the distinctions in the natural sciences, see David C. Logan, "Known Knowns, Known Unknowns, Unknown Unknowns and the Propagation of Scientific Enquiry," *Journal of Experimental Botany* 60, no. 3 (2009), pp. 712–14, https://doi.org/10.1093/jxb/erp043.
59. Sam Loughlin, "Rumsfeld on Looting in Iraq: 'Stuff Happens,'" CNN, April 23, 2003, https://www.cnn.com/2003/US/04/11/sprj.irq.pentagon/.
60. David Corn, "McCain in NH: Would Be 'Fine' to Keep Troops in Iraq for 'A Hundred Years,'" *Mother Jones*, January 4, 2008, https://www.motherjones.com/politics/2008/01/mccain-nh-would-be-fine-keep-troops-iraq-hundred-years/.
61. "America Is Not the World's Policeman: Text of Barack Obama's Speech on Syria," Associated Press, September 11, 2013, https://www.ndtv.com/world-news/america-is-not-the-worlds-policeman-text-of-barack-obamas-speech-on-syria-534239.
62. Jeffrey Goldberg, "The Obama Doctrine," *Atlantic*, April 2016, https://www.theatlantic.com/magazine/archive/2016/04/the-obama-doctrine/471525/.
63. "Death Tolls," *I Am Syria*, accessed August 16, 2020, http://www.iamsyria.org/death-tolls.html.
64. "Refugee Statistics: Global Trends at-a-Glance," United Nations High Commissioner for Refugees, accessed August 16, 2020, https://www.unrefugees.org/refugee-facts/statistics/.
65. Niall Ferguson, "Barack Obama's Revolution in Foreign Policy," *Atlantic*, March 13, 2016, https://www.theatlantic.com/international/archive/2016/03/obama-doctrine-revolution/473481/.
66. Arthur Delaney, "Obama Dings Romney on Russia Remark: The 1980s Are Going to Ask for Their Foreign Policy Back," *Huffington Post*, October 22, 2012, http://www.huffingtonpost.com/2012/10/22/obama-romney-russia_n_2003927.html.
67. David Remnick, "Going the Distance," *New Yorker*, January 27, 2014, https://www.newyorker.com/magazine/2014/01/27/going-the-distance-david-remnick.
68. Board of Governors of the Federal Reserve System, "Share of Total Net Worth Held by the Top 1% (99th to 100th Wealth Percentiles)," retrieved from FRED: Federal Reserve Bank of St. Louis, https://fred.stlouisfed.org/series/WFRBST01134.
69. Anne Case and Angus Deaton, "Rising Morbidity and Mortality in Midlife Among White Non-Hispanic Americans in the 21st Century," *PNAS* 112, no. 49 (December 8, 2015), www.pnas.org/cgi/doi/10.1073/pnas.1518393112; Anne Case and Angus Deaton, "Mortality and Morbidity in the 21st Century," *Brookings Papers on Economic Activity*, Spring 2017, pp. 397–476.
70. CDC Wonder, "Overdose Death Rates Involving Opioids, by Type, United States, 1999–2018," CDC, 2020, https://www.cdc.gov/drugoverdose/images/data/2018-Opioid-Deaths-By-Type-US.png.
71. Holly Hedegaard, Margaret Warner, and Arialdi M. Miniño, "Drug Overdose Deaths in the United States, 1999–2016," NCHS Data Brief No. 294 (December 2017). See also Rose A. Rudd et al., "Increases in Drug and Opioid-Involved Overdose Deaths—United States, 2010–2015," *Morbidity and Mortality Weekly Report* 65 (2016), pp. 1445–52, http://dx.doi.org/10.15585/mmwr.mm655051e1. For the comparison with 1918–19, see Christakis, *Apollo's Arrow*, fig. 16.
72. Bryce Pardo, "Evolution of the U.S. Overdose Crisis: Understanding China's Role in the Production and Supply of Synthetic Opioids," testimony presented before the House Foreign Affairs Subcommittee on Africa, Global Health, Global Human Rights, and International Organizations, September 6, 2018, RAND Corporation, https://www.rand.org/pubs/testimonies/CT497.html.
73. Katie Reilly, "Hillary Clinton's 'Basket of Deplorables' Remarks About Donald Trump Supporters," *Time*, September 10, 2016, https://time.com/4486502/hillary-clinton-basket-of-deplorables-transcript/.
74. Dana R. Fisher et al., "The Science of Contemporary Street Protest: New Efforts in the United States," *Science Advances* 5, no. 1 (October 23, 2019), table 1, https://doi.org.10.1126/sciadv.aaw5461; Dana R. Fisher, *American Resistance: From the Women's March to the Blue Wave* (New York: Columbia University Press, 2019).
75. Michael Lewis, *The Fifth Risk* (New York: W. W. Norton, 2018).

76. Niall Ferguson, "Europe's 'Hamilton Moment' Is a Flop. That's Fine," Bloomberg, July 19, 2020, https://www.bloomberg.com/opinion/articles/2020-07-19/coronavirus-and-the-economy-europe-s-hamilton-moment-is-a-flop.

77. Kissinger, "The Coronavirus Pandemic Will Forever Alter the World Order."

78. White House, *National Security Strategy of the United States of America* (December 2017), https://www.whitehouse.gov/wp-content/uploads/2017/12/NSS-Final-12-18-2017-0905.pdf.

79. Nadia Schadlow, "The End of American Illusion," *Foreign Affairs*, September/October 2020, https://www.foreignaffairs.com/articles/americas/2020-08-11/end-american-illusion.

80. "Central Bank Liquidity Swap Operations," Federal Reserve Bank of New York, accessed August 16, 2020, https://apps.newyorkfed.org/markets/autorates/fxswap.

81. Robin Wigglesworth, "A Solution to the Looming Debt Crisis in Emerging Markets," *Financial Times*, May 3, 2020, https://www.ft.com/content/b97eb604-4f6b-49bc-b350-3287bbde00c9.

82. James Kynge and Sun Yu, "China Faces Wave of Calls for Debt Relief on 'Belt and Road' Projects," *Financial Times*, April 30, 2020, https://www.ft.com/content/5a3192be-27c6-4fe7-87e7-78d4158bd39b.

83. Sebastian Horn, Carmen M. Reinhart, and Christoph Trebesch, "China's Overseas Lending," NBER Working Paper No. 26050 (May 2020), http://papers.nber.org/tmp/15188-w26050.pdf.

84. Gita Gopinath et al., "Dominant Currency Paradigm," NBER Working Paper No. 22943 (December 2016), https://www.nber.org/papers/w22943.pdf.

85. Henry M. Paulson Jr., "The Future of the Dollar," *Foreign Affairs*, May 19, 2020, https://www.foreignaffairs.com/articles/2020-05-19/future-dollar.

86. John Paul Koning (@jp_koning), "Facebook isn't a real threat," Twitter, February 6, 2020, 6:56 a.m., https://twitter.com/jp_koning/status/1225418083323568129. See Huw van Steenis, "The New Digital-Payments Race," Project Syndicate, April 21, 2020, https://www.project-syndicate.org/onpoint/central-banks-digital-payments-by-huw-van-steenis-2020-04.

87. Hiroyuki Nishimura, "China Takes Battle for Cryptocurrency Hegemony to New Stage," *Nikkei Asian Review*, June 14, 2020, https://asia.nikkei.com/Spotlight/Comment/China-takes-battle-for-cryptocurrency-hegemony-to-new-stage.

88. "COVID-19 Treatment and Vaccine Tracker," Milken Institute, August 18, 2020, https://covid-19tracker.milkeninstitute.org/.

89. Manas Mishra and Shounak Dasgupta, "U.S. Narrows List of Promising COVID-19 Vaccine Candidates to About 7," *Financial Post*, June 16, 2020, https://business.financialpost.com/pmn/business-pmn/u-s-narrows-list-of-promising-covid-19-vaccine-candidates-to-about-7-2.

90. Josephine Ma, "Can China Win COVID-19 Vaccine Race with Old School Technology?," *South China Morning Post*, June 18, 2020, https://www.scmp.com/news/china/science/article/3089356/can-china-win-covid-19-vaccine-race-old-school-technology.

91. Tung Thanh Le et al., "The COVID-19 Vaccine Development Landscape," *Nature Reviews Drug Discovery* 19 (April 9, 2020), pp. 305–6, https://doi.org/10.1038/d41573-020-00073-5.

92. Wee Sui-Lee and Elsie Chen, "China Investigates Latest Vaccine Scandal After Violent Protests," *New York Times*, January 14, 2019, https://www.nytimes.com/2019/01/14/business/china-vaccine-scandal-protests.html.

93. Javier C. Hernández, "In China, Vaccine Scandal Infuriates Parents and Tests Government," *New York Times*, July 23, 2018, https://www.nytimes.com/2018/07/23/world/asia/china-vaccines-scandal-investigation.html.

94. Jane Parry, "China Sentences Former Drug Regulatory Chief to Death," *BMJ* 334, no. 7605 (June 9, 2007), p. 1183, https://doi.org/10.1136/bmj.39234.428449.DB.

95. Natalie Liu, "German Decision on Huawei 5G 'Imminent,' Says Ambassador," *Voice of America News*, February 11, 2020, https://www.voanews.com/europe/german-decision-huawei-5g-imminent-says-ambassador.

96. Katy Balls and James Forsyth, "The MP Demanding a New Approach to China," *Spectator*, May 16, 2020, https://www.spectator.co.uk/article/the-mp-demanding-a-new-approach-to-china; Jonathan Schieber, "UK Government Reverses Course on Huawei's Involvement in 5G Networks," *Tech Crunch*, May 23, 2020, https://techcrunch.com/2020/05/23/uk-government-reverses-course-on-huaweis-involvement-in-5g-networks/; "UK Will Pay Price If It Carries Out Decision to Exclude Huawei: *China Daily* Editorial," *China Daily*, May 24, 2020, http://www.chinadaily.com.cn/a/202005/24/WS5eca6650a310a8b241158044.html.

97. Kathrin Hille, "Huawei Says New U.S. Sanctions Put Its Survival at Stake," *Financial Times*, May 18, 2020, https://www.ft.com/content/3c532149-94b2-4023-82e0-b51190dc2c46.

98. Michael D. Shear and Miriam Jordan, "Trump Suspends Visas Allowing Hundreds of Thousands of Foreigners to Work in the U.S.," *New York Times*, July 23, 2020, https://www.nytimes.com/2020/06/22/us/politics/trump-h1b-work-visas.html.

99. Ishan Banerjee and Matt Sheehan, "America's Got AI Talent: U.S.' Big Lead in AI Research Is Built on Importing Researchers," *Macro Polo*, June 9, 2020, https://macropolo.org/americas-got-ai-talent-us-big-lead-in-ai-research-is-built-on-importing-researchers/.

100. Carl Benedikt Frey and Michael Osborne, "China Won't Win the Race for AI Dominance," *Foreign Affairs,* June 19, 2020, https://www.foreignaffairs.com/articles/united-states/2020-06-19/china-wont-win-race-ai-dominance.

101. Lu Zhenhua, Wang Zili, and Xu Heqian, "China and U.S. to Fight for Tech Primacy, Not War: Tsinghua Expert," *Nikkei Asian Review,* May 18, 2020, https://asia.nikkei.com/Spotlight/Caixin/China-and-US-to-fight-for-tech-primacy-not-war-Tsinghua-expert.

102. Ariel E. Levite and Lyu Jinghua, "Travails of an Interconnected World: From Pandemics to the Digital Economy," *Lawfare* (blog), April 30, 2020, https://www.lawfareblog.com/travails-interconnected-world-pandemics-digital-economy.

103. Brose, *Kill Chain.*

104. Michael R. Auslin, "The Sino-American Littoral War of 2025: A Future History," in *Asia's New Geopolitics: Essays on Reshaping the Indo-Pacific* (Stanford, CA: Hoover Institution Press, 2020), pp. 185–228.

105. Richard Haass, "American Support for Taiwan Must Be Unambiguous," *Foreign Affairs,* September 2, 2020, https://www.foreignaffairs.com/articles/united-states/american-support-taiwan-must-be-unambiguous.

106. Brother Mao, "U.S. Punishing Huawei Is a Strategic Trap," *Brother Mao's World* (blog), https://mp.weixin.qq.com/s/X3rYjXgAdtVxA4CE8_5TWg.

107. Grant Newsham, "Can the PLA Get Across the Taiwan Strait?," *Asia Times,* May 13, 2019, https://asiatimes.com/2019/05/can-the-pla-get-across-the-taiwan-strait/.

108. Salvatore Babones, "Boris Johnson's Huawei 5G Decision Is a Massive Mistake," *National Interest,* January 28, 2020, https://nationalinterest.org/blog/buzz/boris-johnsons-huawei-5g-decision-massive-mistake-118016.

109. Graham Allison, "Could Donald Trump's War Against Huawei Trigger a Real War with China?," *National Interest,* June 11, 2020, https://nationalinterest.org/feature/could-donald-trump%E2%80%99s-war-against-huawei-trigger-real-war-china-162565.

110. Steve Blank, "The Chip Wars of the Twenty-First Century," *War on the Rocks,* June 11, 2020, https://warontherocks.com/2020/06/the-chip-wars-of-the-21st-century/.

111. Jenny Leonard, "Lighthizer Says He Feels 'Very Good' About Phase One China Deal," Bloomberg, June 4, 2020, https://www.bloomberg.com/news/articles/2020-06-04/lighthizer-says-he-feels-very-good-about-phase-one-china-deal-kb16qm1v; "China Halts Some U.S. Farm Imports, Threatening Trade Deal," Bloomberg, June 1, 2020, https://www.bloomberg.com/news/articles/2020-06-01/china-halts-some-u-s-farm-imports-threatening-trade-deal.

112. "Foreign Ministry Spokesperson Zhao Lijian's Remarks on Yang Jiechi's Meeting with U.S. Secretary of State Mike Pompeo," Ministry of Foreign Affairs of the People's Republic of China, June 18, 2020, https://www.fmprc.gov.cn/mfa_eng/xwfw_665399/s2510_665401/t1789798.shtml.

113. Michael R. Pompeo, "'Europe and the China Challenge': Speech at the Virtual Copenhagen Democracy Summit," U.S. Department of State, June 19, 2020, https://www.state.gov/secretary-michael-r-pompeo-at-the-virtual-copenhagen-democracy-summit.

114. M5sParlamento, "Luigi Di Maio ospite a TG2 Post Rai 2 24 03 2020," March 24, 2020, YouTube video, 22:31, https://www.youtube.com/watch?v=0W7JRf6qaog.

115. Philip Wen and Drew Hinshaw, "China Asserts Claim to Global Leadership, Mask by Mask," *Wall Street Journal,* April 1, 2020, https://www.wsj.com/articles/china-asserts-claim-to-global-leadership-mask-by-mask-11585752077.

116. Mattia Ferraresi, "China Isn't Helping Italy. It's Waging Information Warfare," *Foreign Policy,* March 31, 2020, https://foreignpolicy.com/2020/03/31/china-isnt-helping-italy-its-waging-information-warfare/.

117. Alan Crawford and Peter Martin, "China's Coronavirus Diplomacy Has Finally Pushed Europe Too Far," *Taipei Times,* April 26, 2020, https://www.taipeitimes.com/News/editorials/archives/2020/04/26/2003735306.

118. Julian Reichelt, "'You Are Endangering the World': BILD Editor-in-Chief Julian Reichelt Responds to the Chinese President Xi Jinping," *Bild,* April 17, 2020, https://www.bild.de/politik/international/bild-international/bild-chief-editor-responds-to-the-chinese-president-70098436.bild.html. See Joseph de Weck, "China's COVID-19 Diplomacy Is Backfiring in Europe," Foreign Policy Research Institute, April 21, 2020, https://www.fpri.org/article/2020/04/chinas-covid-19-diplomacy-is-backfiring-in-europe/.

119. Stuart Lau, "Chinese Foreign Minister Sees Only Limited Diplomatic Gains from European Trip," *South China Morning Post,* September 3, 2020, https://www.scmp.com/news/china/diplomacy/article/3100003/chinese-foreign-minister-sees-only-limited-diplomatic-gains.

120. Laura Silver, Kat Devlin, and Christine Huang, "Unfavorable Views of China Reach Historic Highs in Many Countries," Pew Research Center, October 6, 2020, https://www.pewresearch.org/global/2020/10/06/unfavorable-views-of-china-reach-historic-highs-in-many-countries/.

121. Joseph de Weck and Dimitris Valatsas, "The European Union Will Survive COVID-19," Foreign Policy Research Institute, April 30, 2020, https://www.fpri.org/article/2020/04/the-european-union-will-survive-covid-19/.

122. Victor Mallet and Roula Khalaf, "Macron Warns of EU Unravelling Unless It Embraces Financial Solidarity," *Financial Times,* April 16, 2020, https://www.ft.com/content/d19dc7a6-c33b-4931-9a7e-4a74674da29a.

123. "Europe's Moment: Repair and Prepare for the Next Generation," European Commission Press Corner, May 27, 2020, https://ec.europa.eu/commission/presscorner/detail/en/ip_20_940.

124. Guy Chazan, "German Stimulus Aims to Kick-Start Recovery 'With a Ka-Boom,'" *Financial Times,* June 4, 2020, https://www.ft.com/content/335b5558-41b5-4a1e-a3b9-1440f7602bd8.

125. Timothy Garton Ash and Antonia Zimmermann, "In Crisis, Europeans Support Radical Positions," *Eupinions,* May 6, 2020, https://eupinions.eu/de/text/in-crisis-europeans-support-radical-positions.

126. Ronja Scheler and Joshua Webb, "Keeping an Equidistance," *Berlin Policy Journal,* May 18, 2020, https://berlinpolicyjournal.com/keeping-an-equidistance/.

127. "Inaugural Lecture on Behalf of H. E. Saddam Hussein," in *The Principles of Non-Alignment,* ed. Hans Köhler (Vienna: Third World Centre, 1982), p. 5.

128. Lee Hsien Loong, "The Endangered Asian Century: America, China, and the Perils of Confrontation," *Foreign Affairs,* July/August 2020, https://www.foreignaffairs.com/articles/asia/2020-06-04/lee-hsien-loong-endangered-asian-century.

129. Emile Simpson, *War from the Ground Up: Twenty-First Century Combat as Politics* (Oxford: Oxford University Press, 2012).

130. Hal Brands and Francis J. Gavin, eds., *COVID-19 and World Order: The Future of Conflict, Competition, and Cooperation* (Baltimore: Johns Hopkins University Press, 2020).

131. Ben Thompson, "China, Leverage, and Values," *Stratechery,* May 21, 2019, https://stratechery.com/2019/china-leverage-and-values/; Ben Thompson, "The China Cultural Clash," *Stratechery,* October 8, 2019, https://stratechery.com/2019/the-china-cultural-clash/.

132. Ben Thompson, "The TikTok War," *Stratechery,* July 14, 2020, https://stratechery.com/2020/the-tiktok-war/.

133. Ross Andersen, "The Panopticon Is Already Here," *Atlantic,* September 2020, https://www.theatlantic.com/magazine/archive/2020/09/china-ai-surveillance/614197/.

134. Jiang Shigong, "Empire and World Order," trans. David Ownby, at Reading the China Dream, https://www.readingthechinadream.com/jiang-shigong-empire-and-world-order.html.

135. Barry Eichengreen, Minxin Pei, Kevin Rudd, and Elizabeth Sidiropoulos, "Xi's Weltpolitik," Project Syndicate, August 14, 2018, https://www.project-syndicate.org/bigpicture/xi-s-weltpolitik.

136. Larry Diamond et al., *Chinese Influence & American Interests: Promoting Constructive Vigilance—Report of the Working Group on Chinese Influence Activities in the United States* (Stanford, CA: Hoover Institution Press, 2018), https://www.hoover.org/sites/default/files/research/docs/chineseinfluence_americaninterests_fullreport_web.pdf.

137. Frances Stonor Saunders, *The Cultural Cold War: The CIA and the World of Arts and Letters* (New York: Free Press, 2001).

138. Régis Debray, "The Third World: From Kalashnikovs to God and Computers," *New Perspectives Quarterly* 3, no. 1 (Spring 1986), p. 43.

139. Hoover Institution, "Cardinal Conversations: Reid Hoffman and Peter Thiel on 'Technology and Politics,'" January 31, 2018, YouTube video, 1:31:25, https://www.youtube.com/watch?v=J2klGJRrjqw. See also Ali Yahya, "The Long-Tail Problem of AI, and How Autonomous Markets Can Solve It," Andreesen Horowitz, July 24, 2020, https://a16z.com/2020/07/24/long-tail-problem-in-a-i/.

140. "Chinese Cultural Revolution: The Boy Who Denounced His Mother," *Guardian,* March 29, 2013, YouTube video, 3:35, https://www.youtube.com/watch?v=CCA6ME81RLQ.

141. "China Uses Sci-Fi to Try to Spark a Tech Boom," *Straits Times,* September 22, 2018, https://www.straitstimes.com/asia/east-asia/china-uses-sci-fi-to-try-to-spark-a-tech-boom. See also Rebecca Davis, "China Issues Guidelines on Developing a Sci-Fi Film Sector," *Variety,* August 17, 2020, https://variety.com/2020/film/news/china-guidelines-science-fiction-1234737913/.

142. Liu Cixin, *The Dark Forest,* trans. Joel Martinsen (New York: Tom Doherty, 2015), p. 484.

Conclusion: Future Shocks

1. Stephen M. Kissler et al., "Projecting the Transmission Dynamics of SARS-CoV-2 Through the Postpandemic Period," *Science* 368, no. 6493 (May 2020), pp. 860–68, https://science.sciencemag.org/content/368/6493/860/tab-pdf; Eskild Petersen et al., "Comparing SARS-CoV-2 with SARS-CoV and Influenza Pandemics," *Lancet Infectious Diseases* 20, no. 9 (September 2020), pp. E238–E244, https://doi.org/10.1016/S1473-3099(20)30484-9.

2. Pasquale Cirillo and Nassim Nicholas Taleb, "Tail Risk of Contagious Diseases" (working paper, 2020).

3. Scott Galloway, "The Great Distancing," *No Mercy, No Malice* (blog), August 7, 2020, https://www.profgalloway.com/the-great-distancing.

4. Erik Brynjolfsson et al., "COVID-19 and Remote Work: An Early Look at US Data," NBER Working Paper No. 27344 (June 2020), http://www.nber.org/papers/w27344.

5. Nicholas Bloom, "How Working from Home Works Out," SIEPR Policy Brief (June 2020), https://siepr.stanford.edu/research/publications/how-working-home-works-out.

6. Bruno Maçães, "The Great Pause Was an Economic Revolution," *Foreign Policy,* June 22, 2020, https://foreignpolicy.com/2020/06/22/the-great-pause-was-an-economic-revolution%e2%80%a8/.

7. Sebastian Mallaby, "The Age of Magic Money," *Foreign Affairs,* July/August 2020, https://www.foreign affairs.com/articles/united-states/2020-05-29/pandemic-financial-crisis.

8. Jon Cohen, "Swine Flu Strain with Human Pandemic Potential Increasingly Found in Pigs in China," *Science,* June 29, 2020, https://www.sciencemag.org/news/2020/06/swine-flu-strain-human-pandemic -potential-increasingly-found-pigs-china.

9. Jessie Yeung, Philip Wang, and Martin Goillandeau, "Kazakhstan Denies Chinese Government Report That Country Has 'Unknown Pneumonia' Outbreak More Deadly Than Covid-19," CNN, July 10, 2020, https://amp.cnn.com/cnn/2020/07/10/asia/kazakhstan-pneumonia-intl-hnk-scli-scn/index.html.

10. Dorothy H. Crawford, *Deadly Companions: How Microbes Shaped Our History* (Oxford: Oxford University Press, 2007), pp. 195–96.

11. Marc Galimand et al., "Multidrug Resistance in *Yersinia Pestis* Mediated by a Transferable Plasmid," *NEJM* 337, no. 10 (1997), pp. 677–80.

12. Nick Bostrom and Milan M. Ćirković, eds., *Global Catastrophic Risks* (Oxford: Oxford University Press, 2008), pp. 2–4.

13. World Food Programme, "COVID-19 Will Double Number of People Facing Food Crises Unless Swift Action Is Taken," April 21, 2020, https://www.wfp.org/news/covid-19-will-double-number-people -facing-food-crises-unless-swift-action-taken.

14. "Slowing the Coronavirus Is Speeding the Spread of Other Diseases," *New York Times,* June 14, 2020, https://www.nytimes.com/2020/06/14/health/coronavirus-vaccines-measles.html; Peter Sands, "HIV, Tuberculosis, and Malaria: How Can the Impact of COVID-19 Be Minimised?," *Lancet,* July 13, 2020, https://www.thelancet.com/journals/langlo/article/PIIS2214-109X(20)30317-X /fulltext.

15. James Hansen et al., "Ice Melt, Sea Level Rise and Superstorms: Evidence from Paleoclimate Data, Climate Modeling, and Modern Observations That 2°C Global Warming Is Highly Dangerous," *Atmospheric Chemistry and Physics Discussions* 15, no. 14 (July 23, 2015), pp. 20059–179.

16. IPCC, *Climate Change 2014: Synthesis Report: Contribution of Working Groups I, II and III to the Fifth Assessment Report of the Intergovernmental Panel on Climate Change,* ed. Core Writing Team, R. K. Pachauri and L. A. Meyer (Geneva: IPCC, 2014), https://www.ipcc.ch/site/assets/uploads/2018/02 /SYR_AR5_FINAL_full.pdf. See Christopher R. Schwalm, Spencer Glendon, and Philip B. Duffy, "RCP8.5 Tracks Cumulative CO2 Emissions," *PNAS* 117, no. 33 (August 18, 2020), pp. 19656–57, https://www.pnas.org/content/117/33/19656.

17. David Frame and Myles R. Allen, "Climate Change and Global Risk," in *Global Catastrophic Risks,* ed. Nick Bostrom and Milan M. Ćirković (Oxford: Oxford University Press, 2008), pp. 279–81. See also Bjorn Lomborg, *False Alarm: How Climate Change Panic Costs Us Trillions, Hurts the Poor, and Fails to Fix the Planet* (New York: Basic Books, 2020); Michael Shellenberger, *Apocalypse Never: Why Environmental Alarmism Hurts Us All* (New York: HarperCollins, 2020).

18. Elizabeth Weil, "They Know How to Prevent Megafires. Why Won't Anybody Listen?," *ProPublica,* August 28, 2020, https://www.propublica.org/article/they-know-how-to-prevent-megafires-why-wont -anybody-listen.

19. Chingy Tse-Cheng, "Expert Warns China's Three Gorges Dam in Danger of Collapse," *Taiwan News,* June 22, 2020, https://www.taiwannews.com.tw/en/news/3951673; Keoni Everington, "Videos Show Massive Flooding in S. China, Three Gorges Dam Next," *Taiwan News,* June 23, 2020, https://www .taiwannews.com.tw/en/news/3952434.

20. Jacob B. Lowenstern et al., "Steam Explosions, Earthquakes, and Volcanic Eruptions—What's in Yellowstone's Future?," U.S. Geological Survey and National Park Service (2005), https://pubs.usgs.gov /fs/2005/3024/fs2005-3024.pdf.

21. Milan M. Ćirković, "Observation Selection Effects and Global Catastrophic Risks," in *Global Catastrophic Risks,* ed. Nick Bostrom and Milan M. Ćirković (Oxford: Oxford University Press, 2008), pp. 135–37.

22. Arnon Dar, "Influence of Supernovae, Gamma-Ray Bursts, Solar Flares, and Cosmic Rays on the Terrestrial Environment," in *Global Catastrophic Risks,* ed. Nick Bostrom and Milan M. Ćirković (Oxford: Oxford University Press, 2008), p. 259.

23. Richard A. Clarke and R. P. Eddy, *Warnings: Finding Cassandras to Stop Catastrophes* (New York: HarperCollins, 2018), p. 322. See also "The World Should Think Better About Catastrophic and Existential Risks," *Economist,* June 25, 2020, https://www.economist.com/briefing/2020/06/25/the-world -should-think-better-about-catastrophic-and-existential-risks.

24. Frank Wilczek, "Big Troubles, Imagined and Real," in *Global Catastrophic Risks,* ed. Nick Bostrom and Milan M. Ćirković (Oxford: Oxford University Press, 2008), p. 356f. See also Katsuhiko Sato, "First-Order Phase Transition of a Vacuum and the Expansion of the Universe," *Monthly Notices of the Royal Astronomical Society* 195 (May 1981), pp. 467–79.

25. Nick Bostrom, "The Vulnerable World Hypothesis," Working Paper, v.3.42, Future of Humanity Institute, University of Oxford (2018).

26. Joseph Cirincione, "The Continuing Threat of Nuclear War," and William C. Potter and Gary Ackerman, "Catastrophic Nuclear Terrorism: A Preventable Peril," in *Global Catastrophic Risks,* ed. Nick Bostrom and Milan M. Ćirković (Oxford: Oxford University Press, 2008). See also Clarke and Eddy, *Warnings,* pp. 278f.

27. Ali Nouri and Christopher F. Chyba, "Biotechnology and Biosecurity," in *Global Catastrophic Risks,* ed. Nick Bostrom and Milan M. Ćirković (Oxford: Oxford University Press, 2008), pp. 456f.

28. Martin Jinek et al., "A Programmable Dual-RNA–Guided-DNA Endonuclease in Adaptive Bacterial Immunity," *Science* 337, no. 6096 (August 17, 2012), pp. 816–21. See also Jennifer Kahn, "The CRISPR Quandary," *New York Times Magazine,* November 9, 2015, www.nytimes.com/2015/11/15/magazine /the-cripsr-quandary.html.

29. "Biotech: DIY Disaster Zone," *Financial Times,* June 23, 2020, https://www.ft.com/content/7c0d9214 -938d-4931-868e-e3533b8da70a.

30. Christopher Wills, *Children of Prometheus: The Accelerating Pace of Human Evolution* (Reading, MA: Perseus, 1998).

31. Clarke and Eddy, *Warnings,* pp. 292–99.

32. Eliezer Yudkowsky, "AI as a Positive and Negative Factor in Global Risk," in *Global Catastrophic Risks,* ed. Nick Bostrom and Milan M. Ćirković (Oxford: Oxford University Press, 2008), pp. 201–7. See also James J. Hughes, "Millennial Tendencies in Responses to Apocalyptic Threats," in *Global Catastrophic Risks,* ed. Nick Bostrom and Milan M. Ćirković (Oxford: Oxford University Press, 2008), pp. 79–81.

33. Chris Phoenix and Mike Treder, "Nanotechnology as Global Catastrophic Risk," in *Global Catastrophic Risks,* ed. Nick Bostrom and Milan M. Ćirković (Oxford: Oxford University Press, 2008), pp. 488f. See K. E. Drexler, *Nanosystems: Molecular Machinery, Manufacturing, and Computation* (New York: Wiley Interscience, 1992).

34. Toby Ord, *The Precipice: Existential Risk and the Future of Humanity* (New York: Hachette, 2020).

35. Richard A. Posner, "Public Policy Towards Catastrophe," in *Global Catastrophic Risks,* ed. Nick Bostrom and Milan M. Ćirković (Oxford: Oxford University Press, 2008), pp. 186f. For some creative suggestions on how to overcome this, see Bina Venkataraman, *The Optimist's Telescope* (New York: Penguin 2019), and Margaret Heffernan, *Uncharted: How to Map the Future Together* (London: Simon & Schuster, 2020).

36. Clarke and Eddy, *Warnings,* pp. 356, 362–64.

37. Bostrom, "Vulnerable World Hypothesis," pp. 17–23.

38. Bostrom, "Vulnerable World Hypothesis," pp. 23, 28. Similar arguments have been made by others: Christopher Wills, "Evolutionary Theory and the Future of Humanity," and Robin Hanson, "Catastrophe, Social Collapse, and Human Extinction," in *Global Catastrophic Risks,* ed. Nick Bostrom and Milan M. Ćirković (Oxford: Oxford University Press, 2008), pp. 67, 373f.

39. Bryan Caplan, "The Totalitarian Threat," in *Global Catastrophic Risks,* ed. Nick Bostrom and Milan M. Ćirković (Oxford: Oxford University Press, 2008), pp. 511–14.

40. Yuval Noah Harari, "Why Technology Favors Tyranny," *Atlantic,* October 2018, https://www.theatlantic .com/magazine/archive/2018/10/yuval-noah-harari-technology-tyranny/568330/.

41. Steven L. Aggelis, ed., *Conversations with Ray Bradbury* (Jackson: University Press of Mississippi, 2004), p. 99.

42. Huxley to Orwell, October 21, 1949, in *Letters of Note,* vol. 2: *An Eclectic Collection of Correspondence Deserving of a Wider Audience,* ed. Shaun Usher (San Francisco: Chronicle, 2016), p. 33.

43. Yevgeny Zamyatin, *We,* trans. Natasha S. Randall (New York: Modern Library, 2006), p. 187.

44. Daniel Defoe, *A Journal of the Plague Year* (London: Penguin, 2003 [1722]), p. 218.

Index

Page numbers in *italics* refer to illustrations.